THE NEW
WHOLE30®

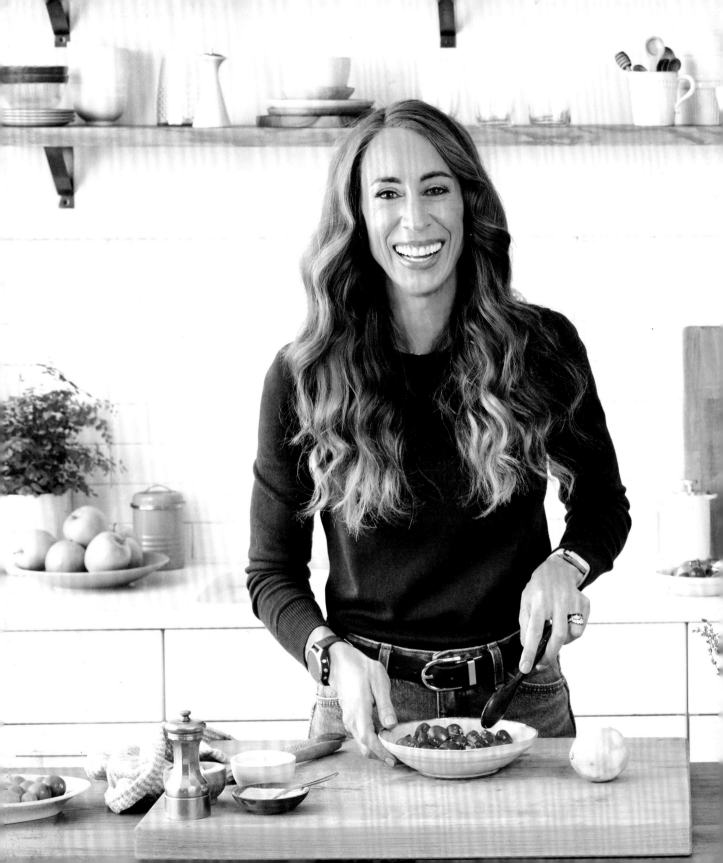

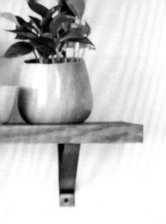

THE NEW
WHOLE30®

THE DEFINITIVE PLAN TO TRANSFORM YOUR HEALTH, HABITS, AND RELATIONSHIP WITH FOOD

MELISSA URBAN

PHOTOGRAPHY BY GHAZALLE BADIOZAMANI

RODALE
NEW YORK

Published in the United States by Rodale Books, an imprint of Random House, a division of Penguin Random House LLC, New York.

Rodale Books is a registered trademark, and the Circle colophon is a trademark of Penguin Random House LLC.

Hardcover ISBN: 9780593235713
Ebook ISBN: 9780593235720

Printed in China

Interior and cover design by Jenny Davis
Food styling by Barrett Washburne and Brett Regot
Prop styling by Vanessa Vazquez

Illustrations on page 98 and 234 by KsanaGraphica/Shutterstock.com and on page 42 by KVASVECTOR/Shutterstock.com

10 9 8 7 6 5 4 3 2 1

First Edition

rodalebooks.com

By Melissa Urban

It Starts With Food: Discover the Whole30 and Change Your Life in Unexpected Ways

Cooking Whole30: Over 150 Recipes for the Whole30 and Beyond

The Whole30 Day by Day: Your Daily Guide to Whole30 Success

Food Freedom Forever: Letting Go of Bad Habits, Guilt, and Anxiety Around Food

The Whole30 Fast and Easy: 150 Simply Delicious Everyday Recipes for Your Whole30

The Whole30 Slow Cooker: All-New Recipes for Your Slow Cooker and Instant Pot

The Whole30 Friends & Family: 150 Recipes for Every Social Occasion

The New Whole30: The Definitive Path to Transform Your Health, Habits, and Relationship with Food

DISCLAIMER

This book presents the research, ideas, and opinions of its author. It is not intended as medical advice, nor as a substitute for medical treatment or consultation with a professional healthcare practitioner. Nothing herein is intended to diagnose, treat, or prevent any disease. This information should only be used in conjunction with the guidance and approval of your physician. Consult your healthcare provider before starting any new dietary or supplement regimen. Your healthcare provider's recommendations always supersede the information found in this book. The Whole30 program is contraindicated for those with a history of disordered eating. The Plant-Based Whole30 is contraindicated for children, or those who are pregnant or nursing. Author and publisher are not responsible for any errors in the URLs or other information contained herein.

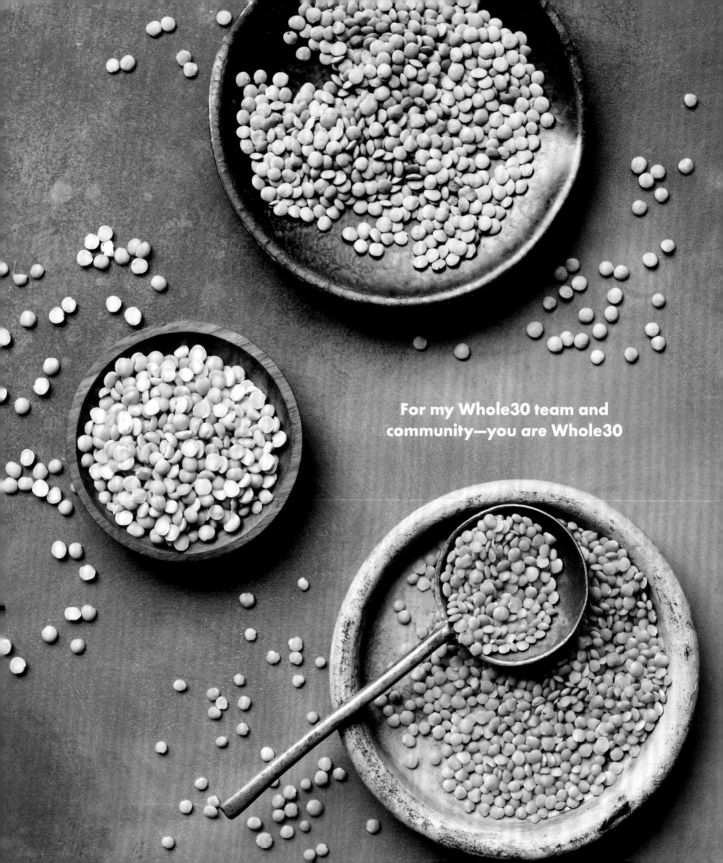

For my Whole30 team and community—you *are* Whole30

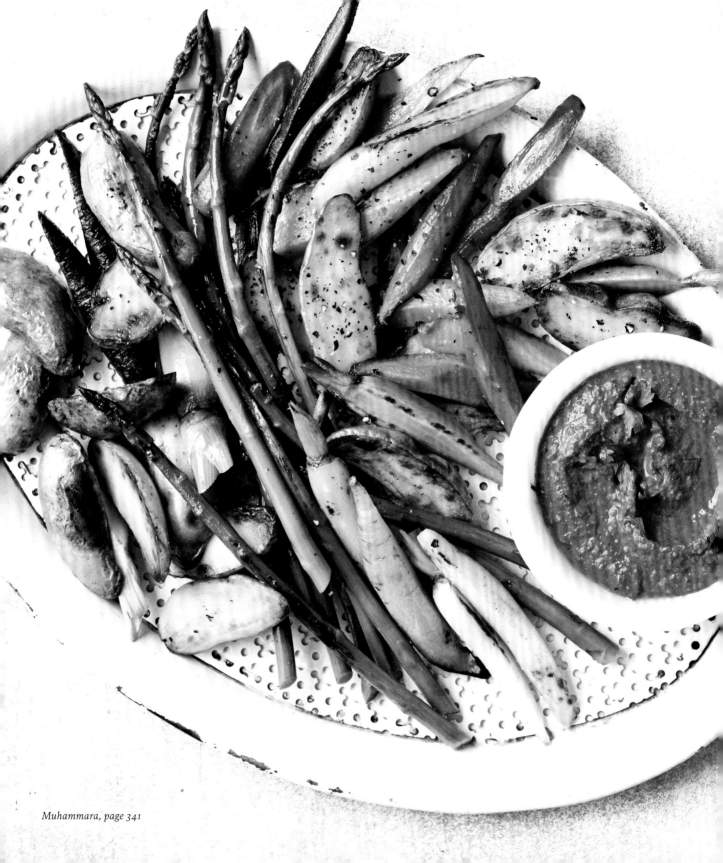

Muhammara, page 341

CONTENTS

PREFACE

On April 21, 2015, I was in midtown Manhattan doing media for the launch of my second book, *The Whole30*. I had finished my interviews and was walking back to my hotel when I heard someone say, "Hey, are you the Whole30 lady?" I'd been recognized in public before, but never in the middle of New York City—and on the day of my book release! I delightedly confirmed, and she immediately launched into the details of her Whole30 success story. I walked away thinking it was an auspicious sign.

It's hard to believe the Whole30 has been around for more than fifteen years, and that book was written *nine* years ago. *The Whole30* would go on to become a #1 *New York Times* bestseller, selling more than 1.6 million copies in North America alone and changing the lives of millions of people just like you. Since then, the Whole30 program has only continued to grow in reputation and influence, cementing it as a well-respected dietary protocol. We've been featured in dozens of major media outlets, you can now walk into any Chipotle and order a Whole30 salad bowl, and I've written six more books about the program—seven, if you count this one.

The Whole30 is obviously here to stay—and yet, a lot has changed in the last nine years. (More than just my last name. Twice, but who's counting?) I've been dreaming about updating *The Whole30* for a few years, but in 2020, I realized the book needed far more than just an update. The Whole30 was ready for a whole new energy, tone, and voice, with fresh content designed to incorporate the sweeping evolution that the brand, the program, and I had undergone.

Plus, we got a few things wrong back then, and it was time to correct that.

Science is gonna science

Science is always evolving, leading us to new understandings of the way various foods and ingredients interact with our bodies. The scientific process is that of observing, asking questions, and seeking answers through tests and experiments, and that often includes challenging previously held beliefs to get further at the truth. The science I shared in *The Whole30* was grounded in the research and hypotheses of the time. I relied on trusted healthcare advisors, medical doctors, and registered dietitians to help me evaluate that research and apply it to the Whole30 Program Rules. To our credit, most of the rules still have a substantial number of current studies supporting them.

Most, but not all.

In some cases, we extrapolated the findings of studies in a more negative way than they deserved. (Hindsight is always 20/20, and everyone has their biases.) In others, the concerns we noted based on earlier research simply didn't bear out upon further study. Today, we have the benefit of nine additional years of scientific evidence. And as we reviewed that evidence, it became obvious that the concerns we held about some ingredients and their impact on the body were overstated. To put it another way, we thought you needed to eliminate these foods for Whole30 success, and it turns out you probably didn't. As a result, you'll find a few new rule changes here to address that issue.

Some of these changes may surprise you, even if you consider yourself health conscious. (Perhaps *especially* if you consider yourself health conscious.) We all have preconceived notions about what is "healthy," based largely on our spheres of influence—our friend group, the media we

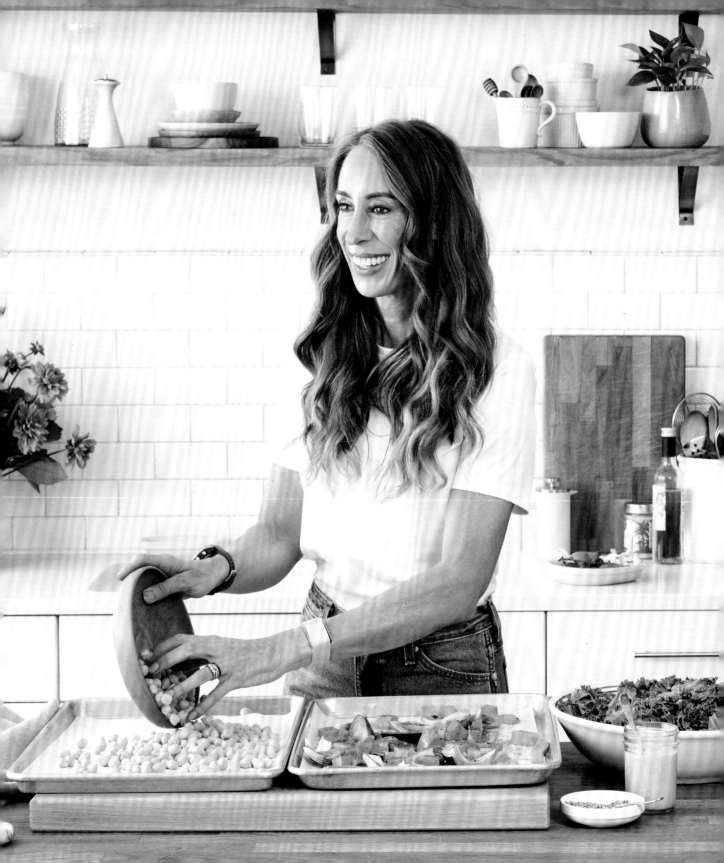

consume, the experts we trust, and our own personal experience. But my goal is to make the Whole30 as successful as possible for as many people as possible, and that means approaching new research with an open mind and a willingness to make changes where needed. I believe it's a good thing when the people you trust to bring you science-backed information say, "We got it wrong, and here's how we're going to fix it"—ideally with references.

So, yes, in this book, some of the Whole30 rules have changed. The good news is that these rule changes add things back *into* the program. To say it a different way, as the result of our research, we're eliminating *less* in this new version of Whole30 and encouraging you even *more* to keep your diet broad, free, and joyful when your Whole30 is over. That's good news!

The goal of the program has always been to eliminate the smallest number of foods while being maximally effective for as many people as possible. Considering that the way foods interact with our bodies is so individual and no two people's "ideal" diet looks the same, this is a tall order. However, I believe that the deep dive we did into the research in preparation for this book helps the Whole30 achieve this goal, with fewer foods and ingredients on the "no" list, more accessibility and options during your 30-day elimination, and an even greater sense of food freedom when your Whole30 is over.

For those of you familiar with the 2015 Program Rules, you can preview a list of rule updates on page 29. (Wine is still a no. I didn't want you to get your hopes up.)

The new plant-powered Whole30

This book also includes the newest addition to the Whole30: our Plant-Based Whole30 program, complete with Program Rules, recipes, and tailored guidance. This is something we've been working on for years, and I'm thrilled to be able to *officially* welcome our vegetarian and vegan friends into the Whole30 community through this new offering.

To be clear, I've always *said* vegetarians and vegans are welcome. In earlier books, I've even offered guidance to adopt Whole30 principles into your chosen dietary framework, even if that included no animal products whatsoever. However, the "programs" we offered weren't exactly comprehensive. Yes, I included some tips and strategies for approaching a Whole30-ish self-experiment from a vegan perspective, but in the end you couldn't *really* do a Whole30 without animal products—and that came through loud and clear in my writing.

I also slipped my own personal biases into those chapters—sometimes strongly. Yes, I said you were welcome in the community even if you didn't eat animal protein. But in the same breath, I suggested you *try* eating meat, because I believed eating meat was necessary for good health.

This belief was driven by my own personal experience, and as a result, so were the biases through which I reviewed the research. I was a vegetarian for many years, as a late teen into my early twenties. I ate eggs and some dairy, but I always struggled with the taste or texture of meat. However, once I started exercising and weightlifting, my body began craving meat again. I tentatively started eating ground beef, chicken breasts, and salmon, and I immediately felt *so* much better. My energy improved, I started building muscle, and my bloodwork showed I was no longer anemic.

Because eating meat worked so well for me, I assumed it was a healthier approach for *everyone*—and my earlier Whole30 writings reflected that. If you tried to be a part of the Whole30 community as a vegetarian or vegan between 2012 and 2016, we probably didn't make you feel very welcome. You may have even gotten the sense that we didn't approve of your choice not to eat animal protein.

(I didn't, to be honest. I was convinced what worked for me would work for everyone. I'm sorry about that.)

Still, I truly wanted those who didn't eat animals to be able to experience the magic of the Whole30 program and community. As I evolved my views and broadened my perspective, I kept returning to the Whole30 mission I've held since day one: that everyone who wants to do a Whole30 can succeed with the program. It became clear that we had to create a whole new version of the Whole30—a program that includes no animal products, supports adequate protein intake and balanced blood sugar, and more than anything, feels respectful, welcoming, and inclusive to those who join.

In 2020, we began sketching out the Plant-Based Whole30 with our registered dietitians and medical advisory board. We spent a year drafting the rules and the supporting documents, resources, and recipes. In January 2022, we ran a beta group of fifty participants through the program, with great success and many learnings. And in March 2022, to great fanfare, the Plant-Based Whole30 officially debuted across our website and in our social media feeds.

Not only does this program serve those who don't eat animals for religious, ethical, financial, or health reasons; it also provides a proven framework for omnivores to explore a more plant-forward or plant-based diet, guiding them to the plant-based foods that work best for their bodies. Launching the Plant-Based Whole30 was a huge step forward in our accessibility and inclusion efforts. Providing *two* well-supported frameworks that respect a broad array of individual values allows more people than ever to access the truly life-changing benefits the program has to offer.

When I was drafting this book's proposal, I knew the Plant-Based Whole30 program had to be included—not as an addendum or an aside, but *equal* to the Original Whole30, featuring just as many resources, guidance, support, and recipes.

More important, however, I wanted this new Whole30 book to be truly welcoming, inclusive, and respectful of your dietary choices.

If you are a vegetarian or vegan who was turned off by the language or tone I shared in the earlier days of Whole30, I understand. I can't take back what I wrote then (as much as I'd like to), but as you keep reading, I think you'll find the Whole30 has evolved, and I'm grateful you're giving us another chance. I think you'll find the acceptance, community, connection, and Whole30 success you've been looking for right here in these pages, and I'm eager for you to experience the life-changing magic of the Plant-Based Whole30 for yourself—no animal products required.

Know better, do better

You may be picking up that I've also gone through a big personal transformation since I wrote *The Whole30*. A baby, a divorce, and a business split in quick succession rocked my world in the years that followed, and I spent the next few years figuring out how to run a business and keep writing books while solo-parenting a toddler every other week.

That time period was one of the most stressful, but also one of the happiest. I spent those years getting to know myself again, after spending so long giving up pieces of myself in an effort to make the marriage work. I put down my armor, no longer needing to show up as "perfect" in my work to overcompensate for how unhappy I had been in my personal life. I began to really *like* myself again, which had a positive impact on my career, health, and personal growth. I learned to show myself empathy and grace, which naturally extended to my other relationships, work, and community. I stopped punishing or shaming myself as a means of "motivation," and I learned how to support myself from a place of kindness. I could still dish out the "tough love" I had become famous for, but the dishing was *much* heavier on the love, as I was far more cognizant of the invisible struggles anyone could be facing at any given moment.

I also became aware of my own privilege, and all the ways in which my path through the world was easier just because of how I was born. Because I am white, straight, able-bodied, and thin, I don't experience the same systemic barriers that other people do. Those barriers (or lack thereof) have helped to make things like going to the gym five days a week or eating whole foods pretty easy for me, while presenting significant hurdles for so many others trying to achieve the same goals. The way I showed up in my community began to reflect this understanding.

At the same time, the Whole30 community has also undergone a big transformation. Up until 2015, I was talking mostly to CrossFitters who had learned about the Whole30 through my personal training blog and other CrossFit gyms. Our community was mostly young, privileged, fit, and disciplined. They responded well to tough love (the tougher the better) and liked the challenge the Whole30 presented. Phrases like "This is not hard," "Just follow the rules," and "No slips, no cheats, no excuses" resonated with and motivated that group.

Today, our community looks *vastly* different. It's exploded far beyond CrossFit, growing to millions of people all over the world. Our demographics now skew older, and many readers have children of their own. Some folks are active, but just as many don't have an exercise routine, and most come to us with burgeoning health complaints. (The top three drivers for doing a Whole30: cravings, digestive issues, and mental health.) Our audience is diverse in nearly every aspect (gender being the outlier; most of our followers are women), and is a much better representation of the world we live in and the complex challenges people face on a daily basis when it comes to food, their bodies, and their health.

My personal growth and the awareness of how our community had changed began to show up in everything I did—and by extension, everything Whole30 did as a business and as a brand. We actively embraced, reflected, promoted, and learned from our community's growing diversity. Our goal became to build new resources, support services, and products *with* our community, not for them. We created new business practices and standards to ensure everyone who came to the Whole30 felt seen, heard, and represented in our work. We partnered with organizations like WANDA (Women Advancing Nutrition Dietetics and Agriculture), the ASPCA (American Society for the Prevention of Cruelty to Animals), and Disability Reframed to further our accessibility efforts. We began meeting regularly to discuss our diversity, equity, and inclusion values, efforts, and projects.

These efforts to include and affirm others take nothing away from anyone else. If you've *always* felt seen, heard, and included in our community, I love that for you, and that certainly won't change. But if you've looked at Whole30 in the past and thought, *I'm not sure this is for me,* I'm really glad you're here, giving me and the program a second look. What you'll find in these pages is more welcoming, supportive, and inclusive than any other version of the Whole30 throughout the years, while still providing the proven structure, tailored support, and expert guidance that has made the Whole30 such a life-changing, powerful experience for so many.

I'm proud of this book, and I'm even more proud of the way the Whole30 brand and program have evolved. Thank you for reading, and for putting your faith in me and us. Let's get to the life-changing part, shall we?

MELISSA URBAN
SALT LAKE CITY, UT, AUGUST 2023

opposite: Seasonal Frittata, page 121

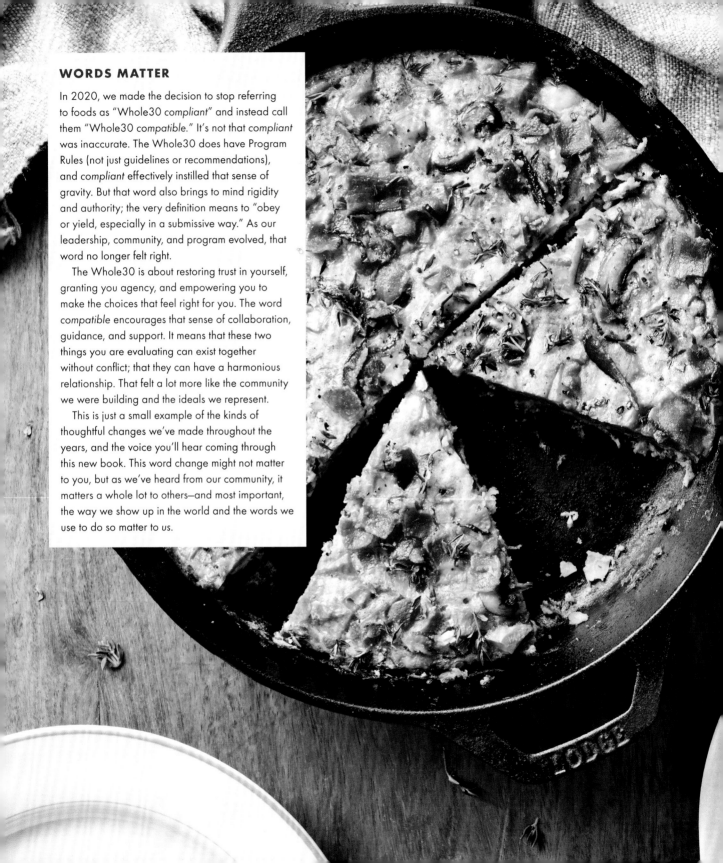

WORDS MATTER

In 2020, we made the decision to stop referring to foods as "Whole30 *compliant*" and instead call them "Whole30 *compatible*." It's not that *compliant* was inaccurate. The Whole30 does have Program Rules (not just guidelines or recommendations), and *compliant* effectively instilled that sense of gravity. But that word also brings to mind rigidity and authority; the very definition means to "obey or yield, especially in a submissive way." As our leadership, community, and program evolved, that word no longer felt right.

The Whole30 is about restoring trust in yourself, granting you agency, and empowering you to make the choices that feel right for you. The word *compatible* encourages that sense of collaboration, guidance, and support. It means that these two things you are evaluating can exist together without conflict; that they can have a harmonious relationship. That felt a lot more like the community we were building and the ideals we represent.

This is just a small example of the kinds of thoughtful changes we've made throughout the years, and the voice you'll hear coming through this new book. This word change might not matter to you, but as we've heard from our community, it matters a whole lot to others—and most important, the way we show up in the world and the words we use to do so matter to *us*.

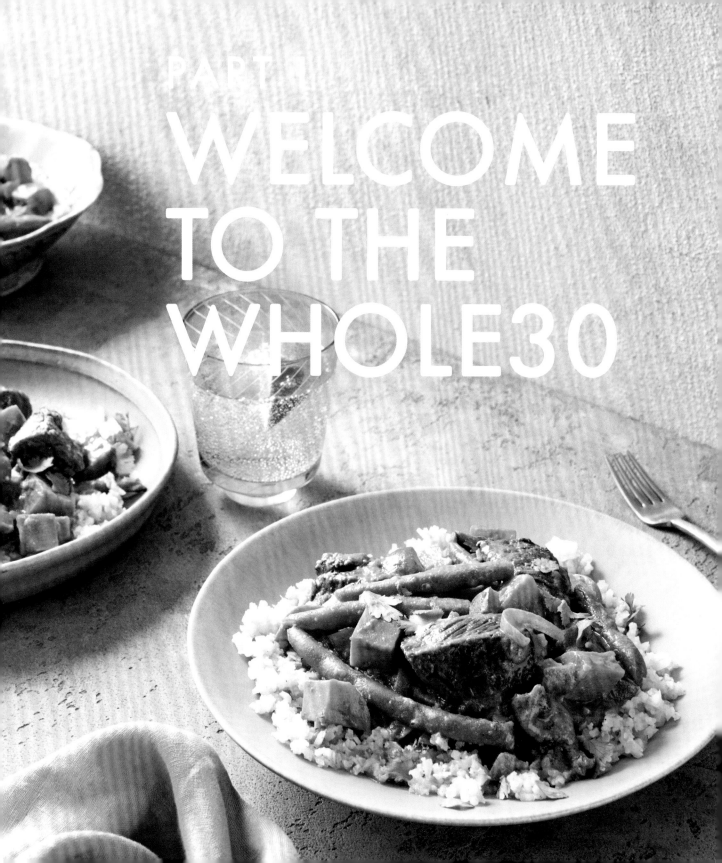

PART I

WELCOME TO THE WHOLE30

The Whole30 started as self-experiment.

In the spring of 2009, a group of friends and I were sitting on the floor of a CrossFit gym, exhausted and hungry after a hard workout. As we ate our snacks, someone brought up the nutrition seminar we had recently attended. The seminar ended with a novel challenge: Give up grains, dairy, legumes, and processed foods, and watch your health and athletic performance dramatically improve. One friend in particular was intrigued by the idea and used the discussion to propose that we try it for a month.

The group hemmed and hawed, wondering out loud if they'd really want to give up their whey protein shakes and beer on the weekend. At the time, I was eating Girl Scout cookies right out of the sleeve. Thin Mints, to be precise. I was the first one to reply. "Sure, I'd be down. When do you want to start?" My friend shot a pointed look at my cookies and said with a smirk, "How about right now?"

I found this *very* rude, but I was always up for a challenge, and my pride was on the line. I sighed deeply, closed the box, and agreed. From that point on, we were both all-in. I had no idea the next 30 days would become the most powerful and transformative of my life.

MY WHOLE30 STORY

In fact, I had already undergone quite the transformation. (This is the part where I say, "Hi, my name is Melissa, and I'm a drug addict.") By early 2000, I was in rehab for the *second* time, desperate to break free from more than five years of addiction. When I was released, I immediately

opposite: Curried Beef with Sweet Potatoes, page 175

joined a gym, hoping that morning workout sessions surrounded by healthy people would help me maintain my recovery. I miraculously stuck with it five days a week, along with my recovery group and therapy sessions.

By 2009, I was unrecognizable. I taught CrossFit classes on the weekends, was writing a successful fitness blog, and was known as the "healthy girl" at my office. If you had asked me how I ate back then, I would have said my diet was *great.* My lunches and snacks consisted of low-fat dairy, whole grains, protein shakes, and low-calorie snack packs. I ate every two hours because if I didn't, I'd get cranky. (I figured I had a high metabolism.) I read every nutrition label, dutifully counted calories, and weighed myself daily.

Sure, I had relentless cravings; I raided the pantry late at night and stuffed my face with sugar, carbs, and cheese on my weekly "cheat day"—but didn't everyone? I wasn't overweight, I stayed active, and I paid attention to what I ate, so I assumed my diet was fine.

My first Whole30 put that assumption to the test.

I expected it would be challenging, but the first few days were *really* hard. I was exhausted, cranky, had a wicked headache, and hated the switch from my morning Dunkin' Donuts Iced Caramel Turbo Latte (don't judge) to black iced coffee. I also had no idea what to eat for lunch, as whey protein shakes and bagels weren't part of the plan. I was determined to stick with it, though, and I started making veggie-packed salads with roasted chicken, salsa, and guacamole. I wasn't much of a cook yet, but it did the trick.

I was surprised at how quickly my taste buds changed. Strawberries became delightfully sweet; I developed a love for avocado, Brussels sprouts, and eggplant (none of which I had eaten before); and I didn't miss my diet soda one bit.

In Whole30 vernacular, these are Non-Scale Victories, or NSVs. They include better energy, deeper sleep, fewer cravings, smoother digestion, less pain, a happier mood—benefits that *aren't* reflected on the scale. See page 44 for a comprehensive list of Whole30 NSVs.

By the end of the second week, it was like someone had flipped a switch. I had *boundless* energy from the moment I woke up until I went to bed—no more 2 P.M. head-on-desk slump. I was sleeping soundly, falling asleep easily, and waking up at 5 A.M. for the gym without an alarm. My stomach was no longer bloated, my skin was gloriously clear, I no longer had midday poop emergencies, and I felt stronger and faster in my workouts. Even my mood was happier—something my boss tentatively asked about at one of our Monday morning meetings: "You seem so . . . *nice* lately. What have you been doing?" These were all totally unexpected benefits, none of which had to do with my weight or body composition.

Before eliminating these foods, I honestly didn't realize how relentless my cravings were, the way my energy levels dipped like a roller coaster throughout the day, that my stomach was always bloated, and how often my digestion moved way too fast. These were everyday occurrences (and had been for years), so I thought they were normal. It wasn't until I started feeling radically better that I realized how comparatively not-great I used to feel.

I couldn't believe that simple dietary changes could make me feel *this* good—but as the days went on and I continued to reap the benefits, I knew I would never go back to the way I used to eat.

Health, habits, and relationship with food

Aside from the physical benefits, the Whole30 brought to light some uncomfortable truths about my relationship with food. Specifically, it highlighted how I was using food the way I used to use drugs: to relieve anxiety, self-soothe, numb my feelings, and show myself love.

In the absence of these foods, I quickly realized I didn't have *any* other coping mechanisms. Feeling lonely? I ate something. Feeling anxious? I ate something. Feeling sad? I ate something. It wasn't always cookies, chips, or chocolate, but it became glaringly obvious how much I used food to distract, avoid, and comfort myself. Now that those foods weren't available, I needed to find other ways to navigate stress and negative emotions.

I learned to sit with my feelings, instead of immediately trying to distract myself from them. I went back to journaling, started confiding in friends and family, opened up more to my therapist, and went for a lot of walks. I found comfort in meal prep, and chopping vegetables became my daily stress relief. My cravings for chocolate and carbs disappeared, in part because of the physiological changes happening in my body and in part because I recognized that covering up my feelings with food didn't actually help—and these other techniques did.

I began making a pot of herbal tea at night. The ritual helped calm me before bed, and I developed a routine of drinking tea and reading before bed instead of snacking and watching TV. Astonishingly, I even stopped thinking about the scale, and I no longer found myself picking apart my body in the mirror. (I wouldn't set foot on the scale again for months, after years of weighing myself daily.)

Finding my food freedom

By the end of my 30 days, I felt like a whole new person—again. I was off the scale and out of the mirror for the first time in my whole life. My cravings were gone, my confidence was up, I felt better than I ever had before, and I knew I had discovered something *big*. I did miss some foods, but I figured bringing back "lite" yogurts, protein shakes, and morning bagels wouldn't affect how I felt *that* much. It wasn't until I started reintroducing them that the full picture emerged.

The low-fat cottage cheese I used to eat daily left me so bloated, it hurt. Whole wheat wraps made my chin break out and also left me bloated. My favorite "lite" yogurts, Diet Pepsi, and iced caramel lattes now tasted sickly sweet. The first whey protein shake I made gave me bubble-guts and diarrhea. What in the Slim Fast was *happening*?

The Whole30 didn't create these issues, but it sure did highlight them. It wasn't until I experienced the "new normal" available to me without some of these foods in my diet that I realized how not-great I used to feel *all the time.* Through this 30-day self-experiment, I had created a blueprint for the foods that worked best for me and could plan my meals accordingly. Dairy was generally not my friend, so I traded whey shakes and cottage cheese for eggs, chicken, and tuna. I stopped eating wheat unless it was really worth it, like when my mom made her famous hermit cookies. I gave up diet sodas forever, never went back to "lite" anything, and even quit caffeine for good—that's how much energy I had.

Equally important, my first Whole30 also helped me figure out the foods that *do* work well for me. Oatmeal, check! Rice, check! Hummus, black beans, tortilla chips, and peanut butter, check! Hot buttered popcorn with lots of salt—big fat hallelujah *check*! These foods felt great when I started eating them again, so I happily reincorporated them into my diet.

That 30-day experiment permanently and profoundly changed my health, habits, and relationship with food and with my body. A few months later, I shared the rules and results on my blog and invited others to try it. I titled the post, "Change Your Life in 30 Days," and a few hundred readers decided to join in. After they reported equally stunning and remarkably similar results at the end of the month, I christened the protocol "the Whole30," and the rest is history.

I've done eight programs since that first one in 2009. My last Whole30 was in 2020, and I probably won't ever do it again. Through repetition, awareness, and documentation of my results, I now *know* how various foods affect me. I've used those learnings to create a personalized, sustainable, joyful diet that allows me to feel my best while enjoying all the foods I love. I no longer need to follow anyone else's food rules, or question whether a food or drink is healthy *for me.* The Whole30 has taught me what works best for my body and to trust myself in those decisions. Thanks to the Whole30, I'll live the rest of my life with no foods off-limits, no morality about food, and no judgments based on what I eat or what I don't.

This is my food freedom.

My story is far from unique. I've heard *thousands* of Whole30 stories over the last fifteen years that all sound something like this: "I had no idea that (fill in food) was impacting my (fill in symptoms) until I did the Whole30. As soon as I stopped eating (food), my (everything) got better! Thanks to the Whole30, I know how to include (fill in food) in my diet in a way that works best for my health and my happiness. It feels like *freedom.*"

The Whole30 doesn't tell you how to eat. I can't do that for you, and neither can anyone else. Instead, the Whole30 provides the framework, structure, and support to help you determine for *yourself* the foods that work best for you, and use that information to create your own version of food freedom.

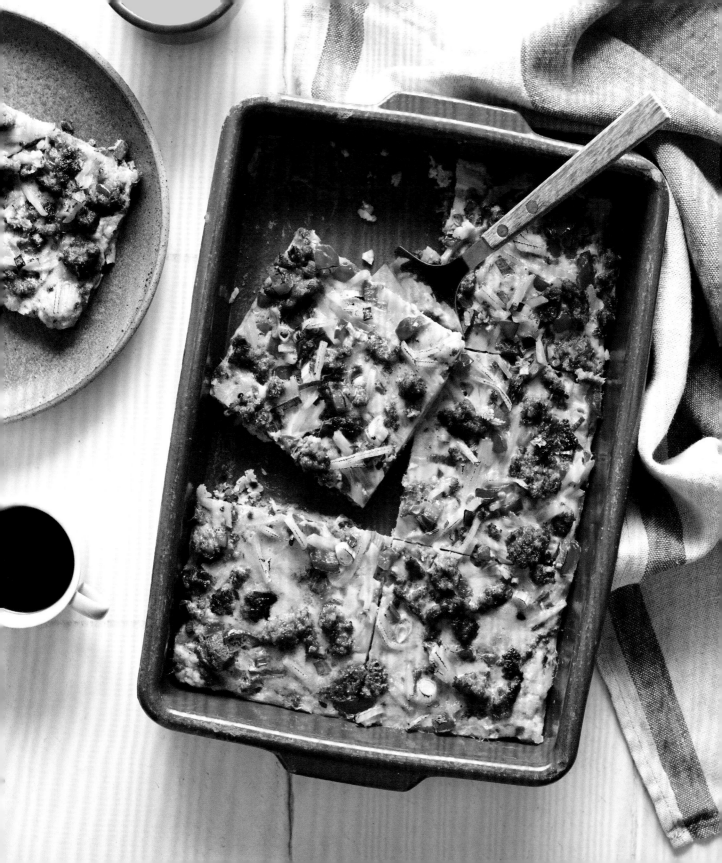

WHAT IS THE WHOLE30?

You've probably heard this incredibly sound nutrition advice from doctors, dietitians, and health experts everywhere: "There is no one-size-fits-all when it comes to diet; you have to figure out what works for you." To which you reply, "Yes, of course, that makes sense. But *how* do I figure out what works for me?"

Whole30 is the answer to "how."

THE WHOLE30 IS A 30-DAY ELIMINATION AND REINTRODUCTION PROGRAM DESIGNED TO HELP YOU:

- Identify food sensitivities and adverse food reactions
- Create new tools to navigate stress and negative emotions
- Restore a healthy relationship with food and your body
- Create a personalized, sustainable, joyful diet based on your learnings

Of course, there's a lot more to it than this.

The Whole30 has been described a number of ways since the program's inception in 2009. For many years, I called it a "reset." That term has no scientific basis—you can't reset your body like you can a frozen video game—but that word does reflect the power of the program and seems to resonate with participants. The Whole30 really *can* feel like you're pushing a hidden Reset button for your body and brain, helping you unlock a new level of "feeling good." Telling people you're doing the Whole30 to reset your health, habits, and relationship with food is an easy way to describe the process, but be prepared in case someone says, "You know that's not a *thing*, right?"

The media have mostly referred to the Whole30 program as a weight loss diet. I don't like it, and

it's inaccurate, but I get it. When I say "diet," what immediately comes to mind? I'm betting it's weight loss—probably accompanied by caloric restriction, deprivation, and a fixation on the scale. Whole30 doesn't neatly fit into that "diet" box, and weight loss is still a $200 *billion* business. Diet culture—which equates thinness with health, values small bodies, and ties our worth to our weight—is *deeply* embedded in our society and our psyches. (See page 60 for more.) Headlines promising to "melt fat," "slim thighs," and "burn calories" continue to dominate, as do ads for fad diets, weight loss hacks, and Ozempic. When a nutrition program like ours doesn't fall into the familiar "eat less to make yourself smaller" framework, the media might not know how to classify it—or they'll purposefully *misclassify* it because "weight loss" is still clickbait.

Case in point: The Whole30 program ranked dead last on *U.S. News and World Report*'s annual "Best Weight Loss Diets" list for many years. I never knew how to respond to media requests for comments. Was I proud to be the worst or annoyed we were even included? (I remain both.)

Despite what you may have read or heard, the Whole30 is not a weight loss diet. The program does not exist to make you smaller, and our structure, support, and language reflect that. While on the Whole30, you won't count or restrict calories. You won't weigh, measure, or track your ingredients or macros. You won't skip meals, control your portions, or replace food with bars or shakes. We'll *never* tell you to ignore or distract yourself from hunger signals. In fact, for 30 days straight, you won't even step on the scale—that's one of our rules. The Whole30 wasn't designed as a weight loss tool; we have much bigger goals in mind.

opposite: Sausage Egg Casserole, page 118

But *will* I lose weight?

I know many people come to the Whole30 with weight loss in mind. In our own surveys, 47 percent of respondents say they desire to change their body composition. If this is you, I don't want you to feel weird or bad about that. (Or guilty, and especially not shameful, like you're doing something wrong for wanting to change your body.) *There is nothing wrong with wanting to lose weight,* and I respect and honor those intentions. I believe the desire to lose weight is value-neutral—neither good nor bad, and always free from judgment.

Weight loss dieting *itself* can be incredibly harmful, though. The mindset and belief system we've been indoctrinated with when we radically cut calories, attach health to thinness, and equate the number on the scale with our worth and value have given most of us an unhealthy relationship with food and our bodies. Unsustainable quick-fix or "yo-yo" diets leave you trapped in a mindset of restriction, deprivation, guilt, stress, and low self-esteem. Repeated cycles of gaining, losing, then regaining weight have serious health consequences. In fact, I suspect many of you are here looking for an alternative, desperate to get off the dieting roller coaster.

To be clear, there *are* healthful ways to lose weight. Those approaches focus on consistency and sustainability, rather than quick fixes and willpower. They encourage personalization to accommodate your lifestyle and preferences. They balance short-term, moderate caloric deficits with long periods of maintenance, promoting the cultivation of lifelong healthy habits. In fact, these sustainable weight loss approaches have quite a lot in common with the Whole30.

Still, the Whole30 is not that. We won't direct you toward weight loss, provide resources to assist you with weight loss, or encourage a caloric deficit

in the name of weight loss. If your *only* goal is to lose a few quick pounds, the Whole30 is probably not the best approach. But wait! Even if this *is* what you came here for, hear me out.

What the Whole30 *can* do is help you create new, healthy habits around food and eating. We can teach you new ways to navigate stress, discomfort, or anxiety that don't involve automatically reaching for chocolate, chips, or wine. We can lead you to increased energy, deeper sleep, fewer cravings, smoother digestion, less pain, and improved self-confidence—in just 30 days. And we can help you release the attachment you have to the scale and the power that scale has held over your feelings of worth and value.

Will you lose weight? The truth is, I don't know, and we don't measure those results in our exit surveys. But if you do, you'll know that you achieved that result through nourishing foods, sustainable habits, and a focus on self-care; and you'll emerge with a personalized plan for turning your learnings into a maintainable lifestyle. And if you don't, how much will it matter if your energy, sleep, cravings, mood, digestion, inflammation, and symptoms are all *dramatically* better?

You've tried the quick-fix weight loss diets. They never work, and they leave you feeling like it's your fault. It's *not* your fault—and there is a different path. Are you willing to take a well-deserved break from the scale and discover the multitude of benefits the Whole30 can bring? Millions of people just like you have trusted the process and describe it as a truly life-changing experience.

Just give us 30 days.

Elimination diet basics

"Reset" and other terms aside, the Whole30 is in fact an *elimination diet* (or to be more precise, an *elimination and reintroduction protocol*), and that's what you should say if your Huberman Lab–loving co-worker asks you why you're passing on the break room donuts. Elimination diets have been around since the 1920s, and many physicians still consider them the gold standard for identifying food sensitivities and intolerances.

In an April 2022 article, the Cleveland Clinic described the Whole30 as "a useful tool to learn more about how your body responds to certain foods."

As with all elimination diets, the Whole30 has two parts: elimination and reintroduction. During *elimination,* you completely eliminate food groups that the scientific literature and our clinical experience have shown to be commonly problematic, for 30 straight days. During this period, you observe how the removal of these foods impacts your energy, sleep, cravings, digestion, mood, chronic pain or fatigue, mental health, and other symptoms. If you are sensitive to any of these foods, this phase allows the body to heal and repair by doing the following:

- Reducing or eliminating cravings
- Promoting a balanced metabolism and blood sugar regulation
- Improving the health of your gut and microbiome
- Calming your immune system (reducing systemic inflammation)

The second phase of the Whole30 is *reintroduction,* which immediately follows elimination and takes at least 10 days. In this phase, you reintroduce the eliminated food groups one at a time, carefully and systematically, into a day of otherwise Whole30 meals. This allows you to "test" the effects of the

WOULDN'T YOU KNOW?

How could you be sensitive to certain foods and not notice? I bet sometimes you *do* notice, but write it off. Before my first Whole30, I thought bloating and diarrhea were normal for my body. (Turns out, it was the copious amounts of low-fat dairy I was eating.)

Much of the time, however, these connections aren't easy to spot. Food sensitivities can contribute to allergies, asthma, migraines, brain fog, fatigue, anxiety, cravings, skin conditions, joint pain and swelling, digestive issues, or other unwanted symptoms in ways that aren't obvious. My friend Alex never connected her swollen, painful joints to gluten until she eliminated and reintroduced bagels, bread, and pasta during her Whole30. Now she is able to avoid the worst of her rheumatoid arthritis symptoms through diet alone.

Almost everyone who completes a Whole30 identifies *something* they hadn't noticed about the way food affects their body—positive or negative. For some like Alex, identifying those connections can be truly life-changing.

reintroduced foods in a controlled environment and observe their impact in all the same areas: energy, sleep, cravings, digestion, mood, chronic pain or fatigue, mental health, and other symptoms.

The elimination and reintroduction process allows you to compare your experience—how you felt without these foods in your diet, and how you felt when you reintroduced them—so you can identify any specific foods or food groups that promote unwanted symptoms.

HOW IT WORKS

Here is a synopsis of how the Whole30 works (whether you're doing the Original or the Plant-Based program), with a breakdown of key elements:

30 DAYS: Whole30's elimination period of 30 days isn't magic, although it is grounded in habit research. According to science, it can take

BEHAVIOR CHANGE AND HABIT RESEARCH

While the goal of an elimination diet is to identify food sensitivities and intolerances, the Whole30 takes it a step further by incorporating principles of behavior change and habit science. As you move through the program, the structure and support can also help you create new habits and stress management tools, and restore a healthy relationship with food.

There are two Whole30 Program Rules that speak specifically to these goals: the Pancake Rule (page 40), and the Scale Rule (page 42). You'll learn more about these goals later in the book. For now, just know that the Whole30 can improve your physical, mental, *and* emotional health, offering synergistic benefits that spill over into every area of your life.

anywhere from 18 to 254(!) days to make a habit stick, depending largely on how emotionally tied you are to that habit. However, one study in 2021 found that, on average, a new habit takes 59 days to solidify.

Creating new habits with food presents a significant emotional challenge, so these habits might take longer to really stick. But asking someone to follow a strict elimination protocol for two months (or longer) isn't reasonable or necessary for our purposes. In our fifteen years of experience, we've found 30 days is the sweet spot. It's long enough for you to see dramatic, life-changing results, but short enough to make the program feel attainable. And when you factor in 10 to 14 days of reintroduction, you're already three-fourths of the way to that 59-day benchmark.

It's also important to note that, like any elimination diet, the Whole30 is *not* meant to be followed long term. Reintroduction is a necessary part of the process; otherwise, you're just restricting a large number of foods with no end in sight. (This also won't get you to food freedom and could put you at risk for nutritional deficiencies and disordered eating habits.) The elimination period may be extended to 45 or even 60 days if appropriate for your context, but it should be followed for no longer than that unless specifically directed by your healthcare provider. (See page 64 for more on this.)

COMPLETE ELIMINATION: During those 30 days, you eliminate the foods on our list, 100 percent. That means *none* of the elimination foods or beverages in question for the full duration of this phase. This isn't me trying to turn Whole30 into boot camp; elimination programs are strict for good reason. To accurately determine what life is like in the absence of these potentially problematic foods, you need to *completely* eliminate them. Eliminating them most of the time (but not completely) won't give you the full picture. Here's an analogy:

Say you've had allergy symptoms off and on your whole life, and your new girlfriend has a cat. After a week hanging out at her place, your allergies seem to be worse; your eyes are itchy and your nose is stuffy all day long. So you tell your girlfriend you

During the *30-day* elimination phase, you *completely eliminate* foods that the scientific literature and our clinical experience have demonstrated to be *commonly problematic,* and pay attention to what happens to your energy, sleep, cravings, digestion, mood, and symptoms. At the end of those 30 days, you *reintroduce* those food groups one at a time and compare your experience. You then use those learnings to design your own personalized, sustainable *Food Freedom plan.*

need a break from the cat—except you still pop over to her place now and then to bring her flowers, watch a show, or have dinner.

Yes, you're *mostly* avoiding her cat, but you're still exposing yourself regularly. As a result, you have no way of knowing whether the cat is really the issue or if it's something else (like your roommate's new cologne, or pollen in the air).

To accurately determine whether you're sensitive to a particular food, you need to completely avoid it and allow your body time (in this case, 30 straight days) to heal from the effects. If you do eat some of the food or drink in question during that elimination period (e.g., pay a quick visit to the cat), healthcare providers recommend *starting your program over* to ensure you get an adequate amount of time away from that stimulus to accurately evaluate its impact. That means if you decide to eat something from the elimination group during your Whole30, I'm going to strongly recommend you start over from Day 1.

Aside from the physiological benefits of strictly adhering to your elimination protocol, habit research shows that black-and-white rules are actually *easier* for the brain to follow. Ambiguity makes it far more likely your brain will try to negotiate or look for loopholes to get the reward. (Anyone who has ever tried to practice moderation knows this; the willpower required to consume "less" sugar, alcohol, or chocolate without concretely defined terms is *tremendous*.) Psychologically, it requires less willpower, executive function, and effort to tell yourself "This food is dead to me for 30 days" than "I'll *try* not to eat this food for a month, but . . . [fill in negotiation tactics and loopholes here]."

I *do* want you to commit to all 30 days of elimination, followed by an equally conscientious reintroduction. I want you to experience the life-changing magic of the Whole30, as millions of others who have trusted the process have experienced. Equally important, though, *I want you to keep this promise to yourself.* The promise of 30 straight days, the promise of listening to your body, the promise of trusting the signals it sends you. You deserve that, especially after so many quick-fix weight loss diets have let you down while making it feel like it was your fault.

You may wonder if you can do it, but I know you can. And if the *only* benefit of your Whole30 is "I made a promise to myself grounded in self-care, and I kept that promise," you will have succeeded. (See page 63 for additional guidance here.)

COMMONLY PROBLEMATIC: Notice I said the Whole30 eliminates foods that are *commonly problematic*. I didn't say *bad, toxic,* or other words wellness influencers like to use to scare or shame people out of eating certain foods.

The Whole30 doesn't eliminate foods because they are bad. *There are no good or bad foods.* In fact, there is no morality associated with food at all—or with you when you eat food. Whole30 eliminates these foods because, according to the science, they *can* be problematic for some, and you won't know if or how they are problematic for you until you eliminate them, reintroduce them, and compare your experience.

However, studies also show that elimination diets come with a sort of confirmation bias, whereby participants tend to believe the foods they eliminate *are* going to prove problematic for them. The placebo effect upon reintroduction can be strong, so keep an open mind during your Whole30 and evaluate your results objectively. These foods are commonly problematic—but they may not be problematic for you, and the experiment is *just* as successful if you discover they are not!

You may find that wheat or dairy doesn't affect you in any negative way. That's a wonderful thing to know and can give you confidence when making food choices in the future. You also may find that wheat or dairy was the hidden cause of your joint pain, allergies, digestive issues, or migraines. That's also wonderful to know, even if it is a bummer. The goal of the program isn't to "prove" that wheat or dairy is unhealthy and should be avoided. It's to help you figure out the foods that work best for you, then empower you to use that information however you choose.

REINTRODUCTION: I know it's *called* the Whole30, but reintroduction is an essential part of the program, and the "Whole40ish" doesn't have the same ring. Reintroduction provides you with the other half of the learning experience: What happens when you bring these eliminated food groups back into an otherwise Whole30 environment?

See page 37 for the Original Whole30 reintroduction schedule, and page 39 for the Plant-Based Whole30 reintroduction schedule.

To go back to our pet analogy, say you avoid your girlfriend's cat for 30 straight days, with no contact whatsoever. And, yay, your sneezing, itchy eyes, and runny nose have vastly diminished! You've got *some* information here: The last 30 days have been a healthy environment for your allergies. But unless you visit the cat again and see what happens, you'll *never know for sure*. Was it the cat? Did your roommate stop using cologne? Or did the pollen levels drop?

Spending time with the cat and observing what happens is the second half of your self-experiment. If you spend a night with the cat and your allergies are back in full force the next morning, now you know and can take action. (Consult an allergist, take over-the-counter medication, limit sleepovers to your place, or say goodbye to your girlfriend.) If you spend the night with the cat and remain allergy free, great news! It wasn't the cat after all, so you can rule that cause out and start searching for other potential triggers.

In the case of the Whole30, if you eliminate these foods and things get better—your energy improves, you start sleeping better, your digestion smooths out, your stomach stops bloating, your skin clears up, your joints stop aching, your migraines cease, or your anxiety calms—that's excellent intel! Something about what you're doing is obviously working.

But let's say on Day 31, you skip the "careful reintroduction" part and dive right back into pizza, beer, ice cream, and peanut butter—and your symptoms reappear in full force. How are you going to know what to blame for what? Was it the gluten or the dairy that made your skin break out and your stomach bloat? Was it the peanuts or the alcohol that gave you the migraine? You've spent the last 30 days giving up foods you love, but because you skipped reintroduction, you've missed *half* the learning experience. That sounds like a terrible deal to me, and I do not want that for you.

So commit to the full Whole30, including a 30-day elimination period *and* a reintroduction phase of 10 days or more. Treat it like a science experiment and pay close attention to the way the "experimental factors" (reintroduced food groups) affect you. Call it the Whole40, if that helps. But hear me clearly: There is no Whole30 without reintroduction, and without reintroduction, *there is no food freedom.*

FOOD FREEDOM PLAN: What happens *after* the Whole30 is over? Quick-fix weight loss diets send you off into the sunset (may the odds be ever in your favor), providing no further guidance on how to take the program and turn it into a sustainable, healthy lifestyle. Spoiler alert: That's because you can't. Those weight loss diets aren't designed to change your habits or emotional relationship with food, even if they claim to. They're not even designed to improve your health! They exist only to make you smaller, with unsustainable crash-diet tactics that "work" only in the short term, if at all.

The Whole30 *isn't* that. With our program, you will discover that the lessons you learn through elimination and reintroduction *will* become the foundation for a long-term, gratifying, healthy (as *you* define it) diet. Hallelujah!

Food freedom is the final stop on your Whole30 journey. This phase is where you use the information you've learned from elimination and reintroduction to create your own personalized, sustainable, joyful diet. After your Whole30, you know better than any diet trend, new study, or magazine article the foods that work best for you—and the foods that don't.

> Food freedom is feeling empowered to choose the foods that feel right for your body, and trusting yourself to make those choices.

But food freedom isn't just a feeling; it's an actual three-part plan outlined in my book *Food Freedom Forever.* Much as with the Whole30 program, my Food Freedom plan provides the structure, guidance, and introspective prompts to help you navigate food choices with ease, comfort, and confidence, *without* being prescriptive. (How could it be? Everybody's food freedom looks different!) There are two simple questions at the heart of your Food Freedom plan: Is it worth it? and, Do I want it?

Based on your Whole30 experience, you'll know how eliminating and reintroducing those foods impacted your energy, sleep, cravings, mood, digestion, pain, inflammation, and other symptoms. Asking "Is it worth it?" helps you evaluate the known consequences of eating this food against the satisfaction, sense of belonging, or pure pleasure of eating it. Remember how I said gluten left me with bloating and breakouts? Asking "Is it worth it?" helped me easily pass on the leftover break-room donuts at work, but enthusiastically enjoy my mom's freshly baked rolls at Thanksgiving.

Only *you* know how to answer that question for yourself, and your "Is it worth it?" barometer will change given your health, your goals, and the context of the food in question. (Ice cream might be worth it on a summer afternoon while on vacation with your family, but not at 10 P.M. on a random Sunday night.)

If you decide the food in question could be worth it, you'll then ask, "Do I want it?" Yes, ice cream is delicious. Yes, you usually enjoy ice cream. But do you *want* ice cream right now? Your Whole30 helped you get back in touch with your body's natural signals: hunger, fullness, craving, or a need for comfort. Tune in to those signals again to honor what your body wants and needs in your food freedom. You may be surprised how often you turn down a "treat" because in that moment, you'd be just as happy without it. (Also, you're an adult with access to transportation and funds. If you decide

SAY YES WITH CONFIDENCE

We've talked a lot about the way various foods may be having a sneaky negative impact on your health. However, the Whole30 is just as much about identifying the foods that *do* work well for you as those that do not.

In the same way, food freedom isn't about always saying no. In your food freedom, you'll also learn to say a confident yes to whatever *you* decide is worth it. Your Yes List may include some, most, or all of the Whole30 elimination groups! You may discover that gluten works well for you, and sourdough becomes your BFF. Or you may decide that some bloating or joint pain is totally worth the joy of eating your favorite ice cream.

What's important is that your elimination and reintroduction experience—not someone else's food rules—will inform your choices going forward, so you can trust yourself to answer "Is it worth it?" and "Do I want it?" in the way that feels the best to you. (Not bad for a month and a half of work, right?)

later that night that you *do* want the ice cream, you can always go get some.)

Much like your Whole30 journey, your Food Freedom plan will be one of a kind. Your uniquely personal reasons for starting the Whole30, the lessons you took from the experience, the observations you made about how foods and food groups work in your unique body, and your collection of Non-Scale Victories will shape your Food Freedom plan. However, there are some big-picture concepts I encourage everyone to embrace:

- **Food freedom is where you live most of the time.** I don't want you to follow the Whole30 rules 365 days a year, or complete multiple Whole30s back to back because you're scared to reintroduce. The purpose of the Whole30 is to *get you to food freedom.*
- **Food freedom decisions are self-care.** No foods are off-limits if *you* decide they are worth it. And if you decide not to eat something, you won't feel deprived, because you made that decision, too—not out of fear or compliance, but from a place of trust and self-care.
- **Food freedom is flexible, not rigid.** Because you're making conscientious decisions in the moment, what's worth it now might not be worth it the next time—and vice versa. Your body, health, goals, and environment are always changing. Your food freedom decisions will evolve gracefully, right along with you.
- **Food freedom gives you the best of all worlds.** In your food freedom, you'll enjoy foods that are culturally significant, play a role in your family traditions, or are just plain delicious—while feeling exactly as good as you want to feel, relying on *your* body to guide your choices.

Let's be realistic, though—one 40-ish-day dietary self-experiment isn't going to completely override years or decades of habits, associations, and behaviors. (That's why I've done the Whole30

more than once.) Even if you are confident in your Food Freedom plan, stress, a vacation, the holidays, a big life change, or a health issue can quickly leave you struggling to feel your best. Under these conditions, it's also common for old habits, negative self-talk, and a contentious relationship with the scale to creep back in.

If this happens to you, don't panic! Just return to the Whole30.

Each time you do the Whole30, you'll learn even more about the way foods work in your current context. Like me, you'll observe more nuance in how foods impact your physical and mental health in ways you might have missed the first time around. You may choose to come back to the program to jump-start a return to the boundless energy, deeper sleep, happier mood, or smoother digestion you experienced earlier from the plan. Or you may choose to use it as a reset (there's that word again) after a vacation, the holidays, or during the transition between summer and back-to-school to help reestablish a routine.

Think of food freedom as a *practice,* not an end state. Your Food Freedom plan involves continuous fine-tuning in the way that serves you best. Stay flexible, show yourself grace, and trust yourself along the way. Should you ever want to return to the structure and support of the Whole30, the program will be here, ready to show you even more about the way foods work in your unique body.

As with everything else, food freedom gets easier with practice. You'll learn to work through your decision-making process faster and with

Medical doctors who prescribe elimination diets for their patients often recommend repeating the elimination and reintroduction period at least once, to confirm their patients' original findings and rule out any placebo effect that may have occurred in the first experiment.

opposite: Roasted Salmon, Asparagus, and Potatoes with Olive-Walnut Vinaigrette, page 162

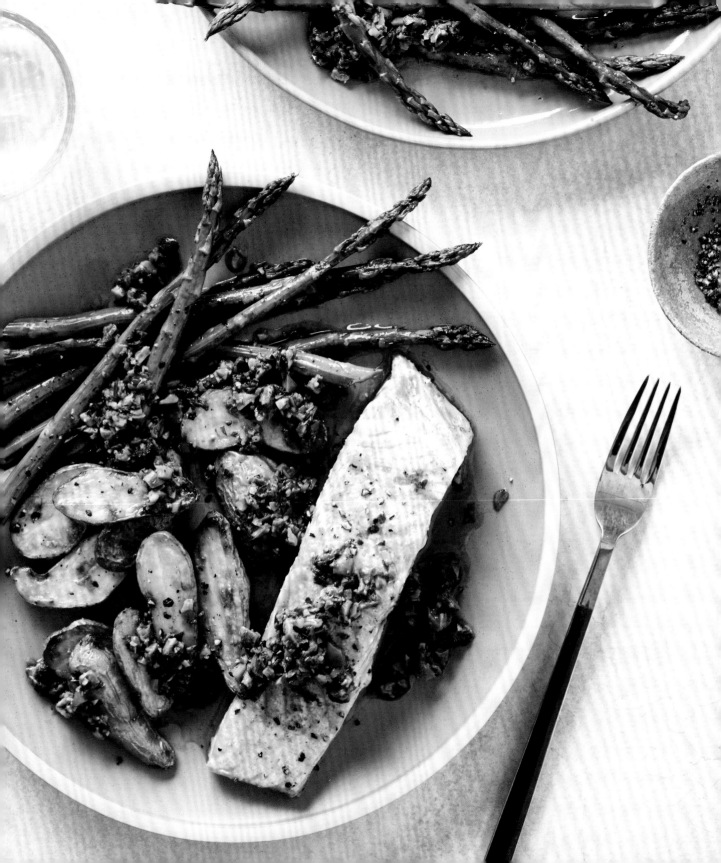

less effort. You'll naturally create new habits that support your healthy lifestyle. You'll continue to build confidence in your Food Freedom plan and in your body, which will spill over into every area of your life. There will be days, then weeks, then months when you'll look back and realize you haven't had to think about it at all—you've just been living it.

Pro tip: Read or listen to *Food Freedom Forever* during your Whole30 reintroduction to help you prepare for this next phase.

That is true food freedom—and it's waiting for you on the other side of your Whole30.

ORIGINAL WHOLE30 VS. PLANT-BASED WHOLE30

The New Whole30 offers two different programs: the *Original Whole30* and the *Plant-Based Whole30*. Where you go from here depends on the track you choose.

ORIGINAL WHOLE30: This is the version I first did in 2009, and it's the one you've likely heard the most about. During the elimination period, the Original Whole30 includes animal protein (meat, seafood, and eggs), veggies, fruit, and natural fats from both plants and animals. It's designed for omnivores, or plant-forward eaters who eat at least two animal-protein sources (like eggs and fish) on a regular basis.

PLANT-BASED WHOLE30: The Plant-Based Whole30 was launched in March 2022, after two years of planning, research, and beta testing. This version of the program is 100 percent vegan and

The Whole30 Mindset checklist

I've found it helpful to give new Whole30'ers a mindset "cheat sheet," especially if you're coming to us from quick-fix weight loss diets. Return to this checklist anytime you find yourself slipping back into a diet mindset or similar behaviors, to remind yourself that this is not that.

☐ The Whole30 is a short-term self-experiment designed to help me learn the foods that work best for me, so I can create my own personalized, sustainable, joyful diet.

☐ The foods I eliminate are not bad or unhealthy; they're just unknown. In my Whole30 elimination and reintroduction, I trust myself to determine how these foods work for me.

☐ No foods are good or bad, and I am not good or bad based on what I eat. Food is not moral, and I will show myself grace as I work to embrace this mindset.

☐ For 30 days, I'll take a break from checking the scale and focusing on body weight, and instead celebrate all the other benefits I'm seeing in my Whole30 journey.

☐ I am making a commitment to myself and the Whole30, including reintroduction. I am worthy of keeping this commitment, and I will advocate for myself during my program.

includes no animal products. The elimination phase of the Plant-Based Whole30 relies on soy and legumes for protein, and includes veggies, fruit, and plant-based natural fats. It's designed for vegans, those who consume little animal protein, and omnivores looking to evaluate how a 100 percent plant-based diet might work for them. As such, the Plant-Based Whole30 reintroduction schedule includes an *optional* track for the reintroduction of animal protein and dairy, if you choose.

Each program has its own set of elimination and reintroduction guidelines. It's important to note that there is no mix-and-match Whole30 option. (That means you can't do the Original Whole30 plus tofu, or the Plant-Based Whole30 plus eggs.) Each protocol was carefully designed to provide balanced nutrition during the elimination phase, while excluding as many commonly problematic food groups as is reasonable. Mixing and matching the plans will likely confuse your results and lead to fewer definitive findings, so unless your healthcare provider advises otherwise, you should follow either the Original or the Plant-Based program exactly as written.

Which program is right for me?

Choose your program based on your current diet, or the diet you want to test. Following are some suggestions to help guide you toward the right plan for you:

· **If you are an omnivore and eat a variety of animal proteins daily** (even if you avoid some, like pork or shellfish), do the Original Whole30.
· **If you are an omnivore and eat at least two animal proteins daily** (like eggs and fish, or chicken and seafood), do the Original Whole30. You can supplement your protein needs with Whole30-compatible plant-based crumbles or "meat" made from pea protein. This will help you identify the plant-based protein sources that work best for you during reintroduction.
· **If you are a vegetarian and eat only eggs and/or dairy**, do the Plant-Based Whole30 and follow the reintroduction track that includes

animal products, reintroducing only the sources you choose.
· **If you are vegan and are considering including animal protein and/or dairy in your diet**, do the Plant-Based Whole30 and follow the reintroduction track that includes animal products, reintroducing only the sources you choose.
· **If you are a vegan and will not eat any animal products**, do the Plant-Based Whole30 and follow the plant-based reintroduction protocol.
· **If you are an omnivore and want to evaluate how a 100 percent plant-based diet would work for you**, do the Plant-Based Whole30 and follow the reintroduction track that includes animal protein and dairy.

WHOLE30 PROGRAM RULE CHANGES

If you've been following Whole30 since the original book was published in 2015, you'll find some rule changes reflected in this book—some of which you may already be aware of and some of which are relatively recent. Before you review the current Program Rules, here is a quick history of those rule changes and the research behind them. Of note, these rule changes all allow *more* foods in the elimination phase and take nothing else away. This is great news, as it means today's Whole30 is more inclusive and accessible than ever. But if you're new to the Whole30, you might be less interested in the program's history, so feel free to skip ahead.

Coconut aminos as an exception to the "no added sugar" rule (2017)

Coconut aminos first came on the scene in 2013, and have since exploded in popularity as a soy sauce substitute. The first company to release the product (Whole30 Approved partner Coconut Secret) detailed the ingredients as "organic coconut 'sap' aged and blended with sun-dried, mineral-rich sea salt."

As other brands released their own products, their ingredient panels varied, sometimes listing coconut sap, but also coconut nectar, coconut blossom nectar, or coconut syrup, the last of which sounded like sugar. So we spent a month researching and consulting with several experts in the manufacturing process. What was the difference in the way these ingredients were phrased, and how *were* the aminos made?

Turns out the coconut nectar is harvested from the coconut flower blossoms, not the tree itself, as the word *sap* might indicate. From there, you can do a few things with the nectar: brew it with sea salt and water, ferment it, and turn it into aminos; dry it and allow it to granulate, turning it into coconut sugar; or sell it as coconut syrup, a liquid sweetener.

That means that technically *all* aminos are derived from a sugar source. However, unlike the other two forms of coconut nectar (sugar or syrup), aminos are not a sugar substitute. (I can't imagine pouring coconut aminos into your morning coffee.)

As a result of this research, and because this product clearly does not fall under the "no added sugar" rule, we've made all coconut aminos an exception to that rule during elimination, even if the word *nectar* or *syrup* is listed in the ingredients.

Botanical extracts as an exception to the "no alcohol" rule (2019)

Botanical extracts (like vanilla, blueberry, or cinnamon extract) are made by placing a raw material, such as vanilla beans, in alcohol and water. This extracts elements from the raw material into the liquid mixture to yield the end product: vanilla extract.

Extracts (especially those that are certified as organic) are held to the highest quality standards for all flavorings, including artificial and natural flavorings. As such, labeling is comprehensive and transparent compared to other forms of flavoring. As for the alcohol in these extracts, it is always distilled (thereby rendering it gluten free, regardless of the starting material). And while extracts generally contain a high percentage of alcohol (vanilla extract is 35 percent or more, for example), all botanical extracts sold on the market have been deemed "nonpotable," meaning you're definitely *not* drinking them.

The point of elimination on the Whole30 is to avoid foods or drinks that are commonly problematic, promoting cravings, hormonal imbalance or blood sugar dysregulation, digestive issues, or inflammation. Given the new understanding we have of how botanical extracts are derived and labeled, we simply don't have concerns. And as we don't eliminate things just for the sake of leaving them out, we've made this rule change.

As such, botanical extracts (such as vanilla extract, lemon extract, or lavender extract) are allowed during your elimination phase, even if the label on these products lists alcohol.

Peas as an exception to the "no legumes" rule in the Original Whole30 (2021)

While peas are technically a legume, we've rarely (if ever) seen them present problems upon reintroduction. Most varieties of peas are lower in FODMAPs (fermentable oligosaccharides, disaccharides, monosaccharides, and polyols) than other legumes, and the Cleveland Clinic confirms that pea protein is a hypoallergenic protein source (unlikely to cause an allergic reaction).

Upon consulting with our advisory group of medical doctors and registered dietitians as part of our annual review of the Original Whole30 Program Rules, we concluded there was no scientific or clinical standing to continue to eliminate peas as part of the Original Whole30. As such, you may enjoy all forms of green, yellow, and split peas during your Whole30 elimination.

MSG is no longer eliminated (2021)

We made this rule change in December 2021, and boy, did it attract attention. Statistics show that today, 47 percent of Americans still believe MSG is harmful, while the vast majority of credible scientific and medical evidence says otherwise.

Monosodium glutamate (MSG) is a flavor enhancer added to restaurant foods, canned foods, soups, deli meats, chips, and other foods. It's best known for its use in Asian cooking, particularly Chinese cuisine, and the collection of symptoms known as "Chinese restaurant syndrome" that many inaccurately claim results from its consumption.

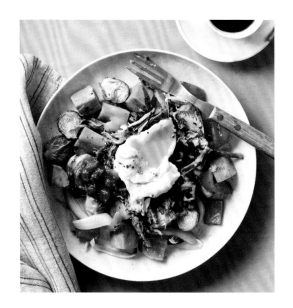

For decades, we were led to believe that MSG is harmful for health, promoting headaches, heart palpitations, numbness, and other neurological effects. However, systematic reviews of the data have shown that the negative associations with MSG were rooted in racism and questionable research that date back to the 1960s. In fact, decades of research have *not* found a strong connection between MSG and the symptoms people may associate with consuming it, and do *not* demonstrate causal evidence of MSG being problematic when consumed in a normal dose. In general, the studies of MSG have been found to be unreliable and inconsistent, often using extreme, excessive dosages that don't mimic eating in the real world.

Between the lack of verifiable science to back up these claims and the compelling evidence that Chinese restaurant syndrome is in fact rooted in racism and xenophobia, the Whole30 no longer calls for avoidance of MSG during your 30-day elimination.

Veggie and Shredded Pork Breakfast Hash, page 124

The Pancake Rule has modified language (2023)

The Pancake Rule has been in place (under a few different monikers) since the inception of the Whole30 in 2009. This rule was designed to eliminate "comfort food" re-creations made with technically compatible ingredients, to help participants reduce cravings, develop new habits, and restore a healthy relationship with food. (See page 40.)

In 2015, the Pancake Rule included:

Pancakes, bread, tortillas, biscuits, crepes, muffins, cupcakes, cookies, pizza crust, waffles, cereal, granola, ice cream, potato chips, French fries, and this one recipe where eggs, date paste, and coconut milk are combined with prayers to create a thick, creamy concoction that can once again transform your undrinkable black coffee into sweet, dreamy caffeine.

In 2015, however, the food landscape was *very* different from how it looks today. It was hard to find tasty store-bought gluten-free baked goods, dairy-free cream cheese and queso had yet to take off, and cauliflower had not yet realized its full potential as pizza crust or pretzels. The Pancake Rule called out these foods without needing to be super-specific as to their ingredients because you couldn't walk into your local grocery store and find Siete almond-flour tortillas or potato chips fried in avocado oil. Most of these re-creations were happening in your own kitchen, as you tried your best to make versions of banana bread, pizza crust, and, yes, pancakes.

Over the years, grain-free, dairy-free baked goods, pasta, cheese, and other products have *dramatically* evolved. Every year, we would have at least three or four discussions around a specific new product that challenged the boundaries of the Pancake Rule. (Plantain chips, cauliflower gnocchi, coconut wraps, and grain-free crackers were heavily discussed in the Whole30 HQ Slack channels.)

The Whole30 program recommendations, tone, and voice were also evolving. We (and I) were shifting away from the tough love we were known for and toward a more understanding, empathetic, inclusive approach. I began emphasizing that we wanted to eliminate as few foods as possible, without sacrificing results. As a result, the degree to which we explored this rule in particular was intense. In fact, we debated whether the rule was still in the best interest of the program. (When we review the Program Rules, *nothing* is off-limits. We are always testing our own assumptions.)

After weeks of discussion, we agreed the Pancake Rule *is* still integral for Whole30 program participants' success. In follow-up community surveys, you agreed. In a 2023 survey of 1,100 Whole30 alumni, 89 percent said their Whole30 would not have been as successful without the Pancake Rule. One participant wrote, "I *always* try to find a loophole in the system. Without the Pancake Rule, I wouldn't have achieved the same degree of behavior and identity change." Another said, "This was the one rule that most helped me examine my relationship with food." One woman shared, "I no longer binge on comfort foods. The Pancake Rule did that."

However, the rule needed a language refresh, so we've revised it to be even more specific about the foods that fall within this rule. In this new version, we have left a few foods out.

The new rule reads (emphasis added):

All baked goods *made from alternative flour* (bread, tortillas, wraps, crackers, pizza or pie crust, biscuits, pancakes, crepes, waffles, muffins, cupcakes, cookies, and brownies); pasta or noodles *made from alternative flour;* cereals *made from alternative flour;* chips (including *potato, sweet potato, tortilla, plantain, taro, or cassava* chips); French fries or tots.

To summarize the differences:

- **Alternative flour:** This language makes this rule more specific to flour-based products and allows products that are just protein and/or veggies. (For example, flour- or starch-free egg-white wraps, coconut wraps, or the aforementioned egg-and-banana "pancake" are now compatible with the elimination phase.)
- **Chips:** Previous language made it hard to know *which* chips were and were not compatible. This rule specifies specific potato and potato-like chips, but it leaves you free to enjoy other fruit and veggie chips, like apple, kale, and coconut.
- **Other changes:** The Pancake Rule language previously didn't allow for 100 percent (no added sugar) fruit pops or sorbets; grain-free granolas made from nuts and seeds; and whole dates used in smoothies or other beverages like coffee. Current language allows for these foods during elimination.

This new language satisfies the spirit and intention of the Pancake Rule while reincorporating fruit, veggies, nuts, seeds, and protein in creative ways that can add excitement, flavor, and convenience to your Whole30 elimination phase. It also addresses some past criticisms of this rule, which (as an example) pointed out the inconsistency in allowing fruit—but not if it's frozen in a rectangular shape.

Fair. We're happy to correct this.

Carrageenan is no longer eliminated (2024)

Carrageenan is a gelling agent, thickener, and emulsifier made from seaweed. While its origins are natural, it's been a controversial ingredient over the years. It used to be found in many foods, from deli turkey to almond milk. Today, you won't find it in nearly as many products, probably because consumers have been leery of its potential negative impact on health.

Some researchers believed that carrageenan had the potential to negatively impact the microbiota and gut barrier, and to promote increased inflammatory activity. To add to the confusion, some experts claimed the negative health effects of *degraded* carrageenan (a form not used in food) could also apply to food-grade carrageenan. Out of an abundance of caution, we took a conservative stance and added carrageenan to our elimination list.

The safety of carrageenan in the food supply has been the subject of much debate, although research directly assessing the effects of food-grade carrageenan in humans is very limited. However, review of the current science does not demonstrate enough of a risk to your blood sugar regulation, digestive health, or immune system to continue to restrict this additive as part of the Whole30 elimination phase. (To be honest, this rule change won't affect your Whole30 experience much if at all, as so many brands have already eliminated carrageenan from their formulations.)

However, if you have inflammatory bowel disease or other chronic digestive disorders, you may still choose to avoid carrageenan during your Whole30, as there is some evidence that in this specific context, avoidance may help reduce inflammation.

Added sulfites are no longer eliminated (2024)

Sulfites occur naturally in many foods (like kimchi, sauerkraut, balsamic vinegar, and red wine vinegar) and beverages (like wine) as a by-product of fermentation. Sulfites are also added to processed

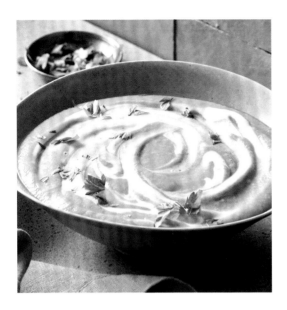

review did not cite any evidence demonstrating that sulfites are harmful to the health of the general population when consumed in recommended amounts, and no statements were made that indicate sulfites should be completely avoided by individuals who are not sensitive. As such, you are no longer required to eliminate added sulfites during your Whole30 elimination phase.

You won't find many Whole30-compatible foods with added sulfites—perhaps in dried fruits, or bottled lemon or lime juice (in the form of potassium metabisulfite). So this rule change won't much affect your Whole30, if at all. Added sulfites are also easy to avoid on the program if you have asthma, or simply prefer to buy products without this specific additive.

Cooking oils are no longer eliminated, regardless of their source (2024)

"Seed oils" is an umbrella term used to describe seed and vegetable oils that are relatively higher in omega-6 polyunsaturated fatty acids (PUFAs). Examples include sunflower, safflower, corn, soybean, and grapeseed oils. Additionally, canola and rice bran oil are often included in discussions of seed oils, despite their lower content of omega-6 relative to other fatty acids.

The Whole30 has *never* taken an elimination stance against seed oils. Since the earliest documentation of the Program Rules in 2009, canola, sunflower, safflower, and grapeseed oils have always been compatible with the program.

However, via association with their respective food groups, other seed oils *have* been part of the Whole30 elimination phase. These include soybean

foods like dried fruits and vegetables, seafood, juices, and meat products to preserve food flavor and color, inhibit bacterial growth, and reduce food spoilage.

The FDA classifies sulfites as "generally recognized as safe," but does cite them as a potential food intolerance. In addition, food processors are required to declare the presence of sulfites in foods when the concentration exceeds 10 parts per million or greater. Sensitive individuals may experience gastrointestinal disturbances, skin rashes, headaches, and respiratory symptoms when consumed. Asthmatics tend to have higher rates of sulfite sensitivity than the general population. Because of these concerns, added sulfites (but *not* those naturally occurring) were part of the Whole30 elimination phase.

Studies examining the effects of sulfites on human health are scarce. No studies were found that directly compared the effects of a sulfite-containing diet to a sulfite-free diet. However, our

Creamy Sweet Potato–Ginger Red Lentil Soup, page 291

and peanut oils (because we eliminate legumes on the Original Whole30), and corn and rice bran oils (because we eliminate grains on both programs).

We eliminated these oils in part to make it easier to follow the Program Rules. Eliminating grains from all sources is an easier rule to convey than "eliminate all grains *but* these three or four exceptions." (To be clear, there have never been concerns that soybean oil, peanut oil, or corn oil would trigger a food sensitivity. By the time these beans or seeds are processed down to an oil, the amount of protein left is incredibly low and highly unlikely to trigger a response.)

We did have concerns, however, that consumption of seed oils might have adverse health consequences. Our healthcare advisors and the references I reviewed when writing my earlier books agreed that seed oils promote systemic inflammation and metabolic disease. In fairness, the science appeared compelling. In truth, the references relied almost purely on observational and mechanistic data. This type of research cannot be extrapolated to the general population. What happens in a carefully controlled lab setting is completely different from what happens in a highly complex biological system. (This is why we have randomized controlled trials, or even better, meta-analyses of RCTs, to eliminate as much "noise" as possible and determine the true effect in actual humans.)

In addition, the message conveyed to the public often wasn't that the *over*consumption of seed oils or the consumption of seed oils *in the context of a diet full of ultra-processed foods* was problematic. What was shared—and what you'll mostly still hear today—are blanket statements like "seed oils are inflammatory," or even "seed oils are toxic," without any context or nuance.

At the time, given how strong the science looked and the recommendations of our advisors, it seemed logical to direct Whole30'ers toward oils

with more heart-healthy monounsaturated fats, and away from seed oils in our Program Rules.

In 2023, we employed an outside research team to provide an unbiased review of the current science to determine if consumption of seed oils is a risk factor for disease independent of calorie intake, omega-3 intake, and diet quality. The evidence is quite clear that oils rich in omega-6 polyunsaturated fats can be included as part of a healthy diet, do not have a meaningful effect on inflammation, and may even *reduce* the risk of chronic disease.

This conclusion does come with some caveats, however. In general, seed oils are best incorporated into a diet already low in ultra-processed foods (but to be fair, *any* ingredient is more health-promoting when included in that context). Seed oils high in omega-6 fatty acids should also be balanced with an adequate intake of omega-3 fatty acids from fatty fish, nuts, and seeds, and perhaps in conjunction with targeted supplementation. In addition, to minimize the risk of oxidation, seed oils should be used for cooking at lower temperatures (not high heat) and should not be reheated.

Given these findings, and in the context of the Whole30 elimination phase—which includes no ultra-processed foods, many whole-food sources of omega-3 fatty acids, and a variety of oils appropriate for high-heat cooking—we see no reason to continue to eliminate *any* cooking oils on the Whole30. Allowing these additional oils back into the elimination phase also serves to make the Whole30 more accessible, as these oils offer a lower-cost alternative to more expensive oils like extra-virgin olive oil or avocado oil.

Visit whole30.com/program-rules-changes to read articles related to all our Whole30 Program Rule changes throughout the years.

THE ORIGINAL WHOLE30 PROGRAM RULES

PHASE 1: Whole30 elimination—30 days

During your 30-day elimination, you'll eat meat, seafood, and eggs; vegetables and fruit; natural animal and plant-based fats; and herbs, spices, and seasonings.

    Following is a list of the food and beverage groups you'll eliminate in the first phase of the Original Whole30. To accurately identify specific food sensitivities, commit to the complete elimination of these groups for 30 straight days.

ADDED SUGAR (REAL OR ARTIFICIAL)

This includes agave nectar, brown sugar, cane sugar, coconut sugar, date syrup, high-fructose corn syrup, honey, maple syrup, molasses, monk-fruit extract, stevia (Truvia), saccharin (Sweet'n Low), sucralose (Splenda), aspartame (Equal, NutraSweet), erythritol, and xylitol. The only exception is fruit-juice concentrate.

ALCOHOL (WINE, BEER, CIDER, LIQUOR, ETC.)

This includes wine, Champagne, beer, hard cider, hard kombucha, vodka, rum, gin, whiskey, tequila, and so on, in any form (drinking, as an ingredient, or for cooking).

GRAINS (WHEAT, OATS, RICE, CORN, QUINOA, ETC.)

This includes wheat, rye, barley, farro, triticale, oats, corn, rice, millet, bulgur, sorghum, sprouted grains, and pseudo-cereals like quinoa, amaranth, and buckwheat. This also includes wheat, corn, or rice in the form of bran, germ, or starch.

LEGUMES (BEANS, LENTILS, SOY, AND PEANUTS)

This includes beans (black, red, pinto, navy, garbanzo/chickpeas, white, kidney, lima, fava, cannellini, adzuki, mung, and cranberry, plus black-eyed peas); lentils; peanuts and peanut butter; and nearly all forms of soy (soy sauce, miso, tofu, tempeh, edamame, soy protein, soy milk, or soy lecithin). Exceptions include green beans and most peas (see the Fine Print, following).

DAIRY (MILK, CHEESE, SOUR CREAM, YOGURT, ETC.)

This includes cow's, goat's, or sheep's milk products like milk, cream, cheese, cottage cheese, kefir, yogurt, sour cream, ice cream, or frozen yogurt. Exceptions include ghee and other forms of clarified butter (see the Fine Print, following).

THE PANCAKE RULE (BAKED GOODS, PASTA, CEREAL, CHIPS, AND FRIES)

This includes all baked goods made from alternative flour (breads, tortillas, wraps, crackers, pizza or pie crusts, biscuits, pancakes, crepes, waffles, muffins, cupcakes, cookies, and brownies); pasta or noodles made from alternative flour; cereals made from alternative flour; chips (including potato, sweet potato, tortilla, plantain, taro, or cassava); French fries or tots. (See page 40.)

THE SCALE RULE (WEIGHING YOURSELF OR TAKING MEASUREMENTS)

Do not weigh yourself, take body measurements, or analyze your body fat during the 30-day elimination period. (See page 42.)

THE FINE PRINT (EXCEPTIONS)

These foods *are* allowed during the Original Whole30 elimination phase:

- Green beans
- Most peas (sugar snap, snow, green, yellow, and split peas)
- Ghee and other forms of clarified butter
- Cooking oils (regardless of their source)
- Coconut aminos
- Alcohol-based botanical extracts (such as vanilla, lemon, or lavender)
- Cane, Champagne, red wine, rice, sherry, and white wine vinegars
- Iodized salt (which contains dextrose as a stabilizer)

PHASE 2: Whole30 reintroduction—10+ days

Immediately following elimination, you'll reintroduce these food groups one at a time, returning to the elimination phase for 2 to 3 days in between. Reintroduce each ingredient into an otherwise Whole30 meal for all your meals that day, with the exception of alcohol. Include enough of the reintroduced food group to properly challenge your system. (See page 83.)

ADDED SUGAR (OPTIONAL)

Spend one day adding some form of sugar to all your otherwise Whole30 meals. (For example, honey in your tea, sweetened coffee creamer, honey mustard dressing, maple-cured bacon, sweetened almond butter.) Return to the Original Whole30 elimination phase for 2 to 3 days.

LEGUMES

Spend one day adding beans, lentils, peanuts, and/or soy in any form to all your otherwise Whole30 meals. Return to the Original Whole30 elimination phase for 2 to 3 days.

NON-GLUTEN GRAINS

Spend one day adding rice, corn, oats, quinoa, buckwheat, etc., in any form to all your otherwise Whole30 meals. Return to the Original Whole30 elimination phase for 2 to 3 days.

DAIRY

Spend one day adding milk, cream, cheese, cottage cheese, kefir, yogurt, sour cream, etc., to all your otherwise Whole30 meals. Return to the Original Whole30 elimination phase for 2 to 3 days.

GLUTEN-CONTAINING GRAINS

Spend one day adding gluten-containing grains (wheat, rye, barley, farro, etc.) in any form (bread, rolls, pasta, crackers, wraps, cereal) to all your otherwise Whole30 meals. Return to the Original Whole30 elimination phase for 2 to 3 days.

ALCOHOL (OPTIONAL)

Spend one day adding 1 to 2 glasses of alcohol (gluten-containing or gluten-free) to one of your otherwise Whole30 meals. Return to the Original Whole30 elimination phase for 2 to 3 days.

THE PLANT-BASED WHOLE30 PROGRAM RULES

PHASE 1: Plant-Based Whole30 elimination— 30 days

During your 30-day elimination, you'll eat beans, lentils, and peas; minimally processed forms of soy; whole forms of plant-based protein powders; vegetables and fruit; natural plant-based fats; and herbs, spices, and seasonings.

Following is a list of the food and beverage groups you'll eliminate in the first phase of the Plant-Based Whole30. *By definition, the Plant-Based Whole30 elimination phase assumes you will also not be eating any animal protein, animal fats, or animal-based dairy.* To accurately identify specific food sensitivities, commit to the complete elimination of these groups for 30 straight days.

ADDED SUGAR (REAL OR ARTIFICIAL)

This includes agave nectar, brown sugar, cane sugar, coconut sugar, date syrup, high-fructose corn syrup, honey, maple syrup, molasses, monk-fruit extract, stevia (Truvia), saccharin (Sweet'n Low), sucralose (Splenda), aspartame (Equal, NutraSweet), erythritol, and xylitol. The only exception is fruit-juice concentrate.

ALCOHOL (WINE, BEER, CIDER, LIQUOR, ETC.)

This includes wine, Champagne, beer, hard cider, hard kombucha, vodka, rum, gin, whiskey, tequila, and so on, in any form (drinking, as an ingredient, or for cooking).

GRAINS (WHEAT, OATS, RICE, CORN, QUINOA, ETC.)

This includes wheat, rye, barley, farro, triticale, oats, corn, rice, millet, bulgur, sorghum, sprouted grains, and pseudo-cereals like quinoa, amaranth, and buckwheat. This also includes wheat, corn, or rice in the form of bran, germ, starch.

SOY (HIGHLY PROCESSED FORMS)

This specifically includes soybean oil, textured soy protein, textured vegetable protein (TVP), soy protein isolate, or soy protein concentrate.

THE PANCAKE RULE (BAKED GOODS, PASTA, CEREAL, CHIPS, AND FRIES)

This includes all baked goods made from alternative flour (bread, tortillas, wraps, crackers, pizza or pie crusts, biscuits, pancakes, crepes, waffles, muffins, cupcakes, cookies, and brownies); pasta or noodles made from alternative flour; cereals made from alternative flour; chips (including potato, sweet potato, tortilla, plantain, taro, or cassava); French fries or tots. (See page 40.)

THE SCALE RULE (WEIGHING YOURSELF OR TAKING MEASUREMENTS)

Do not weigh yourself, take body measurements, or analyze your body fat during the 30-day elimination period. (See page 42.)

THE FINE PRINT (EXCEPTIONS)

These foods *are* allowed during the Plant-Based Whole30 elimination phase:

- Rice found in fermented soy (listed as an ingredient in miso or tempeh)
- Cooking oils (regardless of the source)
- Coconut aminos
- Alcohol-based botanical extracts (such as vanilla, lemon, or lavender)
- Cane, Champagne, red wine, rice, sherry, and white wine vinegar
- Iodized salt (which contains dextrose as a stabilizer)

PHASE 2: Plant-Based Whole30 reintroduction— 6+ days

Immediately following elimination, you'll reintroduce these food groups one at a time, returning to the elimination phase for 2 to 3 days in between. *Note, the Plant-Based Whole30 includes the option to reintroduce animal protein and/or dairy, if you choose.* Reintroduce each ingredient into an otherwise Plant-Based Whole30 meal for all your meals that day, with the exception of alcohol. Include enough of the reintroduced food group to properly challenge your system. (See page 83.)

ADDED SUGAR (OPTIONAL)

Spend one day adding some form of sugar to all your otherwise Plant-Based Whole30 meals. (For example, honey in your tea, sweetened coffee creamer, honey mustard, sweetened almond butter.) Return to the Plant-Based Whole30 elimination phase for 2 to 3 days.

NON-GLUTEN GRAINS

Spend one day adding rice, corn, oats, quinoa, buckwheat, etc., in any form to all your otherwise Plant-Based Whole30 meals. Return to the Plant-Based Whole30 elimination phase for 2 to 3 days.

ANIMAL PROTEIN (OPTIONAL)

Spend one day adding beef, bison, lamb, chicken, turkey, wild game, pork, fish, shellfish, and/or eggs to all your otherwise Plant-Based Whole30 meals. Return to the Plant-Based Whole30 elimination phase for 2 to 3 days.

ANIMAL-SOURCED DAIRY (OPTIONAL)

Spend one day adding milk, cream, cheese, cottage cheese, kefir, yogurt, sour cream, etc., to all your otherwise Plant-Based Whole30 meals. Return to the Plant-Based Whole30 elimination phase for 2 to 3 days.

GLUTEN-CONTAINING GRAINS

Spend one day adding gluten-containing grains (wheat, rye, barley, farro, etc.) in any form (bread, rolls, pasta, crackers, wraps, cereal) to all your otherwise Plant-Based Whole30 meals. Return to the Plant-Based Whole30 elimination phase for 2 to 3 days.

ALCOHOL (OPTIONAL)

Spend one day adding 1 to 2 glasses of alcohol (gluten-containing or gluten-free) to one of your otherwise Plant-Based Whole30 meals. Return to the Plant-Based Whole30 elimination phase for 2 to 3 days.

THE PANCAKE RULE AND THE SCALE RULE

As mentioned on page 22, there are two Whole30 Program Rules that speak specifically to the goal of creating new habits, developing effective tools for navigating stress and discomfort, and reestablishing a healthy relationship with food and your body. Both rules are grounded in the science of behavior change and habit research, and both have proved integral to Whole30 success, as reported by thousands of people who have completed the program.

The Pancake Rule

Since the creation of the Whole30 program in April 2009, we've had a rule that says: *Do not re-create baked goods, pasta, cereal, chips, or fries with Whole30-compatible ingredients.* We call it the Pancake Rule because this was the food that participants tried to re-create most often in the earliest days of

In a 2023 survey of 690 Whole30 participants, 53 percent reported their primary motivation for starting the program was reducing sugar cravings. At the end of their Whole30, 94 percent said they achieved that goal.

Whole30. Back then, it was just an egg and a banana smashed together into a pancake-like patty. Now, grain-free recipes are *far* more elevated, featuring an assortment of alternative flours, baking soda, natural sweeteners, and dairy-free milks.

This rule is a bit of a different animal. It's still grounded in science, but in psychology and habit research, not biochemistry or physiology. The premise is simple: If you want to change your habits, you have to actually *change your habits.* If you spend all 30 days of the elimination phase trying

to re-create the baked goods and comfort foods you came into the program eating, what are the chances you'll come out of the program with new healthy habits and fresh tools for navigating stress or discomfort? (Spoiler alert: Zero.)

Most of the research in this area has been done with alcohol and alcohol addiction. Researchers have studied the role environmental cues like smells, sounds, visual prompts, and taste can play in triggering cravings and relapses. They've discovered that smell cues *alone* may be enough to trigger cravings. Other environmental cues can also elicit a conditioned response that likely plays a role in relapses—an effect to which I can personally testify.

Granted, sugar and alcohol are not the same, although recent studies confirm that food addiction, particularly with ultra-processed foods, is very real. Studies in humans demonstrate that sugar and hyperpalatable foods can induce cravings and light up the same reward centers in the brain as do alcohol, nicotine, and other drugs, provoking a similar dopamine "seeking" response. Many who come to the Whole30 self-report as being "addicted" to sugar. And if you *feel* addicted to sugar

SO MUCH FLOUR

The Pancake Rule can help you identify food sensitivities, too! Many of these grain-free re-creations contain a heap of alternative flour (like cassava, almond, or tapioca), which many people find disruptive to digestion. Eliminating these foods can also help you reduce gas, bloating, and other digestive issues, and allows you to evaluate how these grain-free re-creations work in your system during reintroduction.

or sweetness, this may make your food cravings vulnerable to the same environmental cues.

As we know that visual cues, taste, and smell can provoke or promote cravings, it's reasonable to assume it will be much harder for you to reduce cravings and change your habits if you spend the next 30 days eating foods that look, taste, and smell just like the comfort foods you came into the program eating. (Our fifteen-plus years of experience and surveys done with Whole30 alumni support this theory.) The Pancake Rule is designed to help you discover other ways to relieve anxiety, self-soothe, navigate stress, and show yourself love—strategies that soon become habits and will serve you long after your Whole30 is over.

Habits often become so ingrained that we maintain the action even though we're no longer benefiting from it. (Anyone in a love-hate relationship with late-night sugar or after-work wine can confirm.) According to habit research, once these neural patterns are grooved, they aren't easily removed. The good news is that they can be *replaced* with something new—a new behavior, a new mindset, or a healthier substitution. Your Whole30 is the perfect time to imprint a new habit over an old one that is no longer serving you.

This is where the Pancake Rule comes in. Yes,

In a June 2023 survey of more than 1,100 Whole30 alumni, 89 percent said their Whole30 would not have been as successful without the Pancake Rule.

a cassava-flour tortilla chip may be made with Whole30-compatible ingredients, but *your brain doesn't know the difference.* It just knows that it's late; you're bored, anxious, lonely, or stressed; and you're giving in to a craving for reasons that aren't related to hunger. Your brain *doesn't care what the chips are made of.* It just knows they smell, taste, and look just like tortilla chips. It knows chips are easy and rewarding. And it remembers that this is how you

READ YOUR LABELS

When you're evaluating foods for the Pancake Rule, look for alternative flours, starches, or powders in the ingredient list (like cassava flour, almond flour, tapioca starch, arrowroot powder, or potato flour). That's a key indicator that your pasta, tortilla, or pizza crust isn't compatible with the Whole30. But those wraps made with egg whites, spices, and no flour at all? Wrap away!

pass the time between 8 and 10 P.M., when you're tired-but-wired and need to self-soothe.

Now apply that same concept to coconut oil–fried potato chips, almond flour pancakes, "paleo" brownies, and cauliflower pasta. Without the Pancake Rule, you could spend the entirety of your Whole30 still numbing, distracting, comforting yourself, and relieving stress in the same way, with *the same foods.* And that keeps you stuck in those habits, experiencing the same overpowering cravings and without *any* incentive to develop new coping strategies.

That's not much of a reset, now, is it?

The Pancake Rule calls out specific food *re-creations*—situations in which you're trying to make your Whole30 foods look, smell, taste, and feel just like your comfort foods. (It's like swapping your favorite beer for a nonalcoholic beer. Same bottle, same taste, same smell . . . and all the same habit cues.) It's perfectly acceptable, however, to *replace* the bun on your burger with lettuce or the pasta under your marinara with spaghetti squash. (That's the equivalent of trading your beer for an unsweetened iced tea or a sparkling water.)

Here's another good rule of thumb: If the food or drink is *just* the vegetable or protein, it's good to go. That means your jicama taco shells, dried apple "chips," or zucchini noodles are A-okay.

Finally, yes, the Pancake Rule applies to *everyone* on the Whole30. Even if you "don't have a problem" with pancakes, as so many of you have told me. Trust the process and the program, as millions of people have done before you with great success. This rule is just as important to your Whole30 results as the others. And if you have no emotional ties to pancakes, it shouldn't be hard to avoid them for 30 short days, right?

The Scale Rule

The Scale Rule has also been in place since the earliest days of Whole30, and is important to the spirit and intention of the program. In fact, this rule, more than any other, may help you shift your mindset away from quick-fix weight loss dieting.

The rule states: *No stepping on the scale, taking body measurements, or analyzing body fat during your 30-day elimination period.* And yes, it's an official Program *Rule,* not just a suggestion. You might have come to Whole30 wanting to lose weight, and as I've said, we honor that intention. But this rule is just as integral for your Whole30 success as the others.

First, you already know there is so much more to health than the number registering on that $20 hunk of plastic. In fact, contrary to what diet culture has taught you, your weight doesn't say *anything* about your health! The most commonly reported Whole30 benefits—more energy, better sleep, fewer cravings, smoother digestion, less pain—can't be measured by the scale, but that number can quickly overshadow all of those benefits. Here's an interaction I've had more than once with people as they finish their Whole30:

Them: The Whole30 didn't work for me.

Me: Oh, no! What happened?

Them: Well, I'm sleeping better, my energy is through the roof, my skin is glowing, and my joints aren't swollen anymore—but I only lost two pounds.

Me: 😐

HOW CAN I STAY MOTIVATED?

Since you're not using the scale to measure progress, you'll have to find other ways to stay motivated on the Whole30.

- Start with your "why," and look for related victories. If your "why" was to spend more quality time with your kids, look at small improvements in patience, energy levels, or sleep as a sign you're moving in the right direction. (See page 46 for more on "finding your why.")
- Review the Non-Scale Victory (NSV) checklist (page 44) and note any victories you've achieved, no matter the size. Even noting that you kept your promise to yourself for one more day can feel hugely rewarding.
- Check your wearables, like your WHOOP band, Apple watch, or Oura ring. Seeing your sleep, heart rate variability, resting heart rate, recovery scores, or athletic performance improve over the course of the month confirms that your hard work is having a positive impact.
- Look to your support group for encouragement, accountability, tough love, or positive reinforcement. Seeing your efforts through other people's eyes can help to quiet the doubting voice in your head and may help you spot NSVs you didn't even notice!

It turns out the fastest way to sabotage all those I'm-doing-it, proud-of-myself, this-is-really-working feelings is . . . weighing yourself. And do you really want to risk that sense of pride, self-confidence, and success 24 days into your Whole30?

The truth is, very few people have a healthy relationship with the scale, and that number can dramatically influence your behavior, self-esteem, and mindset. (How many of us have vowed to eat less, punished ourselves with exercise, said something mean to ourselves, or noticed our mood plummet after stepping on the scale? All of us, I'm

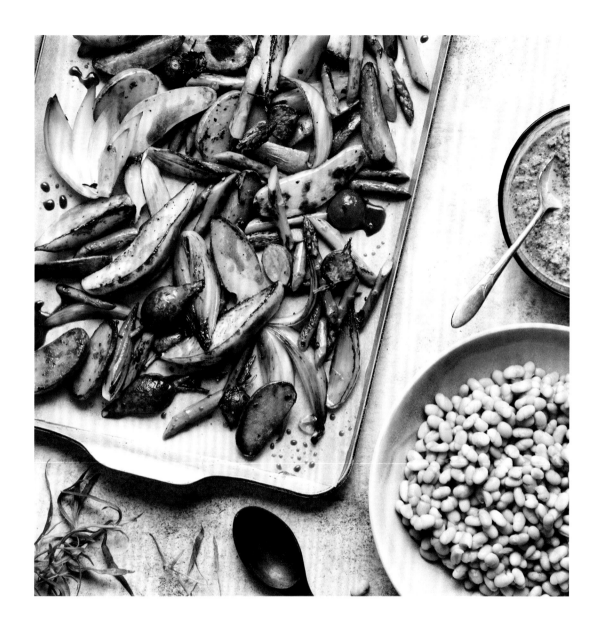

betting.) By taking the scale out of the equation, the Whole30 will help you change your definition of success and bring a multitude of Non-Scale Victories into the spotlight—where they belong!

So we're gonna get rid of that evil plastic overlord for the next 30 days and focus on all the *Non-Scale Victories* you can realize through your Whole30 elimination and reintroduction. (It's a long list.) For more on weighing yourself when your Whole30 elimination is over, see page 86.

Roasted Veggies and White Beans with Zhug, page 260

Non-Scale Victory checklist

PHYSICAL (INSIDE)
- ☐ Fewer PMS symptoms
- ☐ Fewer menopause symptoms
- ☐ Increased libido
- ☐ Healthier gums
- ☐ Less stomach pain
- ☐ Less diarrhea
- ☐ Less constipation
- ☐ Less gas
- ☐ Less bloating
- ☐ Improved regularity
- ☐ Fewer colds and flus
- ☐ Fewer seasonal allergies
- ☐ Fewer migraines
- ☐ Fewer asthma attacks
- ☐ Less acid reflux/GERD
- ☐ Less heartburn
- ☐ Less chronic pain
- ☐ Less tendonitis/bursitis
- ☐ Less shoulder/back/knee pain
- ☐ More mobile joints
- ☐ Less painful joints
- ☐ Improved temperature regulation
- ☐ Improved blood pressure
- ☐ Improved cholesterol
- ☐ Improved circulation
- ☐ Improved blood sugar regulation
- ☐ Improved medical symptoms
- ☐ Reduced or eliminated medications
- ☐ Recovering faster from injury or illness
- ☐ Improved HRV
- ☐ Improved resting heart rate
- ☐ More "green" recovery days per your wearable

PHYSICAL (OUTSIDE)
- ☐ Glowing skin
- ☐ Clearer skin
- ☐ Improvement in eczema or redness
- ☐ Longer, stronger nails
- ☐ Stronger, thicker hair
- ☐ Brighter eyes
- ☐ Fresher breath
- ☐ Whiter teeth
- ☐ Less bloating
- ☐ More defined muscle tone
- ☐ Clothes fit more comfortably
- ☐ Wedding ring fits better

MOOD AND EMOTION
- ☐ Happier
- ☐ More outgoing
- ☐ More patient
- ☐ More playful
- ☐ More optimistic
- ☐ Laughing more
- ☐ Less anxious
- ☐ Less stressed
- ☐ Handles stress better
- ☐ New tools for managing stress
- ☐ Fewer mood swings
- ☐ Improved emotional regulation
- ☐ Feeling empowered in your food choices
- ☐ Improved mental health
- ☐ Improved body image
- ☐ Improved self-esteem
- ☐ Improved self-confidence
- ☐ Improved self-efficacy
- ☐ Fewer symptoms of anxiety and/or depression

FOOD AND BEHAVIORS
- ☐ Healthier relationship with food
- ☐ Practicing mindful eating
- ☐ Reads food labels
- ☐ Eats to satiety
- ☐ Listens to your body
- ☐ No longer quick fix or crash dieting
- ☐ Eats more vegetables
- ☐ Eats more protein
- ☐ Cooks more/enjoys cooking more
- ☐ More confident in the kitchen
- ☐ More at ease around food
- ☐ New strategies to comfort yourself
- ☐ New ways to show yourself love
- ☐ No longer uses food as punishment
- ☐ No longer ignores hunger
- ☐ Can identify cravings versus hunger
- ☐ Fewer sugar or food cravings
- ☐ New strategies to navigate cravings
- ☐ Less guilt or shame around food
- ☐ Less negative self-talk
- ☐ Aware of diet culture influences

BRAIN FUNCTION, SLEEP, ENERGY

- [ ] Improved attention span
- [ ] Improved performance at job or school
- [ ] Improved memory
- [ ] Less brain fog
- [ ] Fewer ADHD symptoms
- [ ] More productive
- [ ] Less anxious
- [ ] Sleeping more
- [ ] Falling asleep more easily
- [ ] Sleeping more soundly
- [ ] No longer need a sleep aid
- [ ] Less "snoozing"
- [ ] Wakes feeling refreshed
- [ ] Less snoring
- [ ] Fewer night sweats
- [ ] More consistent sleep cycles
- [ ] Improved sleep metrics per your wearable
- [ ] Fewer night cramps
- [ ] Higher energy levels
- [ ] More consistent energy
- [ ] More energy in the morning
- [ ] No more midday energy slump
- [ ] More energy to play with your kids
- [ ] More energy to exercise
- [ ] More energy to socialize
- [ ] More energy at work or school
- [ ] No longer "hangry" between meals
- [ ] Feels energetic between meals
- [ ] Drinks/needs less caffeine

SPORTS, EXERCISE, AND PLAY

- [ ] Started moving or exercising
- [ ] More consistent with exercise
- [ ] Improved fitness levels
- [ ] More athletic
- [ ] Improved strength
- [ ] Improved mobility
- [ ] Improved flexibility
- [ ] Faster reaction time
- [ ] Hit a new "personal best"
- [ ] Recovers more effectively
- [ ] Trying new activities
- [ ] Walking more
- [ ] Taking more steps
- [ ] More "green" recovery days per your wearable
- [ ] Playing more with kids or dog
- [ ] Spending more time outside
- [ ] Improved coordination
- [ ] Better balance

LIFESTYLE AND SOCIAL

- [ ] Created new food habits
- [ ] More knowledgeable about nutrition
- [ ] Reads food labels
- [ ] Made new recipes
- [ ] Established meal prep habits
- [ ] Feel supported by family and friends
- [ ] Made new health-conscious friends
- [ ] Joined a new community
- [ ] Works effectively within your food budget
- [ ] Created other health goals
- [ ] Feel closer in your relationships
- [ ] Feel more connected to yourself
- [ ] People notice you seem different
- [ ] People come to you for Whole30 advice
- [ ] More confidence socializing
- [ ] More confidence holding boundaries
- [ ] More confidence advocating for your needs
- [ ] Added (or gaining interest in) new lifestyle habits

PLANNING AND PREPARATION

I love the enthusiasm of those who declare, "I'm going to start the Whole30 *right now*!" But please, slow your roll. From experience, I can tell you taking time to plan and prepare sets you up for much greater success in the program. Habit research shows that when people get excited and jump from contemplation straight into action (skipping over the preparation phase), they're less likely to see the change through. As you'll hear over and over again, when it comes to the Whole30, planning and preparation are key.

Here is my updated five-step approach to planning and preparing for your Whole30. Follow these steps whether it's your first Whole30 or your fifth! Your health context, motivations and goals, and environment are always changing. You will set yourself up for greater Whole30 success, deeper insights, and a less stressful elimination if you take at least a few days to prepare.

Step 1: Find your "why"

Habit-change experts often talk about finding your "why" and using that as an anchor, helping you stay on track with your commitment. But what does that even *mean*? What is a "why"? Why do you need one? How do you find it? And how can you use it?

A "why" is your own internal motivation for pursuing a specific behavior or course of action. A good "why" comes from inside and happens when you create space to be self-aware and introspective. A good "why" is not going to come from external pressures. It's not the thing you think you *should* be doing based on other people's expectations; it's something you *want* to do, based on your own goals and desires.

Having a "why" is mission critical for any habit change, especially a challenging commitment like the Whole30. A solid "why" provides stability and direction, especially when things get stressful or chaotic. Think of it like your North Star, guiding your behaviors and decisions over the course of your elimination and reintroduction. Without a solid "why," it would be easy to get overwhelmed or feel indecisive. You'd be tempted to give in to peer pressure or to abandon your commitment when the going gets tough.

To start the process of finding your "why," ask yourself two questions:

- What would give me a sense of satisfaction or fulfillment at the end of my Whole30?
- What problem or challenge is emotionally motivating me to join the Whole30?

Next, complete the associated exercise. Make a list of all the benefits that could come as a result of this effort. Use the Non-Scale Victory checklist on page 44 as a guide, or focus on the second question and describe the opposite of the problem or challenge you're facing now. For example, if you're battling uncontrollable cravings, you'd write, "Feeling free and comfortable around all foods." If you're struggling with energy, you'd write, "Feeling energized and motivated to play with the kids, cook dinner, and go for walks." Be generous with what you believe can happen, and allow yourself to tap into your emotional side. The more closely connected you are to your "why," the more strongly it will ground you during your Whole30.

Then, pick the three to five benefits that excite you the most, and take each of those a step further by asking yourself, "So what?" What do each of these benefits mean for your health, happiness, and quality of life? Imagine you believe the Whole30 could bring you fewer cravings. Ask yourself, "So what?" Perhaps that means less time spent thinking about food, fewer internal battles of willpower, a greater satisfaction with your meals, and less negative self-talk. Or maybe you think the Whole30 will give you more energy. So what? When you dig deeper, more energy means more quality time spent with your kids, the motivation to exercise, feeling more productive during your workday, and a desire to be more social.

Once you have reached this level, circle a few that emotionally resonate the hardest and will have the biggest impact in your life. *This* is your "why"! It's okay to have more than one, but you don't want a dozen. Choose just a few that are the most important and that will resonate the strongest when you need to return to them.

Write your "why" statements down on Post-it notes and stick them in strategic places around the house, like on your bathroom mirror, nightstand, and refrigerator. Or create an iPhone screensaver of your "why" so you'll be reminded of it often. Share your "why" with the people who want to support you, so they can better understand your motivations and desires. Most important, return to your "why" any time you feel stressed or uncertain in your commitment. Your "why" is the anchor for the promise you made to yourself. Hold on to it when things get tough.

Step 2: Choose your start date

You can start a Whole30 any day of the year, although many people choose the first of the month for ease and camaraderie. (We run group Whole30s around the first of the month, too.) But before you circle that date with a red pen, take these factors into account:

- Allow at least a few days before your program starts for planning and preparation, especially if this is your first Whole30. Most people allow 1 to 2 weeks for this phase.

- Build in at least 10 days at the end of elimination for reintroduction. Leaving for vacation on Day 31 will make it hard (if not impossible) to properly reintroduce.
- If you've got a big vacation, an important athletic event, or your own wedding in your imminent future, plan to start your Whole30 *after* those events. Navigating the Whole30 for the first time under those conditions could prove incredibly challenging, and I'd hate for you to miss the pasta in Italy, a first-place finish, or your own wedding cake.

However, you *don't* have to reschedule your Whole30 around a family dinner, a business lunch, a trip to visit your in-laws, or a party with friends. In fact, I encourage you to use those opportunities to take your Whole30 skills out on the town! Include those situations in your Whole30 plan, and use them to build confidence when unexpected events arise in the future. (See page 76 for tips on how to stay social on the Whole30.)

Step 3: Build your support team

Habit research finds that succeeding with a commitment as big as the Whole30 requires accountability and support. For many, the Whole30 will be a radical change to how you eat and perhaps how you socialize in the coming month. It's important to your Whole30 success that you feel supported by your friends, family members, and co-workers.

The first thing you'll want to develop is your Whole30 "elevator pitch," so you can quickly describe the program to others and dispel any preconceived notions. Try something like:

The Whole30 is a 30-day elimination and reintroduction program designed to identify hidden food sensitivities and help me figure out the foods that work best for me.

Once you've established a common understanding of the program, share your personal reasons for taking on the Whole30. These reasons can range from the physical ("I hope to find out if something I'm eating is contributing to my knee pain") to the emotional ("I've been struggling with cravings and emotional regulation, and I'd like to learn other ways to navigate stress"), to the relational ("I don't like how tired I am all the time, and I'd like to have more energy for me, and for you and the kids.").

Get as personal as is appropriate for your relationship with that person. Your boss likely doesn't need (or want) to hear about your bouts with diarrhea, but you should certainly explain to your spouse the degree to which your digestive distress is making you uncomfortable, and how this change could be helpful for those issues.

Then *ask* for support. People often skip this step, assuming that sharing the commitment is enough. But your loved ones aren't mind readers, and it will be helpful for all of you if you share your needs and expectations clearly. Be specific here! If you need your co-workers not to pressure you to have a drink at happy hour, say so. If you want your spouse to share encouraging words as they notice positive changes, ask for that. If you'd like your best friend to check in once a week for accountability, choose a day together. You may need different things from different people, and your loved ones would probably be thrilled to know the specific actions they can take to support you.

Of course, you can always count on me and the Whole30 community for support, too. See our Resources, starting on page 352, for all the ways we can help to guide you through the program, keep you motivated, hold you accountable, and cheer you on to Whole30 success.

HOW TO SHARE WHOLE30 WITH FRIENDS AND FAMILY

You can't *make* a friend or family member do the Whole30 with you, but you stand a much better chance of enticing them to join you if you follow these three principles:

1. **Share your motivations in a relatable fashion.** Telling a friend who doesn't exercise, "I'm hoping the Whole30 will help me cut my 5K time," probably won't have an impact. But if that same friend also has trouble sleeping, saying, "I'm hoping the Whole30 can help me sleep better—there's data to prove that it can," might make her ears perk up.

2. **Keep the focus on what you will be eating, not the elimination list.** Try, "I've got these three recipes planned for next week—look at this chili!" Bonus if you invite them over for dinner one night.

3. **Remember, their health is their business.** Lead by quiet example, but don't ever pressure, cajole, or try to shame anyone into doing the Whole30. They don't have to do the program to support you, and seeing your Whole30 results may prompt them to look deeper into the program.

Step 4: Get ready to eat!

Now it's time to get your pantry and fridge Whole30 ready. You may feel confident enough to skip this step and play things by ear—but please don't. This is where Present You sets up Future You for success, knowing there will be stressful days, busy days, social pressures, and temptations ahead. There is no such thing as being "too prepared" for the Whole30, so at the very least, let's organize your pantry, plan your first few days of meals, and hit the grocery store.

- **Clean out your pantry.** Donate the foods you won't be eating, bring them into the office break room, or box them up in the garage and save them for reintroduction. I know you feel confident now and are wondering, "Do I really need to do this?" But cleaning out your pantry when things feel easy is setting yourself up for success when things get hard. Habit research shows that the more distance between you and temptation, the easier it is to resist the pull, so get those Oreos out of there.
- **Doing the Whole30 alone?** Dedicate one drawer in your fridge, an out-of-the-way cabinet, and a plastic storage tote in your pantry for your family's cookies, yogurt, and bread. You don't want to have to reach around the chips or chocolate every time you're looking for a can of coconut milk.
- **Plan 3 to 7 days of Whole30 meals.** A meal plan sets you up for Whole30 success, helps you make the most of your budget, and reduces stress. Don't forget to plan some on-the-go foods, too! See page 104 for Original Whole30 ideas, and 239 for Plant-Based Whole30 ideas.
- **Head to the grocery store.** Use your meal plan to make a shopping list, then restock your pantry and fridge and shop for your meals. Sticking to the list saves time and money and prevents food waste.

Meal planning is critical for the Whole30. Yes, even if you ate "pretty healthy" before you started, and even if you've previously done the Whole30. The Whole30 is unique, and it may take time to feel comfortable preparing meals in the elimination phase. What will you eat for breakfast if you're not pouring a bowl of cereal? What will you have for lunch if everyone else orders pizza? What will you make for dinner if you get home from work late, tired, and cranky?

Meal planning not only reduces stress and increases your chance of success, it's also good for your budget. Buying only what you need will also help you reduce food waste, considering most foods you're eating on the Whole30 are fresh and perishable.

Some people plan a week of meals all at once, using Sunday to shop, prep, and cook. Others prefer more flexibility or can shop more often, and plan just 2 or 3 days of meals at a time. You can do it any way you want! The important thing is to assess your schedule, budget, and kitchen skills, then create a meal-planning routine that works best for you. (See "How do I create my Whole30 meal plan?" on page 71.)

I'm also going to add "toss your scale" to this section, because this is another matter of housekeeping. Since you won't be weighing yourself for 30 days (see page 42), it's good practice to remove *that* temptation too, just like you did with the Oreos. Hide it in the basement, stick it in the garage, move it to a lesser-used room, or donate it. It turns out that "out of sight, out of mind" is grounded in behavior-change science. Give Future You the peace of *not* having to step around it every time you take a shower.

Step 5: Plan for challenges

There is a 100 percent chance you will face unexpected challenges during your Whole30. Peer pressure, social events, late nights at the office, and life stresses could easily derail your Whole30 commitment. But they won't! Because you're going to have a *plan*! Are you seeing a theme here?

Habit research shows that when you're up against stress, discomfort, or negative emotions, the brain gravitates to what is *easy* and *rewarding*. Today, that might mean wine, carbs, or chocolate. On the Whole30, those choices aren't an option. You're going to need a plan—ideally, more than one—for handling challenging circumstances.

IF/THEN PLANS

Studies show you are *two to three times* more likely to succeed with your habit change if you incorporate "If/Then" planning. Habits have three parts: the cue, the routine, and the reward. If/Then statements establish a strong link in your brain between the cue (If) and the routine (Then). That link makes it easier to notice the cue when it occurs and prompts you to automatically follow the new routine you've designed for that situation.

Here, I use the If/Then structure to help you create plans for meeting common Whole30-related challenges. You can also use *The Whole30 Day by Day*'s guided journal prompts to create and document these plans.

First, anticipate the obstacles you might face during your Whole30. Be thorough here! It's better to have a plan for a scenario that doesn't arise than be caught in the moment without a plan. Common challenges include peer pressure, business lunches, family dinners, birthday parties, travel delays, or long days at work.

Then, use If/Then statements to create a plan for each circumstance. Here are a few to get you started:

- **Peer pressure:** IF my co-workers pressure me to order a drink, THEN I'll say, "I'm not drinking right now—I'm good with sparkling water," and change the subject.
- **Business lunches:** IF I'm invited to a work lunch, THEN I'll study the menu ahead of time, call the restaurant with questions, and decide in advance so I can order confidently.

- **Family dinners:** IF we're invited to my in-laws' for dinner, THEN I'll offer to cook for them at our house instead, or say, "I'm doing a Whole30 right now, and it's important that I stick with it— can I help you plan the menu or bring a dish?"
- **Birthday parties:** IF I get to the party and someone offers me cake, THEN I'll say, "No cake for me today, thanks."
- **Travel delays:** IF my flight is delayed or I get stuck in traffic, THEN I'll snack on the meat sticks (Original Whole30)/lupini bean snacks (Plant-Based Whole30) and pistachios I keep in my bag.
- **Long workdays:** IF I don't have time to meal prep, THEN I'll reheat my Whole30 leftovers or one of the Whole30 prepared meals from my delivery that week.
- **General pushback:** IF someone gives me a hard time about my "crazy diet," THEN I'll say, "Actually, I feel great—let's talk about something else," then change the subject.

You can see how thinking through these If/Then plans can help you sail through potential Whole30 challenges! Now you know to always have a glass of sparkling water in your hand at social gatherings (and bring your own to parties), to pack some snacks in your work *and* travel bags, to make meals big enough for leftovers, or to sign up for Whole30 meal delivery. (See page 353 for resources.) Record your If/Then plans in a journal or the Notes app on your phone, and add to them as new opportunities present themselves.

THE WHOLE30 TIMELINE

Whether you heard about the Whole30 from a friend, a social media post, or a podcast, you're likely curious about what you can expect while on the program. After watching millions of people go through the Whole30 since 2009, I have a pretty good idea of what your Whole30 journey will look like. (In fact, most Whole30 alumni say our timeline is "eerily accurate.")

While there is no one universal Whole30 experience, here is a weekly timeline designed to help you preview the journey, plan for challenges, and make the most of your Whole30 learnings along the way.

Pre-Whole30: Planning and preparing

Most people start preparing for their Whole30 at least a week before their program begins. Veterans of the program may find they need only a few days to get ready, while those new to the program (especially those coming from a Standard American Diet and/or with less cooking experience) may want to begin earlier.

Your Day 1 experience is greatly influenced by your dietary choices in the days leading up to your Whole30. Cramming in all the sugar, alcohol, bread, and ice cream you can before your program starts may set you up for headaches, crankiness, cravings, and lethargy. I can't tell you what to do, but maybe don't do that.

For even more insights, tips, success strategies, and daily tracking of your Whole30 journey, from elimination through reintroduction, pick up a copy of *The Whole30 Day by Day*.

In contrast, many people "soft-launch" their Whole30 by making small changes ahead of their start date, easing the transition from their current diet to the Whole30 elimination phase. This is a *fantastic* idea, and makes your progression more of a graceful leap than a fall off a cliff. Consider easing your way into the program by conscientiously eating less sugar and fewer processed foods, cutting back on alcohol consumption, and adding more protein, vegetables, fruit, and/or healthy fats to your plate.

Days 1–7: Adaptation

Welcome to the Whole30! You've begun a journey that has changed the lives of millions of people just like you. While you'll likely experience lots of wins even in your first week, it will also be a period of physical and mental adaptation.

On Day 1, most people feel excited, energized, and confident. The newness and excitement of the Whole30 can help you breeze through your first day, but this week can be challenging. Headaches, fatigue, crankiness, and cravings are common during this phase of the program, and you may feel like you're thinking about food a *lot*.

Physically, your body may be struggling to adjust to the decrease in sugar and carbohydrates. (The Whole30 is not low-carb by design, but a whole foods–based approach is generally lower in carbohydrates than a diet that includes lots of ultra-processed foods.) The process of *fat adaptation*—a metabolic adjustment in which your body is able to effectively utilize fat as fuel—starts in just a few days, but it can take 2 to 3 weeks to notice the effects. Though you're eating plenty of dietary fat on the Whole30, an abrupt decrease in added sugar and processed carbs can leave you feeling lethargic, headachy, and brain-foggy until your metabolism adjusts.

Cravings for the foods or drinks you've eliminated can also leave you feeling cranky, fidgety, and easily irritated. If you're used to using food or alcohol to distract, numb, or self-soothe in the face of stress or negative emotions, losing this coping mechanism can feel unsettling and uncomfortable. However, the Whole30 will help you develop other ways to navigate stress, discomfort, and negative emotions as your program progresses. With the support of our community and your friends and family, you'll quickly learn to recognize and navigate these feelings in a way that doesn't involve automatically reaching for a food or beverage.

It's also possible that your digestion will experience a period of adaptation to less sugar, more fiber, more healthy proteins and fats, and more vegetables. You may experience bloating, constipation, or loose stools as your gut, microbiome, and digestive enzymes adjust and learn to process these new foods more effectively. Other health conditions, like acne or joint pain and swelling, may also remain stubbornly persistent this week.

Rest assured, it's not all rough roads! Many people also report improvements in digestion, decreased joint pain, fewer migraines, less inflammation, reduced anxiety, better sleep, and/or fewer cravings once they get through the first few days.

Your best strategies this week are to take a nap or go to bed early; swap your workout for a walk or an easy yoga class; drink lots of water; eat Whole30 foods *whenever you're hungry* (don't limit calories or meals); and keep reminding yourself of your Whole30 "why." Don't forget to keep up with your meal planning, including emergency and on-the-go foods, and your If/Then plans (see page 50)!

FOOD DREAMS

It's common to experience food dreams while on the Whole30. People report dreams about eating chocolate, drinking wine, or ordering fast-food burgers. Given all the planning and preparation you've done, and how big a change the Whole30 is for most, it makes sense that you'd have food on the brain. If you wake up feeling guilty or feeling like you blew your Whole30, shake it off! (And maybe set the intention that the next time you have a food dream, you'll enjoy the heck out of it.) However, if at any point your Whole30 starts to feel like it's taking your mental health in an unhealthy direction, or you're *too* preoccupied with food, please discontinue the program and consult a therapist or healthcare provider.

Days 8–14: Adoption

Heading into Week 2, your body and brain may still be adjusting to this new way of eating. However, you may start noticing that some things are already feeling better, easier, and more comfortable.

It might feel more routine to grocery-shop, meal-plan, and cook your Whole30 meals. Many people report a newfound sense of kitchen confidence thanks to the program, and couples and families enjoy spending more time in the kitchen together. Discovering new foods, ingredients, and delicious recipes can also feel motivating and rewarding.

By the end of this week, you may find you're falling asleep easier, staying asleep longer, and waking with more energy. You may no longer need a midafternoon caffeine boost, as your energy, productivity, and focus improve. You should experience fewer cravings as you discover new ways of navigating stress, begin to create new habits, and continue to eat to satiety. Your taste buds can adjust quickly, and many people discover

THE HARDEST DAYS

This is also the week—specifically Days 10 and 11—that people are statistically most likely to quit their Whole30. (We call them "the hardest days.") By this point, the newness of the program has worn off, and though you've made it through most of the unpleasant physical milestones, you've yet to experience significant benefits. This in-between place can leave you feeling impatient, anxious about whether or not it will be worth it, or tempted to self-sabotage. To help you stick with the program, here are three tips from successful Whole30ers:

1. Have a strong "why," and focus on your long-term goals.
2. Be willing to sit with emotional discomfort and seek other ways to self-soothe (like journaling, movement, and meditation).
3. Lean on your in-person and online support systems for encouragement, support, and accountability.

Prepare yourselves for these days, because if you can see them through, things get *much* easier, and you may discover the Whole30 magic really starting to kick in.

a newfound appreciation for the sweetness and flavors found in fruit, vegetables, herbs, and spices. (We hear "Wow, strawberries taste so sweet" a *lot*.)

Many people find that after some initial digestive discomfort, they have less gas, bloating, constipation, diarrhea, and digestive distress at this point in the program. You may also start to notice a pronounced reduction or improvement in symptoms like acne or eczema, allergies, asthma, migraines, joint pain and swelling, chronic pain, or anxiety.

Days 15–21: Smooth sailing

By the third week, most people are noticing small (or big) Non-Scale Victories (NSVs) in many areas of their lives. (They *all* count.) Many people report their sleep has dramatically improved. Your energy will likely be higher, steadier, and more reliable. People may accuse you of being "strangely happy." You might notice your focus is sharper or easier to sustain, and you feel more creative. Your cravings are probably nonexistent or dramatically diminished. Your clothes or rings may be fitting more comfortably. Your skin might be glowing, your joints may feel less painful, your weekend runs may be easier, and your sinuses may feel clearer.

Most people also report feeling self-confident and capable at this point in their journey. Teaching yourself new cooking skills, maintaining your commitment, and learning how to set and hold boundaries around food and drink are all huge confidence boosters, and carry over into your career, relationships, and other healthy habits.

Of course, this may not happen like magic in your third week. There are a *huge* number of factors that influence which benefits you see and when, including your health context, past dietary habits, and current life stressors. If you hit this point and aren't seeing or feeling the dramatic changes others have reported, that doesn't mean you're doing it wrong. (There's a reason it's not called the "Whole20.")

Trust the process; stay on the lookout for small, gradual improvements to keep you motivated, and celebrate the wins you *are* seeing. Don't be afraid to lean on your support system here! Asking friends and family for the positives they've noticed from your Whole30, soliciting a favorite Whole30 recipe on your Instagram, and sharing how you're feeling with others can help you stay more closely connected to the experience, and committed to seeing the experiment through.

Days 22–30: Home stretch!

This is the point when you might lose track of what day you're on, because your Whole30 feels second nature. The NSVs continue to roll in, and though you're excited to reintroduce the foods you've been missing, you already know you'll take a lot of what you've learned so far into life after your Whole30.

Start thinking about reintroduction this week, to ensure you have a solid plan in place *and* to remind yourself that the Whole30 isn't over until you've completed a thorough reintroduction.

It can be tempting to end your program a few days early ("27 is as good as 30, right?"), but remember—you committed to the Whole30, and many report the last few days bring even more noticeable Non-Scale Victories. It's also tempting to dive right back into pizza, beer, and ice cream on Day 31, which is why we encourage you to plan your reintroduction schedule now. The Whole30 can teach you so much about how foods work for you, but not until you eliminate *and* reintroduce them carefully, then compare your experience.

Finish this week by revisiting all your favorite Whole30 meals, planning your reintroduction schedule, shopping for the first few foods or beverages you'll be reintroducing, and for extra credit, start reading or listening to *Food Freedom Forever* to prepare you for the next phase of your Whole30 journey.

MORE THAN 30?

You may be considering extending your elimination phase beyond the 30 days. There are good reasons for considering an extension—and other instances in which I'd *discourage* you from extending your elimination. See page 64 for more guidance.

Days 31–40+: Celebration and reintroduction

Take the time to celebrate your Whole30 accomplishment! You made a promise to yourself, and you kept that promise. You've learned a whole host of new healthy habits; cultivated effective tools to self-soothe, navigate stress, and relieve anxiety; expanded your kitchen and cooking skills; and improved your self-confidence and self-efficacy. Revisit your Non-Scale Victory checklist (page 44) and see how many NSVs you can check off today!

You'll spend the next 6 to 15 days (perhaps longer) in reintroduction, bringing back one food group at a time, then returning to the elimination phase for 2 to 3 days in between each reintroduction group. During this time, you'll get to enjoy the foods and drinks you've missed, while paying attention to how the reintroduction of these foods impacts your energy, sleep, digestion, mood, cravings, aches and pains, and health conditions. (See page 37 for the Original Whole30 reintroduction schedule, and page 39 for the Plant-Based Whole30 reintroduction schedule.)

The more time you spend here, the more opportunity you'll have to learn how these foods work in your body, which will inform your Food Freedom plan and help you make choices that feel good.

You'll be most successful here if you plan your reintroduction as carefully as you've planned your elimination: day by day, and meal by meal. Journal your experience and record how the reintroduction of each food impacts your physical and mental health. (Bonus: You can use your *Whole30 Day by Day* journal to track your reintroduction experience, too!)

Stay closely connected to the Whole30 community during reintroduction, and even into your food freedom. Continuing to share your

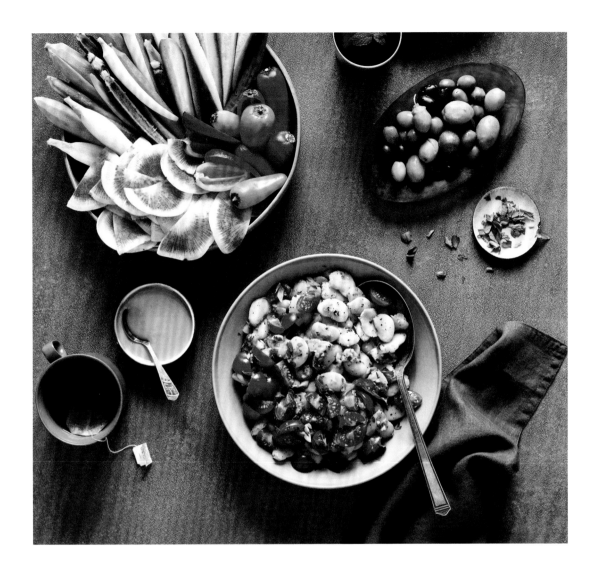

Whole30 journey can motivate and inspire others, while keeping you firmly entrenched in your healthy habits.

YOUR MILEAGE MAY VARY

No two people's Whole30 experience is the same. You may find you breeze past some of these phases while being stuck in others for longer than you anticipated, or you might skip certain phases altogether. In addition, the Whole30 program alone may not be able to provide the benefits you were hoping to see. If you discover your Whole30 experience varies widely from this timeline, or the improvements you hoped to see just aren't appearing, please consult your healthcare provider or registered dietitian for more specialized guidance.

Egyptian-Inspired Butter Beans with Veggies, page 251

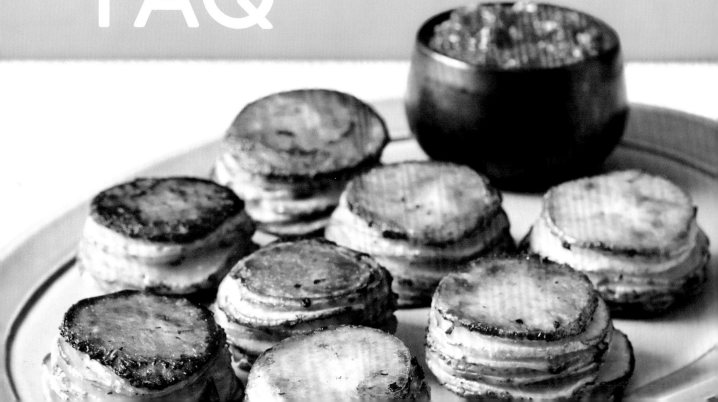

PART 2
THE
WHOLE30
GENERAL
FAQ

This FAQ section applies to both Whole30 programs (Original and Plant-Based) and is designed to answer your questions about the structure, support, and guidelines for the program. Overachievers may want to skim through this entire section before getting started, so as to be prepared for any circumstance. Others might want to dive right into the Program Rules, coming back to the FAQ if and when a question pops up. If you're ready to go, head to page 36 for the Original Whole30 Program Rules, and page 38 for the Plant-Based Whole30 Program Rules.

"CAN I HAVE . . . ?"

Can I have _____ on the Whole30?

Whether you're doing the Original or the Plant-Based program, you'll have to read your labels, menus, and ingredient lists carefully to ensure the item in question is compatible with your elimination phase. This applies to foods, beverages, prepared meals, restaurant menus, and even supplements!

Visit our website (whole30.com) for a detailed, evergreen list of "Can I have?" ingredients and products for both the Original and the Plant-Based programs. Following are three high-level tips for ensuring a product, food, recipe, or menu item is compatible with the program.

1. **Read the Whole30 Program Rules.** (See page 36 for Original; page 38 for Plant-Based.) Read them a few times, including the details of the Pancake Rule (page 40). The better you know the rules and what's included in each food group on the elimination list, the easier it will be to determine compatibility.

2. **Read your labels.** If every ingredient is compatible and it's not part of the Pancake Rule, then the product is compatible! But if it contains something listed in the elimination phase, even as the very last ingredient, it's out for your Whole30.

3. **Focus on the ingredients.** Remember— added sugar is about the *ingredient list*, not the *nutrition label*. Even if the "added sugar" line is rounded down to 0 grams, if you see monk-fruit, erythritol, honey, or any other form of added sugar (other than fruit juice or fruit juice concentrate) in the ingredient list, that food is not compatible.

READ YOUR RECIPES, TOO

Unless you find the recipe on our website, in our books, or on a Whole30 social media feed, you'll have to read the ingredient list carefully to ensure the ingredients are compatible with your program. Be conscientious about sub-ingredients, too! If a recipe calls for bacon, mustard, or broth, make sure you purchase Whole30-compatible items for your dish. (That means no added sugar, white wine, or cornstarch.) With experience, you'll learn how to quickly make recipes Whole30 compatible by omitting certain ingredients (like the cheese on top of chili), substituting ingredients (like using coconut aminos in place of soy sauce), or making creative swaps (like "sandwiching" your protein between slices of sweet potato instead of a bun).

opposite: Crispy Potato Stack, page 317

Can I take supplements?

If you're currently on a supplement regimen, continue to take them as directed by your doctor or dietitian, even if those supplements contain ingredients not compatible with your Whole30 program. Your healthcare provider's orders always supersede Whole30 Program Rules.

Though supplements are not required for either Whole30 program, there are a few our healthcare advisors generally recommend taking to help support a whole foods–based diet. Those supplements include:

- **Vitamin D$_3$:** This vitamin-that's-actually-a-hormone plays a role in maintaining the balance of calcium in your blood and bones, offers immune support, and could even play a role in mental health. Depending on your personal health history, your skin's melanin content, and your geographic location, you might not get enough even with regular sun exposure, especially in winter. If lab testing to determine your levels isn't available, consider starting with 2000–3000 IUs (50–75µg) per day. Studies show doses of up to 5000 IUs a day are well tolerated and safe.
- **Magnesium:** This mineral has many functions, including supporting muscle and nerve function and energy production. It also plays a role in vitamin D absorption. Deficiencies can even affect your mental health and brain function. While many Whole30 foods like leafy greens, nuts, and seeds are magnesium-rich, you may choose to supplement. Typical supplement doses range from 125 to 600 mg per day, and several different forms are available: *Magnesium glycinate* is often used to support deeper sleep, *magnesium citrate* is a form that can also support regularity, and *magnesium l-threonate* is touted for its brain-supporting benefits.

- **Probiotics:** Gastrointestinal (gut) challenges are common—and they happen to be a reason many people do the Whole30 in the first place. However, unless your healthcare provider is prescribing specific probiotics based on lab tests, we recommend waiting until reintroduction is over to introduce probiotics. This will allow you to first evaluate whether your Whole30 improves any of the digestive symptoms you've been having. Our healthcare advisors generally recommend a mix of three strains: *Lactobacillus* and *Bifidobacterium; Saccharomyces boulardii;* and a soil-based probiotic.
- **Multivitamins:** While multivitamins aren't a one-step solution, they are usually low cost, unlikely to cause harm, and could help shore up nutrient deficiencies. Look for a Whole30-compatible multivitamin with folate (instead of folic acid) and vitamin K$_2$ to aid in vitamin D absorption. (If you're doing the Plant-Based Whole30, also look for B$_{12}$, zinc, iodine, selenium, and choline.) Pay attention to the amount of vitamin D in your multivitamin if you are also taking a D$_3$ supplement, to ensure your total dose stays in a healthy range.

In addition, if you're doing the Plant-Based Whole30, our registered dietitians suggest additional supplementation:

- **DHA/EPA from algae oil:** DHA and EPA are omega-3 fatty acids, crucial for brain and heart health. These fatty acids are prevalent in cold-water fatty fish but aren't found in plants. However, they can be produced by algae. Experts at the National Institutes of Health recommend supplementing with 200–300 mg of DHA a day.
- **Iron (based on lab results):** While many plant-based foods contain iron, they don't contain

heme iron, the form that is most bioavailable and plays an important role in transporting oxygen throughout the body. Work with your healthcare provider to determine whether iron supplementation is recommended, based on your bloodwork.

Remember, read your supplement ingredients list, too. Avoid supplements with incompatible ingredients like added sugar, artificial sweeteners, cornstarch, or dairy. Visit our website at whole30 .com/whole30-approved for a list of Whole30 Approved supplements.

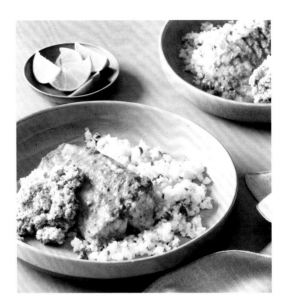

Can I have marijuana or THC?

If your healthcare provider has prescribed medicinal marijuana for a health condition, like anxiety or chronic pain, please continue to follow your treatment plan. (Please also consult with your provider before starting the Whole30, to make sure they approve and can monitor your progress.)

In general, the Program Rules do not accommodate recreational marijuana or THC use in any form during elimination or reintroduction. However, I recognize that "recreational use" doesn't always mean getting stoned and eating a whole bag of Cool Ranch Doritos. Many people use cannabis (THC) for pain management, anxiety, sleep, nausea, and other medical conditions. This may not be "prescribed," but it *is* therapeutic and can prevent pain, suffering, or the need for harsher prescription drugs.

In the context of the Whole30, especially concerning your habits and your emotional relationship with food, the rule that best serves this goal for *most* people is "no marijuana/THC use during elimination and reintroduction." That said, I can't tell you how to balance following the Whole30 Program Rules with keeping your pain, anxiety,

or nausea in check. In the end, only you know whether eliminating THC as part of your Whole30 is in your best interest, and I trust you to make the best decision for you.

Can I smoke or use my nicotine patches?

I would love for you to use your Whole30 as an opportunity to wean yourself off smoking cigarettes or wearing nicotine patches. Many former smokers have told me they used their Whole30 as a smoking-cessation program, and that eliminating added sugar and alcohol at the same time made the process easier.

However, quitting smoking *and* adopting the Whole30 Program Rules could be incredibly stressful, and prove too taxing on your willpower. I trust you to make the decision that is right for you, while encouraging you to use your Whole30 as an opportunity to examine your relationship with nicotine more closely.

Tandoori-Spiced Fish with Apple-Coconut Raita and Coconut-Cauliflower Rice, page 180

DIETS AND ELIMINATION PROGRAMS

What is "diet culture" and where does the Whole30 fit in?

While there isn't one agreed-upon definition of "diet culture," I'll use the one put forth by the National Eating Disorders Association, which says that diet culture:

- Conflates size with health, valuing thinness above all
- Encourages following external rules about when, what, and how much to eat
- Normalizes labeling foods as "good" or "bad"
- Suggests people are more or less good, worthy, or moral based on their body size

Whole30 does its best to provide an *alternative* to diet culture, while allowing people an accessible way to learn more about food and their body. The program's structure, support, and goals are health focused, encouraging participants to celebrate Non-Scale Victories. We don't share the kind of "before and after" photos that conflate health with thinness, nor do we glorify changes in body weight. The Whole30 does not offer specific tactics or guidance for weight loss, and our Program Rules discourage tracking or measuring body weight during the program.

You'll never hear us moralizing any food as "good" or "bad," using words like *clean* or *toxic,* or tying a person's worth or value to their food choices or body. And you don't eliminate food groups on the Whole30 in order to be "healthy." That would imply that the foods we eliminate are inherently

"unhealthy," which isn't true. In fact, the program is not prescriptive, and does not presume to tell you how you should eat going forward.

The Whole30 offers a short-term protocol to guide you through the temporary elimination of foods that are commonly associated with food intolerances and sensitivities. By eliminating them, reintroducing them, and comparing your experience, you'll learn whether *you* tolerate these foods well. Once your elimination and reintroduction are over, we encourage you to take your learnings and apply them in whatever way feels best to you. In fact, we actively *discourage* staying in the Whole30 elimination phase for too long (see page 64), or continuing to restrict foods or food groups unnecessarily beyond elimination.

In addition, the Whole30 doesn't count or restrict calories or portions; rather, it actively encourages participants *not* to track their calories or macros. The program also does not restrict meals or meal timing. During the program, you're encouraged to trust your body's natural signals, eat to satiety, and let your energy, hunger, activity levels, and other factors guide your meal planning.

However, because it's an elimination diet, the Whole30 does involve restriction—and some believe that *any* form of restriction is automatically "diet culture." (I don't agree, but I acknowledge the viewpoint.) Because of that restriction, the Whole30 may not be right for those actively working to resist diet culture and is contraindicated for those with a history of disordered eating, diagnosed or otherwise (see page 69).

In addition, though you won't find diet-culture references in the program, our resources, or our support, many people who do the Whole30 still

KEEP YOUR DIET BROAD AND JOYFUL

Studies show that the unnecessary long-term elimination of foods or food groups could lead to nutritional deficiencies and promote disordered habits or anxiety around food. If you discover upon reintroduction that a food or food group *doesn't* lead to unwanted symptoms, there is no reason to continue to strictly avoid it for "health" reasons. If you don't have a health-related reason to eliminate all gluten grains, dairy, or soy from your diet over the long term, please don't! Continue to enjoy these foods in whatever way feels joyful, sustainable, and satisfying to you.

want to lose weight. If you scan social media or the web looking for Whole30 resources, you *will* find people sharing their Whole30 weight loss, with bikini-clad before-and-after photos and other diet culture–centered content. (To be clear, *we* don't publish content like that—but it's out there, despite all of our resources, guidance, and encouragement to engage with the program the way we intended.)

Any restriction can be triggering and, to be clear, can create disordered eating habits even if none existed before. If you're worried the Whole30 may trigger unhealthy behaviors or associations with food, or if you simply aren't in a place to follow someone else's food rules even temporarily, there are other programs (like intuitive eating) that could be a better fit. But if you're trying to unlearn the harmful tenets of diet culture while supporting your body with foods that make you feel your best, the Whole30 can provide an accessible, supportive, effective place to start.

What are the differences between a food intolerance, sensitivity, and allergy?

A food *intolerance* response takes place in the digestive system and means someone has difficulty digesting or processing components (often a protein or sugar) within the food. An example of a common food intolerance is lactose intolerance: difficulty digesting the carbohydrate component of milk products. A food intolerance is usually caused by the lack of an enzyme needed to digest the food, but it can also be caused by enteric infections, drug or alcohol use, bowel surgery, chronic inflammation, or a digestive disease (like irritable bowel syndrome).

With a food *sensitivity*, an individual experiences either an immune-mediated reaction or a reaction to the food itself, which can generate a multitude of symptoms. Symptoms of food sensitivity arise from a chronic, low-grade inflammatory response. (They are not a result of undigested food, as seen in a food intolerance.) Food sensitivities have no standard medical definition, and to further confuse the matter, the term "sensitivity" is often used interchangeably with "intolerance." (In fairness, a significant overlap between the two can and often does exist.)

While typically less severe, reactions can happen after eating, but can also be delayed; you may not notice symptoms for up to three days after consuming the food. In addition, symptoms of a

Harvard Medical School says the gold standard for identifying food sensitivities is a structured elimination-and-reintroduction protocol.

food sensitivity can be prolonged and body-wide. Most notably, food sensitivities result in digestive issues like abdominal pain, bloating, diarrhea, and acid reflux, but can also lead to headaches, joint pain, fatigue, brain fog, and changes to mental health. This presents a challenge when attempting to pinpoint their source.

A food *allergy* is an adverse reaction arising from a specific immune response after exposure to a given food, even in small amounts. It is mediated by IgE antibodies that trigger an immediate response upon exposure, typically within a few minutes to an hour. In some cases, it can cause a body-wide allergic response known as anaphylaxis, which can be life-threatening.

The most common food allergies in the United States are to cow's milk, wheat, egg, tree nuts, peanut, shellfish, and soy. Please work with your healthcare provider if you suspect or are currently navigating a food allergy. *Do not attempt to reintroduce a food to which you have a known or suspected allergy on your Whole30.* Reintroducing an allergenic food is not safe unless medically supervised.

Can't I just take a food sensitivity test?

You may have heard friends or family members talk about a "food sensitivity" (IgG-based) test they did at home or with their provider. These tests *might* prove helpful in identifying a food sensitivity, but for most people they can cause more confusion than clarity. In fact, organizations including the American Academy of Allergy, Asthma & Immunology and the Canadian Society of Allergy and Clinical Immunology have recommended against using IgG testing to diagnose food intolerances and sensitivities.

These IgG-based food sensitivity tests have not been proven to identify food sensitivities, and often have false positives. Intestinal permeability or frequent exposures to a food can result in multiple foods being erroneously flagged as "culprits" (foods to which you're sensitive). This can result in unnecessary and sometimes excessive restrictions. In addition, these tests can be expensive! By contrast, elimination protocols like the Whole30 offer a free, clear, and effective way to assess which foods may be contributing to symptoms in your body.

Why is the Whole30 so strict?

To accurately determine how certain foods are impacting your body, you need to completely eliminate them for the prescribed period of time. Eating even small amounts of foods to which you are sensitive can disrupt the process and interrupt your healing. Complete elimination, on the other hand, can bring about improvements in any number of symptoms or negative health effects, and makes it easier to identify potentially problematic food(s) during reintroduction.

Rushing through reintroduction can have the same negative consequences. Reintroducing food groups too quickly, or reintroducing too many foods at the same time, will make it hard (if not impossible) to accurately evaluate the impact of these foods, and to know which food contributed to which symptom.

To make the most of your Whole30 self-experiment, completely eliminate all the recommended food groups for 30 straight days, then reintroduce carefully and systematically, one food group at a time, returning to the elimination phase for 2 to 3 days between food groups.

Is there clinical evidence to support the Whole30?

In 2018, Catherine Moring, PhD, RDN, BC-ADM, CDCES, and executive director of the James C. Kennedy Wellness Center in Mississippi, conducted a pilot study with forty-five Original Whole30 participants. Dr. Moring and her team provided education about the side effects of chronic inflammation, the benefits of an elimination diet, and the Whole30 Program Rules and recommendations. They also supported participants by teaching them how to prepare and enjoy minimally processed whole foods without focusing on calorie counting or food restriction.

Dr. Moring's team collected bloodwork and biometrics from the study participants before and after completing a Whole30. Although the results of this cohort study have not yet been peer reviewed or published, Dr. Moring shared this overview of the outcomes with us:

- The average decrease in overall cholesterol was 13.37.
- The average reduction in triglycerides was 24.57.
- The average reduction in LDL ("bad") cholesterol was 6.33.
- The majority of participants (70 percent) experienced lower blood sugar.
- Participants reduced their average blood glucose level by 2.34 mg/dL, from slightly impaired to within normal limits.
- An estimated two-thirds of patients had lower blood pressure after Whole30.

Dr. Moring reported that several participants in the study were able to reverse pre-diabetes. Several others with diabetes were able to reach blood glucose targets. One participant was able to stop taking insulin by the end of their Whole30.

Other Non-Scale Victories reported by Whole30 participants included improved digestion, clear skin, better sleep, fewer medications needed, more energy, less anxiety and depression, reduced pain, improved focus, better moods, and increased self-confidence.

ELIMINATION
What happens if I eat something off-plan during elimination?

If you make an impulsive decision to eat something from the elimination group during the first 30 days, we recommend starting over with Day 1. If that makes you think, "This feels diet culture-y to me," let me explain—then you can decide. There are two important reasons we recommend starting over.

The first is physiological. The purpose of any elimination diet is to allow yourself 30 days in a row without *any* exposure to those potentially problematic foods so you can accurately evaluate how they work in your body. Eating or drinking something to which you might be sensitive interrupts that process and could short-circuit your healing *and* your results. For that reason, the Whole30 recommends committing to 30 full days of elimination.

The second reason we recommend starting over is psychological. Should you give yourself an "out" before you even begin ("I'm doing the Whole30, but maybe not the wine part," or "I'll *mostly* follow the program"), the chances of your successfully completing the Whole30 and experiencing its life-changing benefits drop dramatically. Remember, when things get hard, the brain will always revert to what is easy and rewarding. And when you give yourself an opening like that, you know what comes next: endless mental negotiations, battles of willpower, and justification for doing the easy, rewarding thing, all of which can affect your mood, self-confidence, and self-efficacy. Without your *full* commitment to the program, it could prove much harder to conquer your cravings, employ new effective ways to manage stress, and learn as much as you can about the foods that work best for you.

Your Whole30 success may very well depend on your commitment *now* to follow the program 100 percent, start to finish. (See page 22 as a refresher.) Ultimately, however, you are responsible for your own program. If that recommendation still feels overly harsh, or if you decide that starting over late in your program will do more mental health harm than provide physiological benefit, I once again trust you to make the best decision for you.

What happens if I accidentally eat something off-plan during elimination?

If you read all the labels, avoid all the elimination foods, and *still* consume something off-plan, I do recommend you start over, with some caveats. First, *it happens*—your mom forgets that honey counts as added sugar, you didn't register that your salad dressing included dairy, or you realize halfway through the meal that your mashed potatoes definitely contain butter.

I still want you to experience 30 straight days of elimination, for the sake of learning the most about how foods work for you and giving your body 30 straight days "off" from any potentially problematic foods. (*Especially* if your accidental consumption brought about negative symptoms.) However, I recognize this could be truly demoralizing, and perhaps create more stress than it relieves.

I certainly don't want you to think you "failed," and I promise that the health consequences of eating a little added sugar are not life-or-death. If it feels unfair, demoralizing, or overly burdensome to start over, I trust you to make the decision that is best for you.

Should I extend my elimination beyond 30 days?

I hear this question most often from those who have seen dramatic improvements in a health condition—but I also hear it from people who relished the structure and support of the rules or are nervous about reintroduction.

First, if your healthcare provider advises you to extend your elimination (or make any adjustments to your elimination or reintroduction phase), please follow their recommendations.

If you have chronic pain, chronic fatigue, or an autoimmune condition and have seen improvements during elimination, you might consider extending elimination to 45 or even 60 days, to see if further gains can be achieved through diet alone. Those health conditions may be slower to respond to dietary interventions and may benefit from a longer elimination.

However, if you just enjoyed the structure and rules of the Whole30, that is not a good reason to extend the elimination phase. Remember that continuing to eat according to someone else's rules is not food freedom! If you stay in the elimination phase forever, you'll never know if the food groups you've eliminated might work for you, or be able

"THIS IS NOT HARD"

The original Whole30 Program Rules were famous for one particular tough-love section: "This is not hard. Quitting heroin is hard. Fighting cancer is hard. Birthing a baby is hard. Drinking your coffee black *is not hard.*" That kind of tough-love approach felt organic to me in 2009, because that's how I talked to myself. I didn't show myself grace or have much empathy for myself. I relied heavily on self-shaming and negative self-talk to "motivate" myself. And I had yet to acknowledge any of the inherent privileges that helped me move through the world with less friction—nor did I realize that not everyone's lived experience reflected my own.

If that language still resonates with you today, I get it! I've been told by many that this paragraph alone motivated them to join and succeed with the Whole30. If it works for you, you can keep it—but please, don't use it to shame or berate yourself. Use it in a "You know, that's true! I have done some really hard things, and I know I can do this, too," kind of way.

Still, I wouldn't say it like this to you (or anyone else) today. A lot has happened between then and now, and I'm a different person from who I was in 2009. As I've evolved, I've come to understand that the Whole30 *is* hard. You're undertaking this commitment on top of work, kids, school, household management, health concerns, financial stress, and mental health challenges. Your relationship with food and your body may feel complicated, challenging, or conflicted. Food has been a means of bonding, a coping mechanism, a distraction technique, and perhaps even an enemy. And to simply say "this is not hard" fails to acknowledge the complex realities of the systems we live in, and the very real barriers so many people face when pursuing health efforts.

But here is what I still believe: You *are* powerful—perhaps more powerful than you are giving yourself credit for. I know you *are* doing hard things, which gives you the strength to tackle this challenge, too, with equal parts grit and self-compassion. I know you *are* worthy of keeping this promise to yourself, trusting in yourself and your body and accepting support when you need it. Above all, I am certain you *deserve* to put yourself, your needs, and your happiness first for a change.

Fighting cancer, birthing a baby, or quitting an addictive substance *is* hard. Drinking your coffee black may be hard, too—and that's okay. Allow space and grace for those feelings because that is where you find growth.

The Whole30 can help you take back your power, restore your self-confidence, and bring you the kind of benefits that have a positive impact on *every area of your life.* So yes, this might be hard—but it will also be worth it. More important than that, you're worth it. And you won't be doing it alone; the Whole30 community and I will be with you every step of the way.

to expand your diet in a way that brings you even greater satisfaction. You'd certainly miss out on culturally significant or family-favorite foods during special events or family dinners. And one day in the not-so-distant future, you'd end up purposefully depriving yourself of something that would be delicious and worth it, for no good reason other than "the Program Rules say I can't."

The whole point of the Whole30 is to help you identify the foods that work best in your system and keep your diet as broad, varied, and satisfying as possible. Staying in the elimination phase long term runs counter to the core mission of the Whole30—and that's not what I want for your future. Start your structured reintroduction plan on Day 31, then create your own set of guidelines based on your learnings to incorporate into your Food Freedom plan.

Finally, if you want to extend elimination because you're nervous to reintroduce, take a deep breath. Return to your Whole30 Mindset checklist on page 28, to remind yourself of how the Whole30 is different from the quick-fix weight loss diets you've done in the past. Rest assured that our reintroduction plans are carefully designed to support you, even if you discover a particular food or food group brings on adverse reactions. Remember, you'll return to the elimination phase between each reintroduction group, to ground you if the foods you reintroduce bring on cravings or discomfort. Lean on your support system and our community through this phase, use the last week of your elimination to prepare for reintroduction, and take one step closer to your own Food Freedom plan.

One last note: Unless your healthcare provider directs you otherwise, I don't recommend anyone stay in the elimination phase for *longer* than 60 days. If you desire additional guidance or symptom relief after 60 days of elimination and careful reintroduction, turn to a doctor, functional medicine provider, or dietitian for more personalized guidance.

SPECIAL POPULATIONS

I have a medical condition; can I do the Whole30?

This is the part where I say, "The Whole30 is not a medical treatment protocol, and was not designed to diagnose or treat medical conditions. Your healthcare provider is the only person qualified to answer that question." I'm not a doctor, and it's important that you consult *your* doctor, registered dietitian, and/or therapist to ensure the Program

Rules, duration, and recommendations are a good fit for your health context. If they approve, work with them closely through elimination and reintroduction, so they can continue to monitor your health markers, lab work, and symptoms.

This is especially important if you are currently taking any medication, especially those for a condition like diabetes (type 1 or type 2), high blood pressure, high cholesterol, or an overactive thyroid. Dietary changes can have a quick and significant impact on a number of health markers, which may require ongoing review or adjustment of related medications. It's important that your provider monitors your lab work, medications, and symptoms for the duration of your Whole30.

I have a digestive disorder; can I do the Original Whole30?

Those with digestive disorders (like IBS, IBD, Crohn's, or ulcerative colitis) would benefit tremendously from an elimination program designed and monitored by a qualified healthcare provider. In many cases, the elimination phase in this context is even more robust, and may also include eggs, nightshade vegetables, high-FODMAP fruits and vegetables, and even coffee or spicy foods. Ideally, you'd work with your healthcare provider closely through elimination and reintroduction, so they can continue to monitor your health markers, lab work, supplements or medications, and symptoms.

However, not everyone has access to a provider who can design and monitor their elimination program. The Whole30 can be an accessible way to see if simple dietary changes can provide you with relief from symptoms and improve your overall well-being. If you decide to try the Whole30 (or your healthcare provider prescribes it), there are

DIET DOESN'T FIX EVERYTHING

Diet books and wellness influencers may claim that dietary changes alone can resolve just about any symptom or health condition. (I recently saw a "master class" advertising a cure for nearsightedness; I'm not tossing my contact lenses just yet.) To be clear—that's not true. Yes, the foods you eat have a tremendous impact on your health and how you feel. But dietary changes alone aren't a cure-all. If you're coming into the Whole30 hoping to improve unwanted symptoms, understand that food is just one factor contributing to those symptoms. Your lifestyle, genetics, health history, stress, trauma, systemic barriers, relationships, and environmental factors also play a role.

I share this not to discourage you but to present a *realistic* picture of the role the Whole30 can play in your health, and to dispel the idea that everyone who does the Whole30 is able to toss their meds* or resolve their symptoms. If this is one of your goals, I hope it happens for you! But if it doesn't, know that your Whole30 will provide a fantastic foundation for your healthcare provider's ongoing treatment plans.

*Please don't stop taking any prescribed medications without first consulting with your doctor, no matter how much better you feel.

some small tweaks you could make to support healthy digestion:

- Avoid vegetables and fruits high in FODMAPs (fermentable carbohydrates), as these are poorly absorbed in the small intestine and can worsen digestive symptoms. You can find an Original Whole30 low-FODMAP shopping list at whole30.com/whole30-and-fodmaps.
- Eat the majority of your vegetables cooked, not raw. (Think soups, stews, and sautés, not big bowls of salad.) This can help ease their passage through your digestive tract.
- If even low-FODMAP fruits bring on digestive distress, try eating them in smaller quantities, or avoiding fruits with seeds or rough exteriors (like berries).

If you find your digestion gets worse on the Whole30 or you experience other negative symptoms, please discontinue the program and speak with your healthcare provider.

Note: The Plant-Based Whole30 is not recommended for those with digestive disorders. The beans, chickpeas, lentils, and soybeans necessary for adequate protein intake contain high amounts of fiber and FODMAPs (fermentable carbohydrates), which can worsen symptoms.

I'm pregnant; can I do the Original Whole30?

Check with your OB/GYN or qualified healthcare provider first. If they approve, work with them closely through elimination and reintroduction, so they can continue to monitor the health of you and your baby.

That having been said, our medical advisory board says the Original Whole30 is generally safe during pregnancy. If your doctor approves, you may need to adjust our meal template to include more meals and/or snacks. You can make meals smaller and more frequent if food aversions, morning sickness, or late-stage pregnancy symptoms make it hard to eat full meals. You may also need to modify the Scale Rule, if your provider wants to talk with you about your weight.

For our registered dietitian's detailed recommendations for doing the Original Whole30 while pregnant, visit our website at whole30.com /whole30-pregnancy.

Note: The Plant-Based Whole30 is not recommended for those who are pregnant.

I'm nursing; can I do the Original Whole30?

Check with your OB/GYN or qualified healthcare provider first. If they approve, work with them closely through elimination and reintroduction, so they can continue to monitor the health of you and your baby.

That having been said, our medical advisory board says the Original Whole30 is generally safe while nursing, and many parents have discovered that their baby eats more, sleeps better, is less fussy, and has fewer rashes or breakouts during elimination.

A parent's biggest concern is maintaining milk supply during the Whole30. Milk supply is determined by a variety of factors, including how often you nurse, how thoroughly you empty during each feeding, how much you're sleeping, and your overall stress levels. However, calories, macronutrients, and nutrition play a big role, too. Make sure you're using our meal template recommendations as *minimums* to ensure adequate intake of protein, carbohydrates, and healthy fats. Do not limit your consumption of any Whole30 foods. You may also need to adjust our meal template to include more meals and/or snacks to ensure you and your baby are eating enough.

In a survey of 600 Whole30ers who started the program while nursing, 90 percent said their milk supply either remained stable or increased during their elimination phase.

Above all, listen to your body and trust your instincts. If the Whole30 proves too stressful, or you notice the program is having a negative impact on your milk supply or your baby, please discontinue the program and speak with your healthcare provider.

For more detailed recommendations for doing the Original Whole30 while nursing, visit our website at whole30.com/whole30-nursing.

Note: The Plant-Based Whole30 is not recommended for those who are nursing.

Can my kids do the Original Whole30 with me?

Many parents consider bringing their kids along on their Whole30 journey in an effort to make meal planning easier, introduce more whole foods into their diets, or identify foods that may be contributing to their health symptoms. However, the Whole30 (or any form of strict dietary restriction) comes with inherent risks, especially for children.

If your child doesn't have a health condition or a specific reason for doing an elimination diet, I recommend *against* putting them on a strict Whole30. Children and teens are especially susceptible to the negative effects of diet talk, body and weight talk, and restrictive dieting behaviors. Though it might feel easier if everyone in the house does the program with you, you can streamline

FLYING SOLO

If you're doing the Whole30 without your kids, be conscientious about how you talk about the program and your goals, especially in front of your kids. Frame the Whole30 as a short-term "self-experiment" (or with older kids, "elimination program"), leaving the word *diet* and all the corresponding associations out of the discussion. With older kids, you might say, "My allergies have been awful this year, and I'm curious if some of the foods I'm eating could be making them worse." For young children, keep it even more simple: "This is what I want to eat. Everyone can choose the foods that look good to them today."

meal planning and introduce more whole foods into your child's diet without requiring them to strictly adhere to every tenet of the Whole30.

If your child does have a health condition or symptoms you hope could be alleviated with a dietary intervention like the Whole30, first discuss the program with your pediatrician or family doctor. Ideally, you'd want your child's elimination protocol to be designed and monitored by a doctor or registered dietitian. For many families, however, this requires a level of privilege (money, time, and resources) that is simply not available. Many parents have found that the Whole30 offers an accessible way to identify the food sensitivities contributing to their child's acne or eczema, allergies, asthma, attention deficits, digestive distress, or behavioral issues. You can then share your observations with your child's doctor at their next appointment.

According to our medical advisory board, the Original Whole30 is safe for children as a short-term elimination protocol, as long as meals are carefully planned by the parent. However, if your child has any form of picky eating, make sure that your child will be able to eat enough of the foods on the Whole30 to meet their nutritional needs. If at any point you believe your child's Whole30 is creating stress or negative feelings around food, eating, or their bodies, discontinue the program and speak with your pediatrician or child therapist.

For more detailed recommendations on doing the Whole30 with children, visit our website at whole30.com/whole30-kids.

Note: The Plant-Based Whole30 is not recommended for children. In addition, the Whole30 is not recommended for children with a history of disordered eating, or those predisposed to eating disorders.

I have an eating disorder (or am in recovery from an eating disorder); should I do the Whole30?

In a word, no. *The Whole30 is not recommended for those with a history of disordered eating, diagnosed or otherwise.* In this context, any form of restriction can be triggering. In fact, any program that restricts foods, food groups, calories, or meals can create a dysfunctional relationship with food, eating, and your body.

The Whole30 has worked incredibly well for millions of people. For some, however, the very same protocol has created or resurrected disordered eating thoughts, patterns, and habits. Yes, I said *created;* the program's strict nature and the elimination of many food groups at once can lead to disordered eating behaviors, even if none were present prior. I share this not to scare you, but to raise awareness that food restriction of any nature does pose that risk.

If you have a history of disordered eating, there are other programs (like intuitive eating, the "plate by plate" approach, or a specific plan designed by a registered dietitian) that may be a better fit. If you still think the Whole30 could be helpful, please speak with your therapist, counselor, or qualified healthcare provider first. If they approve, work closely with them throughout your program so they can monitor your physical and mental health, and follow all of their recommendations. If you have concerns about your mental or physical health at any point during the program, immediately discontinue your Whole30 and speak with your therapist or provider.

YOUR WHOLE30 PLATE

How do I use the Whole30 meal templates?

While the program does an excellent job of reconnecting you with your body's natural signals (hungry, full, thirsty, craving), it can take time for those signals to come through loud and clear, and for you to learn to trust them. If you've been eating ultra-processed foods, dieting for weight loss, or using food to self-soothe, it's likely you've been getting mixed signals—or tuning those signals out—for years. It can feel scary to trust your body again, and to learn to differentiate hunger from other feelings (like cravings, thirst, or negative emotions).

The Whole30 is *great* at helping you reconnect to your body, recognize those signals, and trust the messages coming through. Unlike a diet full of ultra-processed foods, your Whole30 meals include whole, nutrient-dense foods with built-in satiety signals (like protein, fat, water, fiber, and micronutrients). And since you won't be counting or restricting calories on the program, you won't need to ignore or trick yourself out of noticing hunger pangs. As such, you're encouraged to use your body's signals to design your Whole30 meals, adding as much food to the plate as you need to maintain your energy, activity levels, focus, and satiety; and eating whenever you're hungry.

Our Original Whole30 meal template (page 98) and the Plant-Based Whole30 meal template (page 234) were designed by registered dietitians to give you a starting point for building your Whole30 plate. The meal templates include a healthy balance of protein, fat, and carbohydrates to keep you energized, satiated between meals, and performing well in your job, sport, and life. Following these recommendations also helps you eat a wide variety of vitamins, minerals, and other micronutrients.

Ideally, we encourage you to plan for at least three hours between meals, to allow your body the time and energy to "rest and digest," so your gut can clear that food and prepare for your next meal. In addition, I strongly discourage you from grazing all day, grabbing a hard-boiled egg here and an apple there. When you're constantly eating, your digestive system is constantly working, which can reduce your energy reserves, make you feel sluggish, and potentially contribute to digestive issues.

You'll notice we generally don't recommend protein in ounces or added fat in tablespoons. Our registered dietitians believe that estimating portions using your own body as a guide helps to accommodate for natural body variables like size, muscle mass, and activity levels. As an example, the Original Whole30 meal template recommends 1 to 2 palm-sized servings of protein per meal. If you have big palms (especially if that correlates to a bigger body, an active body, or a body with lots of muscle mass), you'll need to eat more protein at meals than, say, my tiny and largely sedentary grandma. It also helps you estimate the right portion sizes for yourself outside of your own

HANGRY NO MORE

If you're one of those people who get "hangry" if you don't eat every two hours, good news! The Whole30 promotes satiety and fat adaptation, which means that by Week 2 or 3, most people discover that they can wait many hours between meals and still feel focused, energetic, and calm. This is a huge Non-Scale Victory and can really come in handy if you get stuck on the tarmac, work runs late, or the restaurant has an hour wait.

home, at occasions like a brunch buffet or a work potluck.

In addition, we include a range of serving sizes to encourage you to tap into your body's own signals when preparing your meals—and to ensure you're not undereating on the program. If you find you're hungry two hours after breakfast, bump up your protein and/or added fats the next morning. If you find you're just not hungry at all when it comes time for lunch, it's okay to make your meals a little smaller, but don't go *below* our minimum recommendations for protein and added fats. (As an example, your Whole30 meals should not regularly include *less* than a palm-sized serving of protein, or *no* added fats.)

Let your health context, activity levels, and goals dictate the rest. If you're especially active in your job and have a lot of muscle mass, you likely need more protein and fat to feel your best. If you're an endurance athlete, you'll want to ramp up your starchy veggies and fruit with every meal, and perhaps add a pre-workout and/or post-workout meal, too. (See page 76.)

As your Whole30 progresses, use your hunger levels, energy, focus, performance, and schedule to dictate how big your meals should be and how many meals you need each day. After a week or two on the Whole30, you won't need the meal template anymore, and will be relying on your own body to guide you.

Does every meal have to look like the meal template?

Not at all—that would be unrealistic. Use the template as your guide, but your meals can and should be flexible. If a plate full of veggies at 6 A.M. sounds terrible, serve a fruit salad with your egg or tofu scramble, and add extra veggies to later meals

and snacks. If one meal happens to be light on protein because you're on the go or at a business lunch, try to include a little extra protein later that day.

In addition, many of the recipes in this book have the protein, fat, and carbohydrates all together in the dish. For example, if you're making the Shepherd's Pie (page 171) or the White Bean Chili (page 289), just eyeball your serving size, enjoy the meal in a relaxed fashion, and when you're done, let your body signals dictate whether or not you need a bit more.

Also, please don't be precious about this. If you're using the meal templates as a general guideline; eating some form of protein, fat, and carbs with your meals; and eating enough to keep you satisfied, energized, and focused, you're doing great!

How do I create my Whole30 meal plan?

There are a number of ways to meal-plan, and the method you choose will depend on your time, budget, schedule, and familiarity with the Whole30. Here are four options, ranging from "I'll do it all myself" to "do it all for me."

1. **Use your favorite Whole30 recipes.** You can create a meal plan from the thousands of recipes available in our books, on our website, and in our social media feeds. Mark your favorites, then create your shopping list. Doubling your recipe portions so you'll have leftovers helps you skip some of the meal prep and cooking the next day. Replacing homemade dressings, sauces, spice blends, or broths with Whole30 Approved convenience items can help you save even more time.

2. **Use the meal-planning resources on whole30.com.** We know better than anyone how to guide you in a way that fits your

lifestyle, family, budget, and time. Our website features a host of free articles, meal-planning strategies, and inspiration, plus hundreds of Whole30 recipes to get you started. Our resources will help you plan for the whole family or just yourself (plus leftovers). We offer tips for planning a whole week's worth of meals at once, or one day a time to keep things flexible. We'll get you through two hours of batch-prep and cooking on a Sunday night, or teach you how to plan and prep throughout the week. There is no one "right" way to meal-prep, so use our resources to help you discover the flow that works best for you.

3. **Use recipe blueprints.** You don't *have* to cook from a recipe; you can just meal-plan by following basic blueprints. Pick your protein, carbs, and added fats, then add flavor with a dressing, sauce, seasoning, or spice blend. Vary the ingredients based on what you have on hand, what's on sale, or what is seasonal. One example is ground meat or plant-based crumbles mixed with veggies. Brown your meat or crumbles, sauté a big batch of veggies in your cooking oil of choice, then vary your meals by serving each portion over a different base (like cauliflower rice, spaghetti squash, zoodles, or mashed potatoes) and topping it with a different dressing or sauce (try ranch, tomato sauce, salsa and guacamole, or a curry sauce). This can make meal planning even simpler, as it allows you to cook only once while enjoying variety in your dishes.

4. **Let us cook for you.** If you'd rather have some (or even most!) of your Whole30 meals delivered straight to your door—yeah, we can do that. Our Original Whole30 national meal-delivery services ship to the forty-eight contiguous states, with deliveries once or twice a week. Meals are designed by registered

dietitians and prepared by regional chefs, rotate each week for effortless variety, and feature delicious, hearty, guaranteed-compatible ingredients—no label reading required. Don't fret, Plant-Based Whole30ers! We have meal-delivery options for you, too. Visit whole30. com to learn more.

Can I track calories or macros on the Whole30?

Though it's not a Program Rule, I'd *really* rather you not. Tracking calories or macros and weighing your foods are most often associated with weight loss efforts. The very act of logging and counting can immediately put your brain into "eat less" mode, create stress around the number, and distance you from your body's own signals. This can

FOOD JOURNALING

What may be helpful is *food journaling,* which isn't the same as calorie counting. When you food-journal, you note the foods you eat at each meal in a general fashion. (For example, "Ground meat with sautéed peppers, onions, and spinach; cauliflower rice with ranch dressing.") Making general notes of your meal, how it made you feel ("hungry 90 minutes later"), and notes for the future ("more protein") can help you fine-tune your portions, meal frequency, and timing. It can also help you troubleshoot, connecting digestive symptoms like gas and bloating to specific Whole30 foods like cauliflower or cabbage.

The Whole30 Day by Day includes prompts for food journaling during each day of your Whole30, but you can also use a notebook, the Notes app on your phone, or a Google Doc.

take your Whole30 into unhealthy territory, where you're further restricting foods, macros, or calories unnecessarily.

Don't let a calorie-counting app mess with your head; your body knows how much you need to eat better than any calculator on the internet. Let the Whole30 reconnect you with your body, and let those signals (hunger, fullness, cravings, mood, energy, and athletic performance) guide your portions.

I'm not usually hungry in the morning; can I skip breakfast?

There are no Whole30 rules about how many meals you eat or when you eat them. However, I highly discourage skipping breakfast, for a few reasons. First, you *should* be hungry in the morning, considering you've spent the last 8 to 10 hours fasting. If you're not, that's a sign that your stress and hunger hormones (cortisol, adrenaline, ghrelin, and leptin) could be out of balance.

Skipping breakfast can also push your entire eating window to later in the night, leading to pantry raids at 10 P.M. (when willpower is already at your lowest), further disrupting sleep and energy levels. And skipping breakfast puts you at risk for undereating over the course of your day, which would hurt your energy and sleep quality, and increase stress and cravings.

The fastest way to correct this is to eat in the morning, ideally an hour after waking, even if you're not that hungry. And I have one rule that I guarantee will help, but you're not going to like it: no coffee until you've eaten breakfast.

Caffeine has an appetite-suppressing effect. When you wake up and immediately chug a mug

FASTING, KETO, CLEANSES— OH, MY!

Please don't try to combine the Whole30 with other dietary approaches like intermittent fasting, keto, or juice or broth cleanses. Remember, the Whole30 is a dietary self-experiment. If you start experimenting with too many things at once, you won't know what to blame if you start feeling worse, or what to credit if you start feeling better. For the sake of the experiment, focus on your Whole30 *without* further restricting meals, meal timing, or carbs. If you still want to play around with fasting, keto, or other approaches, start another self-experiment when reintroduction is over and compare those results to your Whole30.

(because you wake up feeling *exhausted*), it turns off those natural hunger signals. So you drink more coffee, delay eating even longer, have your first meal around 10 A.M. . . . and find yourself standing in front of the pantry *again* at 10 P.M., feeling tired-but-wired.

The good news is that the Whole30 can help break this cycle, thanks to the enormous benefits it can bring to your energy, sleep, blood sugar regulation, stress levels, and cravings. However, this doesn't happen overnight, and it requires you to meet us halfway. Start delaying your morning coffee until you eat something, even if it's a smaller version of our meal template. Make a conscientious effort to "close the kitchen" after dinner, ensuring your meals and snacks throughout the day were big enough to provide adequate energy and nutrition. Then, happily watch how your energy levels, hunger, and habits evolve over the course of your Whole30.

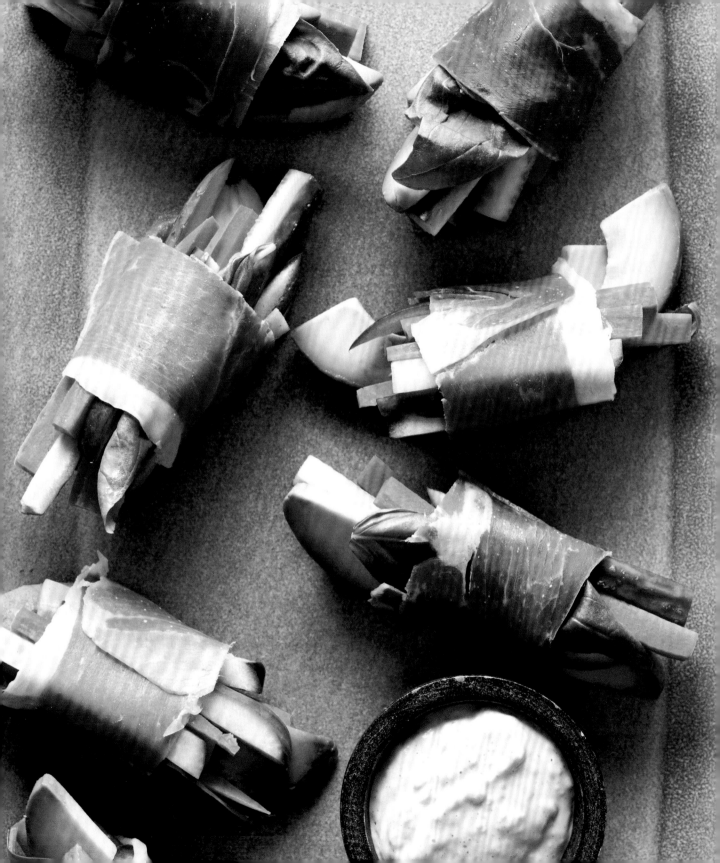

What about snacks?

In older Whole30 books, I recommended against snacking between meals. The suggestion was to make your meals big enough that you didn't need to snack in between, and it was well-intentioned, designed to help your digestive system function more effectively and restore a healthy hormonal balance. If you're able to easily manage this, that's great! You won't have to snack if three to four meals a day leave you satisfied, energized, and focused.

However, today I recognize that your schedule, responsibilities, hunger levels, or activity levels may benefit if (or necessitate that) you eat something between meals. In addition, snacks are a great way to add more energy, protein, and calories in your day, which may be important if you're an athlete or have more muscle mass to support. In that case, please do add snacks or "mini-meals" in whatever way best supports you.

Eating a snack is not the same as grazing, however! Please don't spend your days grabbing a banana here and a handful of pistachios there. Your blood sugar levels, hormones, energy, focus, and satiety all benefit from eating a meal, then allowing your digestive system (and other body systems) a few hours to perform their necessary functions without interruption.

Ideally, snacks should contain at least two of the three macronutrients: protein, fat, and carbs. This will help with satiety, ensuring your snack does tide you over until your next meal. (An apple by itself isn't going to do that as well.) Plan snacks such that you still have a few hours to "rest and digest" before your next meal. And if you find that your stomach is growling every day by 9:30 A.M., use that as a sign to make your breakfast bigger by adding more protein, more fat, or both.

See page 104 for Original Whole30 snack ideas, and page 239 for Plant-Based Whole30 snack ideas.

opposite: Veggie-Stuffed Prosciutto Snack Rolls, page 227

Can we talk about smoothies, too?

We sure can! In the earlier days of Whole30, I strongly discouraged "liquid food" for a number of well-intentioned reasons, but much like with snacking, my thought process has evolved. While there are still benefits to chewing your food (and potential drawbacks to drinking it), smoothies *can* fill an important role in your Whole30.

Smoothies can provide additional protein and energy if you're active in a sport or in your job, or just have higher calorie needs. They can also be a portable, balanced, easy-to-digest source of energy if you're on the go, feeling under the weather, or need something quick to tide you over until your next meal. In addition, smoothies can be a budget-friendly and convenient way to supplement your Whole30 meals, especially if you're using frozen or canned fruit or vegetables.

In general, here are our dietitians' best recommendations regarding smoothies:

- Include all three macronutrients (protein, fat, and carbs) to ensure your smoothie is satiating and balanced.
- Include fruit, but don't make it the star of the show. A fruit-heavy smoothie (especially if it's light in fat and/or protein) can promote blood sugar dysregulation, energy dips, brain fog, and quick hunger.
- Consider including a smoothie *with* a meal instead of *as* your meal. Studies show that drinking meals, even if well balanced in terms of macronutrients, may not be as satisfying or keep you full as long as chewing and swallowing your food.

Look for specific smoothie templates for the Original Whole30 on page 105, and the Plant-Based Whole30 on page 242. (I've also included a smoothie recipe for each program in the recipe sections.)

Do I need a pre-workout or post-workout meal?

If you're a regular gym-goer (but not training competitively), you can likely eat three or four Whole30 meals throughout the day and call it good. In general, significantly altering your meals is recommended only if your workout is more than 60 minutes and at a moderate to high intensity with *continuous/consistent effort.* (A brisk walk, yoga class, short run, or fifteen-minute high-intensity exercise session doesn't require extra nutrition.)

If your context is such that you do need a targeted pre-workout and/or post-workout meal, here are our registered dietitian and sports nutrition coach's general guidelines:

- Pre-workout: Eaten 2 to 3 hours before training (or a smaller portion if you're eating within 1 hour of your workout), focused on protein and high-fiber carbohydrates.
- Post-workout: Eaten within 1 hour of training, focused on lean protein, high-fiber carbohydrates, and plenty of veggies. Protein is specifically important at this meal.

For more specific recommendations, visit our website at whole30.com/whole30-pre-workout -post-workout, or work with a registered dietitian or sports nutrition coach to optimize your pre- and post-workout meals within the Whole30 framework.

WHOLE30 ON THE TOWN

How can I stay social on the Whole30?

It's easier than you think—and I *do* want you to stay social! Gatherings aren't about what's on your plate or in your glass; they are about spending time with people you care about, making memories, and honoring traditions. You can do that with sparkling water in your glass just as easily as Champagne. Here are a few ideas for common social events:

- **Happy hour after work:** Order a sparkling water and lime, and tell anyone who asks, "I'm not drinking right now" or "I'm on a Whole30."
- **Birthday party:** Eat before you go, say, "No, thank you" to the cake and pizza, and BYO LaCroix. Make sure you have emergency food in your bag or car, just in case! If it's a family party, offer to bring a dish, and make something you can enjoy.
- **Dinner with friends:** Suggest a restaurant you know is Whole30-friendly. Plan your order ahead of time, order an unsweetened iced tea or sparkling water, then enjoy the meal!
- **Dinner at Mom and Dad's:** Ask what they'll be making, remind them you're on the Whole30 (if needed), and ask if they can leave the cheese off the salad or the bun off your burger. (Or turn it around and invite them to *your* house, where you'll cook a delicious Whole30 meal!)
- **Date night:** Plan a romantic Whole30 picnic, choose a restaurant you know is Whole30-friendly, or make your date about something other than food. (Try axe-throwing, an evening hike, a gallery stroll, or mini golf.)

How can I dine out while on the Whole30?

Dining out while on the Whole30 has never been as easy as it is today. Most restaurants feature their menus online, offer prominent allergen warnings for gluten or dairy, and are conscientious about dietary allergies or restrictions. At this point, it's commonplace for patrons to ask questions about dishes or ingredients, and for kitchens to make small accommodations.

Still, you'll have to watch out for hidden ingredients. Are the potatoes mashed with cream or butter? Are the eggs scrambled with milk? Does the salad dressing have added sugar? (It almost always does.)

If there isn't a Whole30 Approved restaurant in your area (visit our website to find out), here is an easy plan for dining out while on the Whole30:

- Review the menu ahead of time. (Bonus if you offer to pick the spot, choosing a restaurant that looks Whole30-friendly.) Note the menu options that look promising.
- Call the restaurant during a slower hour (try 2 P.M.) to ask any questions. Explain that you're on a Whole30 right now; most people will know exactly what you're talking about.
- Know your easy swaps! Ask for oil and vinegar instead of salad dressing, request your potato

be baked with a drizzle of olive oil instead of mashed with cream, or get your eggs poached or fried instead of scrambled.
- Confidently pass on the bread basket, order sparkling water with lime, and if anyone asks about the way you're eating, tell them, "Oh, I'll share more after lunch—I don't want to talk about food over food," and change the subject.

Here's my biggest Whole30 pro tip: If you don't make it a big deal, chances are no one else will, either. Go into social situations prepared, and you'll feel far more confident, which lets you spend more time and energy enjoying the meal and the company.

You can find a current list of Whole30 Approved® restaurants and meal delivery companies at whole30.com/whole30-approved.

How do I travel while on the Whole30?

I feel uniquely qualified to answer this question, given I hit the "million mile club" with Delta Airlines last year. (That's *very* different from the "mile high club," just to be clear.) Traveling while on the Whole30 requires (you guessed it) planning and preparation. Some questions to consider:

- What is the form of travel? Flights, train rides, or road trips each have their pros and cons.
- What is the duration of travel? Is it a one-hour flight, a six-hour train ride, or a four-hour road trip?
- Will I be dining out, be provided with meals, or make my own food?
- Will I have access to a fridge, cooler, microwave, and/or kitchen?
- Is there a grocery store nearby, and will I have time to visit it?
- How much and what kinds of foods can I pack with me?

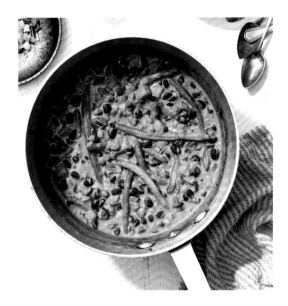

an official Whole30 salad bowl on the menu!) Call ahead and ask the hotel to provide you with a small fridge and microwave (if available) for maximum flexibility, or book a room with a kitchenette.

It's also helpful if your travel companions know you're doing the Whole30. You can offer to help choose restaurants, call the caterer to discuss your group's dietary needs, or alert your co-workers and clients that you won't be ordering drinks with dinner.

What do you mean by "on-the-go" or "emergency" foods?

Planning on-the-go or emergency foods is a huge part of Whole30 success. There will be days when work runs late, your kid's game goes into overtime, you get stuck in traffic, or your flight is delayed. My best tip is to *always* have Whole30-compatible food with you, no matter what. Stash some in your glove box, purse, gym bag, desk drawer, and carry-on for those "just in case" moments. (I have no fewer than three meat sticks on me at all times.)

Planning a three-hour drive to your in-laws' for the weekend is quite easy: Pack a cooler with Whole30 snacks and portable foods, help your in-laws plan meals around your Whole30, and hit the grocery store when you arrive to make sure you have some emergency foods on hand.

Train rides also offer flexibility, as you're not limited to small amounts of liquid, and could pack a small cooler with one or two Whole30 prepared meals, snacks, and drinks.

A flight requires a bit more effort. I know where I can get a Whole30-friendly meal at my local airport, so sometimes I arrive early, eat right before the flight, and make sure I have plenty of on-the-go foods in my carry-on, just in case. (You can also eat a meal right before you leave for the airport.)

If you're traveling for business, research the area near your hotel before you get to the airport. Find a grocery store and have a plan for making a quick run to stock up on essentials. Scope out nearby restaurants and menus, making note of those that look the most Whole30-friendly. (If there's a Chipotle nearby, you're in luck, as they all have

Don't forget to plan for emergency foods at home, too! It's helpful to have leftovers, already-prepared meals, and precooked proteins and veggies on hand in case your Zoom call runs long or you don't have time to meal-plan. I always have a glass storage container with a mixture of sautéed ground meat and veggies in the fridge. (Substitute your favorite plant-based crumbles or beans for the ground meat if you're on the Plant-Based Whole30.) These are easy to reheat and make for a quick meal when topped with a dressing or sauce.

See page 104 for Original Whole30 on-the-go ideas, and page 239 for Plant-Based Whole30 options.

Coconut-Ginger Black Beans, page 268

TROUBLESHOOTING

Is _____ normal on the Whole30?

First, there's no such thing as "normal." Every body is different. Everyone's Whole30 is different. While there are some common experiences during the Whole30, the only ones who can figure out whether your symptoms are of concern for you are you and your doctor.

That having been said, here are some common (although not always pleasant) symptoms you may experience on the Whole30, especially in the first week. (Refer to the Whole30 Timeline on page 51.)

- Headaches (dull)
- Lethargy
- Sleepiness
- Crankiness
- Brain fog
- Cravings
- General malaise
- Breakouts
- Mild digestive issues (bloating, irregularity)

These are particularly common if the Whole30 is a big dietary change for you. In addition, if you have an autoimmune or chronic health condition, it's not unusual for your specific symptoms (arthritic joints, psoriasis, fatigue, etc.) to get worse before they get better, although this usually occurs in the second or third week of the program.

However, these symptoms mostly appear for just a few days, are easily managed, and subside as your body adjusts to the foods you're eating during elimination.

The following symptoms, however, are indicative of something more serious, like a virus or bacterial infection, food poisoning, an allergic reaction, or some other medical issue.

- Nausea, vomiting, or abdominal pain
- Repeated or severe vertigo or dizziness
- Fainting
- Rashes or hives
- Sinus congestion, runny nose, sore throat, or coughing
- Fever

If you experience any of these, please discontinue the Whole30 and speak with your healthcare provider.

Why is my digestion not getting better?

Assuming you don't have a digestive disorder (see page 66), there are a number of reasons why digestion may not improve (or may seem to get worse) during the elimination phase, particularly in the first two weeks.

Any significant change to your diet can create a transient shift in digestion, as your intestinal lining, enzymatic production, and microbiome adjust. If your Whole30 meals contain more fiber than you're used to; if you're eating more cruciferous vegetables, nuts, and seeds; or if your food choices are higher in fermentable carbohydrates, you may experience mild digestive symptoms like diarrhea, constipation, or bloating during the first week or two on the program.

There are small tweaks you can make to your Whole30 program to help your digestive system adjust during elimination:

- Eat more cooked veggies rather than raw, to help ease their passage through your digestive tract. Prepare soups, stews, stir-fries, or sautés instead of big green salads or large crudité plates.
- If you're eating lots of cruciferous vegetables (such as cauliflower, broccoli, Brussels sprouts, or cabbage), try substituting carrots, sweet potatoes, green beans, or squash. (Or simply eat them in smaller quantities.)
- If eating vegetables with every meal is a big change, introduce them in smaller quantities and increase your consumption slowly.
- Eat fruit in smaller portions, rather than large quantities in one sitting.
- If you are constipated, try a gentle, natural solution like prunes (enjoy with caution, as they work quite well) or a magnesium citrate supplement, like Original Natural Calm.
- Keep a food journal (see page 72), and look for links between meals or ingredients and digestive symptoms. It's possible that some of the foods you're eating (like nut butters, tomatoes, or eggs) are contributing to your digestive issues, especially if you're eating far more of them than you're used to.

Digestive enzymes or probiotics can be helpful aids, but I recommend waiting until your Whole30 is over before starting a new supplement, or at the very least, asking your doctor for a specific recommendation tailored to your needs. Taking the wrong type or dose of probiotics can also promote digestive distress, which may complicate your Whole30 findings.

If your digestion isn't improving by the third week of your Whole30, or if at any point your digestive symptoms are concerning, discontinue

See page 243 for additional digestion tips specific to the Plant-Based Whole30.

your program and speak with your healthcare provider.

I'm feeling tired and lethargic on my Whole30—what gives?

The answer to this depends on where you are in your program. This is common for *everyone* in the first five days of the program, as your body adjusts to (potentially) far less sugar than it's used to consuming. Make sure you're eating enough, staying hydrated, and getting enough rest.

If you're active in a sport or in the gym, now is not the time to "suck it up" and press on through your training cycle. Use the first week of the Whole30 as a half-intensity, recovery, or rest period, and give your body time to adjust to this new way of eating. If you're patient here, I promise you'll return faster, stronger, and more energetic.

If you're in Week 2 or 3, it's probably another issue. If you *were* feeling energetic earlier in your program, but now you're back to feeling exhausted and weak, it's probably because you're not eating enough—usually it's a lack of carbohydrates, but it could potentially be a lack of fat, too.

It's great to fill your plate with nutrient-dense vegetables, but all that cauliflower, broccoli, spinach, and asparagus doesn't provide you with much *energy*. If you're not purposefully adding starchy vegetables and/or fruit to every meal and snack, it's likely you're not eating enough to sustain your activity or energy levels. You can get away with that for a little while, but it tends to catch up with people around the halfway mark of their elimination, especially if their training or sport involves high-intensity activity. Here's the bottom line: Whether you're active or not, you *still* need to consume enough calories to maintain your energy.

The good news is that you can test this hypothesis right here and now. Add more carbohydrates and a little more fat to your next meal and snack, and then continue that practice for your next three or four meals. You don't have to double your portions, but you should swap some of those lower-calorie vegetables for potatoes, winter squash, or beets; throw some fruit on the plate; and be generous with your added fats. You should start feeling better immediately—which is your sign to keep that practice up for the remainder of your elimination.

There are other factors that may be contributing to fatigue during elimination:

- **Sodium consumption:** If you've eliminated most processed foods from your diet and you're hesitant to salt your food, you may be too low in this critical electrolyte. This is especially true if you're active, sweat a lot, or spend time outdoors in a hot climate. Unless sodium supplementation is contraindicated, try adding a supplement like LMNT Electrolytes Raw Unflavored to your water bottle, and see if that helps.
- **Caffeine consumption:** Many find they're naturally drinking less caffeine on a Whole30, in part because it's not quite as fun without the creamer and sugar. If this is your context, it's possible you're going through a temporary adjustment as your body gets used to lower amounts in your system. Energy should improve within a day or two (and resist the urge to artificially inflate your energy with more caffeine).
- **Sleep:** This one seems obvious, but if you're having trouble sleeping or sleep has been disrupted by an outside factor (noisy neighbors, a new baby, fireworks), you may feel more tired than usual.
- **Stress:** Stress plays a big role in just about every bodily system. If your stress levels are high

and your nervous system is having a hard time staying regulated, that will translate to feeling tired, down, and distracted.

If you're still feeling tired after making a significant effort to eat more at each meal and considering the other factors listed here, speak with your healthcare provider.

My sugar cravings are intense—help!

Sugar cravings are common, especially in the first week of your Whole30. It's natural to miss the foods you used to rely on for comfort, to relieve anxiety, or to self-soothe. Social situations, environmental cues, and even smells can bring on cravings via association. In addition, if you were eating lots of sugar and now your meals are naturally lower in sugar, you'll likely have a temporary energy-access issue as your body adjusts. This can make you feel tired, headachy, and unfocused, and lead to you crave fast energy (in the form of sugar).

If you discover you're not *really* hungry, take a tip from habit research done with smokers. Studies

HUNGER VERSUS CRAVING

It can be hard to differentiate between a craving and true hunger. Here's my #1 tip for this: Ask yourself, "Am I hungry enough to eat a chicken breast and broccoli?" (If you don't like broccoli, or you're doing a Plant-Based Whole30, substitute any basic protein and steamed vegetable.) If the answer is, "Heck, yes, gimme that chicken breast!," you're legitimately hungry! Go eat a meal or snack. If the answer is, "No, but I'd eat a _____ [fill in crunchy, salty, sweet snacky food here]," you're having a craving, so practice one of my crave-busting techniques.

show that the average craving lasts just 3 to 5 minutes, and that the best way to work through it is to distract yourself. Make a list of short practices that might feel good in a moment of temptation. These might include:

- Tidying or cleaning a small area
- Chopping a few vegetables
- Working on today's crossword or Wordle
- Sending a text or phoning a friend
- Paying some bills
- Reading a few pages of your book

Another technique that works is to do the exact opposite of the above: Commit to sitting with the craving, exploring what you're feeling with curiosity and not judgment. *Wow, all of a sudden, I can't stop thinking about ice cream. Where did that come from?* Maybe you're thirsty. Maybe it's related to the time of day, or the social situation you're in. Maybe you're tired, lonely, anxious, or sad, and ice cream would feel like a pick-me-up. You don't have to solve the mystery, but allowing space for your cravings and exploring what's beneath them might help make them seem less sudden, unpredictable, or powerful.

If you're well into your Whole30 and still experiencing cravings, make sure you're eating enough. Stress is also a physiological driver of cravings. If you've got some stressful things happening, it's natural for your body to respond by craving energy to get you through the crisis.

It's also possible that your cravings aren't slowing down because you're continuing to satisfy

SALAD GOES LAST!

My family has always had the habit of eating our salad *last,* not first, when served a meal. Turns out, this practice is a highly effective way to shift your dessert habit! By ending the meal with something fresh, crunchy, and green, you're sending your body a totally different signal. Ending with a salad interrupts the pattern of "a meal isn't complete until I've had something sweet," so your brain won't have the same associations when the meal is over. If you're coming into the Whole30 with an established dessert habit, try serving a small green salad with dinner, and save it for the end of the meal.

them with Whole30-compatible foods. If you find that replacing your daily cravings with as-close-as-you-can-get Whole30 foods only feeds those cravings, consider using a distraction technique to move through the craving or replacing the ritual of that midafternoon snack or dessert with something totally different but also restorative. Early in my Whole30 journey I got into the habit of brewing a pot of herbal tea after dinner instead of reaching for dessert, and found it a cozy, satisfying replacement.

If at any point in your program, you feel as though you are overly preoccupied with food, starting to develop an unhealthy relationship with food, secretly consuming foods, or binging on foods (Whole30 or otherwise), discontinue your program and speak with a qualified healthcare provider or therapist.

REINTRODUCTION

Do I have to reintroduce?

Yes. (Can I just say that at this point in the book?) Reintroduction is a necessary part of every elimination program. Reintroduction helps you pinpoint the foods that may have been contributing to negative symptoms, like bloating, allergies, pain, or breakouts. This phase will also help you confirm the foods that work well in your body, giving you the confidence to continue eating them with joy, no matter what warnings you may hear from "wellness" influencers on Instagram.

Without reintroduction, you miss *half* the learning experience of the Whole30—and that feels like a major bummer, considering how hard it is to give up the foods you love for 30 days. Be patient, take your time with reintroduction, and use that knowledge to fuel your food freedom. I promise, it'll be worth the extra time.

Do I have to reintroduce food groups in the order you've listed them?

Nope. We've arranged each reintroduction schedule in the order of *least* likely to be problematic to *most* likely to be problematic, based on research and the results of millions of people who have completed the program since 2009. However, you can reintroduce food groups in whatever order you choose. If you really miss oatmeal and rice, reintroduce non-gluten grains first. If you are most looking forward to a glass of wine, reintroduce alcohol first. Just make sure you reintroduce only one food group at a time and you return to the elimination phase for 2 to 3 days between each food group.

What does it mean to "properly challenge the system" during reintroduction?

You want to reintroduce enough of the experimental food to provoke a response, to determine if you are in fact sensitive to that food. You may not notice anything if you add just a splash of milk to your coffee, but that likely isn't enough of a challenge to your digestive and immune systems. Instead, pour a generous serving of milk over fresh berries and grain-free granola, add 2 or 3 ounces of cheese to your salad, and eat a whole container of unsweetened Greek yogurt over the course of your day. These amounts reflect a typical serving size and should be enough to provoke a response if you are sensitive.

Why do I have to return to the elimination phase in between reintroduction groups?

The symptoms of a food intolerance or sensitivity can last for hours or even days. If reintroducing one food group causes negative symptoms (like digestive distress, blood sugar dysregulation, migraines, or a resurgence of allergy symptoms), you need to allow those symptoms to subside before reintroducing *another* food group that might also have a negative impact. This will allow you to accurately evaluate the impact of each group individually.

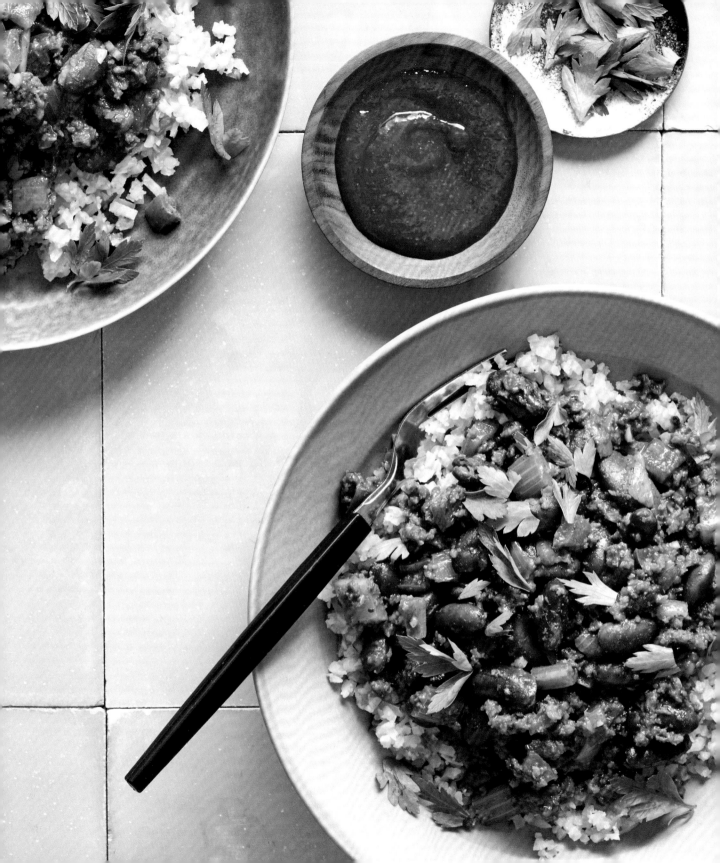

In addition, some symptoms related to a food sensitivity or intolerance (like breakouts, headaches, or joint swelling) may take a day or two to appear. Returning to the elimination phase for 2 to 3 days after each reintroduction group gives you the time to observe any delayed negative effects, should they occur.

Why do you recommend choosing low-sugar options for reintroduction foods?

Most of the foods you'll want to reintroduce likely come with at least *some* added sugar. But reintroducing high-sugar versions of grains or dairy can complicate your observations. Choosing lower-sugar options for these categories helps you evaluate more clearly the impact of that food without a large amount of sugar confounding the results. If you determine that plain yogurt with breakfast has no negative effects, but a few weeks later notice that a sugary yogurt tanks your energy by 11 A.M., you'll know exactly why.

Why is reintroducing added sugar optional, and how would I do that?

Most people don't miss plain sugar as much as they miss sugar *attached* to other foods, like grains or dairy. If that's the case, once you reintroduce low-sugar grains and dairy, you'll have a good benchmark to now compare your mom's chocolate chip cookies or double-chocolate ice cream.

However, if you really want to evaluate the impact of adding sugar all by itself into otherwise

Whole30 meals, these extra three days in the beginning of your reintroduction schedule will help you evaluate how it impacts your energy, mood, hunger, cravings, and other symptoms.

As counterintuitive as it may feel after 30 days of elimination, look for products that *do* contain added sugar for this step. Add cane sugar or a sweetened dairy-free creamer to your coffee, drink a sugary (or sweetened "diet") beverage, top your roasted salmon or tofu with a maple syrup glaze, use condiments like ketchup or salad dressing that contain added sugar, choose a sweetened nut butter, add date paste to your smoothie, or choose honey-roasted pecans instead of plain for your snack. Again, return to the Whole30 elimination phase for 2 to 3 days following this step.

Can I separate out reintroduction groups further?

You certainly can reintroduce corn apart from the other non-gluten grains, or soy apart from other legumes. However, there are pros and cons to this approach.

Pro

- A slower reintroduction schedule will help you more clearly pinpoint the specific foods (not just the food groups) contributing to symptoms.
- If you already suspect a certain food isn't working well for you, a more thorough reintroduction is the perfect opportunity to confirm those findings.
- If you have a chronic illness, pain, or an autoimmune condition, a more gradual reintroduction schedule can help you feel your best, even if multiple foods provoke negative symptoms.

opposite: Creole-Style Red Beans over Cauliflower Rice, page 292

Con

- A longer reintroduction schedule requires you to pay close attention to your food choices for even longer.
- A longer reintroduction schedule may make socializing more challenging, as you'll have to time your reintroduction foods with upcoming events.
- The longer you make this phase, the more likely you will grow impatient and abandon reintroduction altogether, thus losing the benefits.

In summary, the more carefully and systematically you approach reintroduction, the more you'll gain awareness of an individual food's effects. However, for most Whole30ers, the standard reintroduction schedule should suffice. If you do decide to extend reintroduction, remember to return to 2 to 3 days of Whole30 elimination between *each* reintroduced food or food group.

How do I reintroduce Pancake Rule foods?

As grain-free banana bread, cassava-flour tortillas, or potato chips fried in avocado oil *are* made from Whole30-compatible ingredients, you might think, *I'll just eat them as I choose throughout my reintroduction.* However, I encourage you to separate these foods from the rest of your reintroduction schedule and turn them into their own reintroduction category. That means dedicating one day to reintroducing only Pancake Rule foods, then spending 2 to 3 days back on the Whole30 elimination.

In addition, pay close attention to how that paleo banana bread, cassava-flour tortilla, or serving of potato chips makes you feel. It's possible that the high quantity of alternative flour found in many of these foods will mess with your digestion or energy level, or that the return of baked goods, cereal, chips, or fries will bring back cravings.

How do I reintroduce the scale?

You are welcome to weigh yourself once your Whole30 elimination phase is over. But before you step on the scale, ask yourself one question: Will the scale change how I feel about my Whole30 experience, the progress I've made, and the improvements I've noticed?

Imagine stepping on the scale and seeing a number that doesn't reflect what you were hoping for. Now think how that will make you feel. Be honest with yourself.

If that number *won't* sway your confidence, diminish your sense of pride in your Whole30 accomplishments, or tarnish your list of Non-Scale Victories, then by all means check that measurement off your list.

But if a less-than-expected weight loss result is going to have an impact on how you feel about yourself, your efforts, and your Non-Scale Victories, then *don't do it*. The scale doesn't measure confident, strong, proud, energetic, committed, happy, or healthy. Why would you give anything the power to take all that away from you?

What should I be paying attention to during reintroduction?

First, *you might not notice anything at all*. I don't want to predispose you to finding something negative when you bring back gluten or dairy, because it's entirely possible your body does just fine with some or all those food groups. In fact, you may notice that the reintroduction of those food groups leads to improvements in energy, focus, digestion, or other factors. This is especially true if you're active; you may discover that reintroducing rice, oatmeal, or other grains provides a boost to energy, athletic

CHECK YOUR WEARABLES

If you wear a fitness tracker like a WHOOP band or an Apple watch, the data can be a treasure trove of information during reintroduction, too! Look back at your stats during the 30 days of elimination: Did your HRV (heart rate variability), resting heart rate, respiratory rate, sleep quality, and recovery score improve during that period? These are all objective markers of health and can provide tangible proof of the benefits you felt during elimination! Now review and compare the same data after a reintroduction day. These insights can provide you with additional information about the effect of these foods on your nervous system, cardiovascular system, and overall health.

performance, and recovery. In summary, keep an open mind when going into reintroduction, and remember this phase is as much about identifying the foods that *do* work for you as the foods that don't.

That having been said, pay attention to anything that got better during elimination and gets worse again with reintroduction. Specifically, does a reintroduction day or meal bring about issues in any of the following areas:

- **Energy:** Are you back to sluggish mornings, blood sugar crashes, that 2 P.M. "head on desk" feeling, or skipping the gym because you're just too tired? Are your chronic fatigue symptoms back—or did they get worse?
- **Sleep:** Is your sleep more restless, are you struggling to fall asleep, are you waking in the middle of the night again, or back to hitting the snooze button?
- **Cravings:** Are you feeling cravings more often, or experiencing strong cravings again? Are you back to automatically reaching for food to numb, self-soothe, or relieve anxiety? Do you suddenly feel the need for something sweet after a meal or late at night?

- **Digestion:** Are you back to feeling bloated, gassy, constipated, or experiencing diarrhea? Has your acid reflux or heartburn returned? Is your stomach hurting or cramping?
- **Mood and focus:** Have you lost your confidence, happiness, or positivity? Are you feeling more anxious, less motivated, or having trouble focusing? Are you feeling more stressed, or less capable of emotional regulation?
- **Skin:** Did your skin break out? Did patches of eczema, psoriasis, or rosacea reappear or get worse? Are you experiencing hives, rashes, or other skin disruptions?
- **Respiratory:** Are you stuffy, congested, or experiencing sinus pain? Did your asthma or allergies return or get worse?
- **Pain and inflammation:** Are your joints swollen or painful? Did your chronic tendinitis, arthritis, or pain return or get worse? Did you get a headache or migraine?

Some effects will be impossible to ignore, like the time I reintroduced goat cheese and my stomach felt like it was birthing an alien 30 minutes later. Other effects can be more subtle and may require additional "tests" in your food freedom to determine how the food impacts you. This is why I repeatedly say that *reintroduction is a lifelong process.* The more you pay attention to what happens when you eat these foods in your food freedom, the more you'll learn about the foods that work (and don't work) for your body.

In a 2023 beta test of 45 WHOOP users, 91 percent improved their average HRV (a measure of nervous system regulation) during their Whole30 elimination. The average improvement was an astonishing 29 percent.

Can the elimination phase create a food sensitivity?

No, the removal of a food from your diet will not *create* a sensitivity or intolerance in just 30 days if none was there before. However, some people do notice that certain reintroduction foods bother them more than they did before, and there are a few explanations.

First, it's entirely possible that the food in question has always perpetuated negative symptoms, but you wrote them off as "normal." (I can't tell you how many times a Whole30 alumni said to me, "I just assumed everyone had stomach pain after they ate.") However, after the absence of that food and the relief of those symptoms, you're far more *aware* of the impact when you reintroduce it. I always experienced digestive distress when I ate dairy, but cheese and yogurt were part of my daily routine, and I just accepted the bloating and diarrhea as a fact of life. It wasn't until I stopped eating dairy, and the bloating and diarrhea went away, that I realized I didn't have to live with those symptoms.

However, the removal of these foods from your diet, even in the short term, *can* impact your gut microbiome and the enzymes your body was producing to help you digest those foods. Take lactose, the sugar found in dairy products. Most adults are already poor digesters of lactose, as our bodies produce very little of the enzyme required to digest it. Our gut bacteria can help us digest lactose, but when you stop eating dairy, your body downregulates enzymatic production and that gut bacteria population even further. When you reintroduce high-lactose foods (like milk or soft cheese) a month later, you may discover your body has less capacity to digest it, which can lead to unpleasant symptoms. (This can happen with other foods, too, like grains and legumes.)

Again, you haven't *created* an intolerance—and for many, this is just a temporary state. Research finds that reintroducing these foods in smaller quantities more regularly can encourage your gut microbiome and enzymatic production to adjust, helping you tolerate these foods better. (Of course, lactose isn't the only component of food that can be problematic; you may be reacting to the milk proteins, casein and whey.)

This serves to reinforce the idea that reintroduction is a lifelong process! If you really miss dairy but experience negative effects during Whole30 reintroduction, see if repeated reintroduction of smaller amounts eases those symptoms. Or test a goat's-milk or sheep's-milk cheese against cow's milk to see if the source makes a difference. Or test a lactose-free milk or cottage cheese to determine if it's the protein components you're reacting to. Continue to pay attention every time you eat dairy (as an example), and see if your ability to digest it improves with repeated exposure, stays the same, or gets worse—all valuable information for your food freedom.

If I experience a negative reaction during reintroduction, should I give up that food forever?

Not unless the reaction is so problematic you have no desire to repeat it. During her first Whole30, my friend Alex (who has rheumatoid arthritis) discovered that gluten made her joints swollen and painful—but she still eats gluten. She's just conscientious about how often, how much, and when she chooses to enjoy it. The box of donuts on the break-room counter—not worth it for her. But her mom's famous Christmas Eve lasagna—*totally* worth it.

You always get to decide the role any food or food group plays in your food freedom. If the food in question is special, culturally significant, or just plain delicious, you may choose to keep eating it and deal with the consequences. Or, like Alex, you may choose to moderate when, how often, and how much you consume it, so you can feel your best most of the time. Or you may decide the effects just aren't worth it, and happily send that food off into the sunset, never to be missed again (because *you're* the one who decided it wasn't worth eating, given the consequences).

In addition, food sensitivities can improve or even disappear with time. Case in point: I can now enjoy goat cheese in a salad once in a while—no more alien babies! Your body, microbiome, gut health, immune system, activity levels, stress levels, and environment are always evolving. It's entirely possible that the post-Whole30 dietary changes you make in your food freedom can better prepare your body to tolerate these foods—or at least reduce their negative impact. (Can I beat the "reintroduction is a lifelong process" drum here again?) Just because you have a negative reaction now doesn't mean you always will. If you really miss the food in question, continue to "test" it in your food freedom—you may be pleasantly surprised.

If I experience no negative effects when reintroducing, can I consider that food "good to go" from now on?

I'd recommend against it—at least for a while. You may not experience immediate digestive distress, breakouts, joint pain, or other symptoms, but sometimes repeated exposure to that food, or eating that food in larger quantities, can bring out symptoms, subtle or not so subtle.

I can eat a typical amount of wheat just fine. If I have a sandwich on regular bread, eat the bun on my burger, or have a slice of birthday cake, I don't have many noticeable effects. If I eat wheat for two or three days in a row, however, it's a different story. My stomach becomes painfully bloated, my skin breaks out (either on my chin or forehead—never in between), and mentally, I find myself in a major funk. Maybe high doses of wheat mess with my brain chemistry, or maybe I just don't feel good, which makes me depressed. Either way, I've learned that if I want to feel my best, I need to modulate how often and how much I consume products containing wheat.

I know this because I've repeated this "experiment" hundreds of times since my first Whole30, and I've paid attention each time I've said yes to the bread, bun, or cupcake. The first time I felt a little down and unmotivated after eating cupcakes too many days in a row, I took note. The fifth time it happened (I *really* like cupcakes), I knew I could rely on my body's signals—too much wheat (especially when combined with sugar) doesn't feel good.

Conversely, I can confidently say that my body *loves* rice and oatmeal. Every time I've reintroduced those foods, I've noticed smooth digestion, improved energy, great focus, and better performance in the gym or on the trail. After conducting *that* experiment hundreds of times with the same results, I can now say with all certainty that those foods do work well for me, and I consider them part of my everyday diet, with no caveats.

Reintroduction is—say it with me—*a lifelong process*. It's wonderful when a food or food group you enjoy doesn't bring on immediate negative symptoms. But please do continue to pay attention when you eat that food, in an effort to better understand your body and how that food interacts with your physical and mental health.

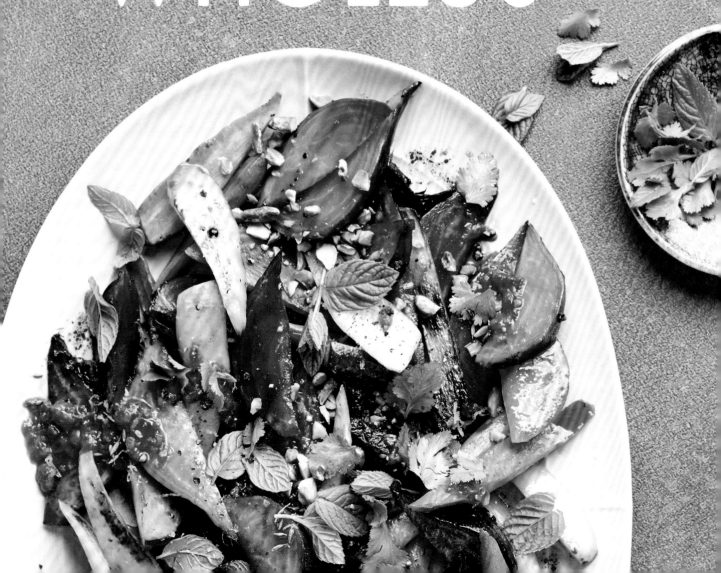

PART 3
COOKING
WHOLE30

My Whole30 cooking philosophy is this: You don't need to cook complicated meals from fancy recipes; all you need are fresh ingredients and basic kitchen techniques. In fact, my go-to meals today are mostly "ingredient meals"—no recipe required. If I'm in the mood for meat, I'll mix cooked ground chicken with sautéed veggies, spoon it over spaghetti squash, and top it with a tomato sauce. If I'm in a plant-based mood, I'll scramble some tofu with greens, tomatoes, and roasted sweet potatoes, then top it with avocado and add a side of berries or melon.

I didn't even know what spaghetti squash was before my first Whole30. I had never eaten an avocado. I hadn't cooked bacon, or Brussels sprouts, or Swiss chard. In fact, one of the most common testimonials I hear from Whole30 alumni is, "The Whole30 taught me how to cook." Making Whole30 meals does require some kitchen skills, but I promise, *anyone* can make the recipes in this book, even if you don't know your small dice from your julienne.

KITCHEN TOOLS AND GADGETS

Described here are some gadgets and tools to help you plan, prepare, and cook your way through the Whole30. You probably have many of these in your kitchen already, but if not, you don't have to stock up all at once. You can purchase tools as you have the budget for them or when a new recipe catches your eye. Or you can cook your way through most of the book by getting creative with the tools you have on hand. That one cutting board you have will be working hard, but the point is that it will work.

opposite: Moroccan Carrots and Beets, page 321

POTS AND PANS: There's a lot to consider here, from stainless steel to enameled nonstick to cast iron. Would you rather buy a matching set or have individual pieces based on your needs? Would you rather stock up all at once or buy one piece at a time? At minimum, you'll want a 3- to 4-quart Dutch oven for making soups, stews, and chilis; and one small (1- to 2-quart) stockpot for making sauces. You could start with just two shallow pans—one nonstick skillet and one oven-safe skillet. If you have room for one more, look for a high-sided sauté pan with a cover, handy for dishes like Coconut-Cauliflower Rice (page 180) or Coconut-Ginger Black Beans (page 268).

KNIVES: I know you have knives, but do you have *Whole30-worthy* knives? Investing here will make your Whole30 meal prep 100 percent more enjoyable. There's a different kitchen knife for practically any task, but you really need just two: a paring knife and an 8-inch chef's knife. Look for knives that are all one piece (not a separate blade and handle that have been joined together), and if you are able, spend more here. This is one investment that will pay back every time you cook. (Don't forget a knife sharpener, too, to keep those blades fresh.)

CUTTING BOARDS: You'll be chopping, slicing, and dicing a lot on your Whole30, so make sure you have a good cutting board (or three). You've got three materials to choose from—wood, plastic, and rubber—and each has its pros and cons. I like upcycled plastic boards, as they're eco-friendly, a snap to clean, and fast-drying. You could also look for bamboo (or maple, if you want to splurge) or rubber if you don't mind washing them by hand. Buy a few sizes, so you don't have to break out your biggest board just to mince a clove of garlic.

BAKING SHEETS: You won't be making cookies on the Whole30, but you will be roasting lots of vegetables and meats in the oven. Make sure

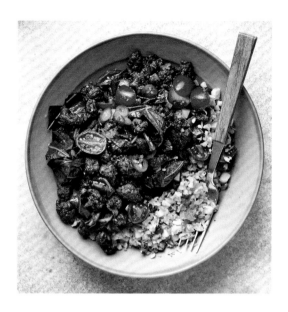

INSTANT POT

An Instant Pot is a multifunction electric pressure cooker that doubles as a slow cooker. These have become very popular, in part because of how quickly and easily they work. (You can bake a potato in just 15 minutes!) They offer multiple cooking functions, including rice cooking, steaming, and sautéing, which may help you make the most of your budget and your counter space.

you have at least two large rimmed baking sheets (also called sheet pans), so you don't crowd your sweet potatoes when they're roasting.

STRAINER: A strainer allows you to drain water from boiled vegetables or broths, and doubles as a steamer when placed inside a stockpot. It's nice to have two strainers—one with fine mesh to filter out smaller particles of food and a larger one (also called a colander) with bigger holes for draining larger foods or for steaming.

FOOD PROCESSOR: This sounds like an expensive tool, but there are a number of options to fit any budget. You can go big and get a gorgeous model that will handle up to two heads of cauliflower at a time; choose a smaller, more cost-effective machine perfect for small batches of dressings or sauces; or something in between. It's all up to your budget—and available counter space. (Note, food processors are different from blenders. Blenders work best for liquid mixtures, while food processors chop, shred, and puree solid ingredients to the desired consistency.) If you're cooking for

one, you may be able to get away with a mini food processor. However, these process foods only in small batches (usually 2 to 3 cups at a time), so if you're doubling the Sausage and Cauliflower Grits recipe (page 117) for a family of four, that small motor will be working awfully hard. However, that doesn't mean you need an expensive, professional-grade appliance. There are plenty of 7- to 10-cup food processors selling under $100. (Some are even combination blender/food processors, saving you money and counter space.)

SLOW COOKER: Slow cookers do the work for you, cooking delicious meals while you sleep, work, or otherwise live your life. These vary wildly in price, from a $40 basic model to fancier versions for $200 and up, but you don't need to break the bank. Look for a larger size (7 quarts) so you can double recipes to have leftovers, and make sure you can program it for maximum convenience. (Mine has a Warm feature that keeps the dish warm between cooking and serving.)

SPIRALIZER: Vegetable noodles are an easy way to add variety to your Whole30 meals in a manner that's fun for the whole family. This little machine cuts your zucchini, cucumbers, butternut squash, and sweet potatoes into long noodles quickly and easily, saving you money on pre-cut noodles at the grocery store. You can find them for under $40, and it takes under a minute to spiralize an entire zucchini.

Somali-Inspired Beef and Collards Sauté, page 179

MEASURING CUPS AND SPOONS: You'll need at least one basic set of measuring cups and spoons, but I highly recommend doubling up, as you'll be using them a lot. It's also helpful to have a larger (3- to 4-cup) glass measuring cup with a pouring spout for larger quantities of broth.

MEAT THERMOMETER: This is one of the most important tools for the budding chef. Cooking meat and poultry to just the right point—not raw, not overdone, just tender—takes time, attention, and lots of practice, but using a meat thermometer is cheating in a good way. Look for an instant-read device that you can insert directly into the meat to determine if done; you should be able to find one for around $10.

PARCHMENT: Parchment is moisture-resistant paper that is specially treated for oven use. It will keep your baking sheets clean, and your delicate meats and veggies will release from the baking sheet with ease. At about $3 a roll, this is a great investment for easy Whole30 kitchen cleanup. Buy any brand at any grocery store.

GARLIC PRESS: Mincing garlic is one of my least favorite tasks—and *lots* of recipes call for minced garlic. For under $20, you'll never have to mince again. Just peel the clove, put it in the press, and squeeze.

CITRUS SQUEEZER: Squeeze all the juice out of your lemons or limes without giving yourself a hand cramp. That's all this tool does, but it's enough.

MICROPLANE: You'll find citrus zest in many of the recipes in this book. Zest (which comes from the peel of citrus fruits like lime, lemon, orange, or grapefruit) adds a surprising amount of flavor to a dish. This special grater sells for under $10 and can quickly zest citrus or grate spices like ginger or nutmeg.

FOOD STORAGE CONTAINERS: With all the food prep and meal planning you'll be doing, you'll need plenty of containers to store those leftovers, extra dressings and sauces, and freezer meals. I love glass storage containers, but you can use plastic, silicone, and stainless steel, or recycle empty pickle or mayonnaise jars. Make sure you have a good number, and plenty of different sizes.

COOKING AND RECIPE TIPS

Before you dive in to the delicious recipes, starting on page 107 for the Original Whole30 and on page 244 for the Plant-Based Whole30, here are some helpful hints for cooking your way through any recipe in this book.

Read the recipe

I know you want to jump right in and start cooking, but the only time I ever mess up a recipe is when I don't take the time to read it *before* I start cooking. Read the ingredients, the instructions, and the tips all the way through, then read it again. Look for ingredients that aren't familiar, kitchen tools you may not have, and prep and cooking times. (There is nothing worse than getting halfway through the prep and realizing the protein needs to marinate for 2 to 4 hours.)

Read your labels

While I've done my best to specify "Whole30-compatible" for many ingredients in these recipes, remember that not every broth, bacon, or mustard is going to fit your Whole30 elimination phase. When you're evaluating ingredients for your recipe, make sure you read *all* your labels—

right down to the spices. If there is cornstarch in the broth, added sugar in the bacon, or white wine in the mustard, choose another product for that dish.

Mise en place

This is a French term that means "putting in place," and it's key to staying organized and precise in the kitchen. (It also makes cleanup much easier—bonus!) Before you start cooking, lay out your ingredients on a clean section of the counter. Do all your chopping, measuring, and prepping (like rinsing and draining beans) first. If all the dry spices go in at the same time, those can be put in the same small bowl. If the veggies cook at the same time, chop them all, then add them to a different bowl.

When all your ingredients are laid out, measured, and ready to be added to the dish at the right time, *then* you can start cooking. I know it seems like extra work, but it makes the cooking process so much faster and smoother; ensures the ingredients you need are ready when you need them; and will help you catch an ingredient you might have forgotten in your first read-through.

Cooking times

Our recipe team tested all these recipes and instructions *many* times, but your mileage (and cooking times) may vary, based on a number of factors. A steak, piece of salmon, or chicken breast may take longer to cook based on its thickness. Veggies may take shorter or longer to cook based on how small or large you cut them. Beans may cook faster if you soak them for a long period of time.

In addition, some ovens run hotter or colder than the temperature setting. When your temperature setting says 375°F, your actual oven temp might be 365° or 380°F. (You can use an oven thermometer to help gauge this.)

Also, altitude has a big impact on cooking times! With higher elevations, foods require longer times to boil, steam, simmer, or bake. The recipes in this book reflect cooking times at sea level, so if you live at 4,500 feet (as I do here in Salt Lake City), you may need to adjust.

Essentially, practice *in your own kitchen* makes perfect. Follow the recipes to the letter if you're unfamiliar with cooking, and taste or test along the way to evaluate the doneness, finding the cooking times that work for your environment, oven, and preferences. I even make comments in the margins of my favorite recipes, noting ingredients I leave out, amounts I like to double, and cooking times I have adjusted. And remember, as with the Whole30, cooking gets easier as you gain experience and confidence.

Cooking oils

In our recipes, we generally call for specific cooking oils, like extra-virgin olive oil or avocado oil. You are always free to use whatever oil or cooking fat you have in your pantry. However, some oils and fats (like coconut oil or lard) impart more flavor than others, which may not lead to the desired result. In addition, substituting some cooking fats for oils may not produce the anticipated texture. For example, for the Quick Cauliflower Rice recipe (page 189), subbing avocado oil for ghee might produce a looser, more oily consistency.

In general, don't overthink it! If you have the capacity, buy a few different cooking oils and fats, and learn which works best for your tastes in each recipe. I love roasting sweet potatoes in duck fat or avocado oil, but coconut oil isn't my favorite flavor profile. But if there's coconut milk in the dish itself, then I'll choose coconut oil to sauté my veggies.

You can also cook your way through the Whole30 with just one or two oils. Extra-virgin olive oil, avocado oil, and a cultured oil like Zero

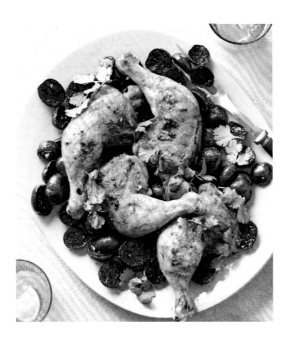

Acre Farms are the most versatile. All are great for cooking, as well as making dressings, sauces, and marinades.

Expand your food horizons

The recipes here are reflective of our diverse community and feature a wide range of ingredients from around the globe. In the tips and recipe headnotes, you'll learn about the history and origins of Aleppo pepper flakes, za'atar, xawaash, and zhug; and read about dishes from all around the world, like ful medames, larb, shawarma, Estofado de Ternera a la Catalana, and chana masala.

If some of these flavors are new to you, get excited! You're about to discover a breadth and depth of spice, heat, sweetness, and smokiness that your current pantry may not include. Also, don't be intimidated. You can find all the ingredients for these dishes at your local grocery store or health food market, or on Amazon; we also include suggested substitutions or "make your own" versions, which work perfectly fine, too.

As with all Whole30 cookbooks, the recipes here are creative, hearty, and full of flavor, but simple enough for anyone to pull off, even if you're new to cooking. Build up your spice collection as you go, visit your local cultural markets for hidden gems you can't find at your local grocer, and enjoy your exploration of the recipes you'll find here.

IMPROVISE AND MAKE IT FUN

If you're new to cooking, recipes can be super helpful, giving you a path to deliciousness without any guesswork. But don't be afraid to play around with your ingredients! Unlike baking, cooking doesn't have to be precise. If you like more greens in your dish, add some spinach or chard. If you don't have the specific veggies we call for in our Seasonal Frittata (page 121), substitute whatever is in your fridge. If you like it spicy, add more cayenne or double the jalapeño. If you don't love garlic, *leave it out.* (In some circles, this would send you right to jail, but we're not fussy like that.)

Involve the whole family in choosing a recipe, chopping the veggies, and measuring the ingredients, even if they're not doing the Whole30 with you. Make meal prep part of your post-work wind down by playing fun music, listening to a podcast, or chatting with your spouse. Try new veggies, and experiment with new spice blends and flavors. Share your meals on social media and connect with other Whole30ers for recipe inspiration.

Your Whole30 can help you connect to your food in a whole new way—joyful, expansive, creative, and deeply gratifying. So get out there and start cooking! You've got 30-plus days of delicious, satisfying, hearty Whole30 meals waiting for you.

Peruvian-Inspired Roast Chicken and Potatoes with Green Sauce and Broccolini, page 161

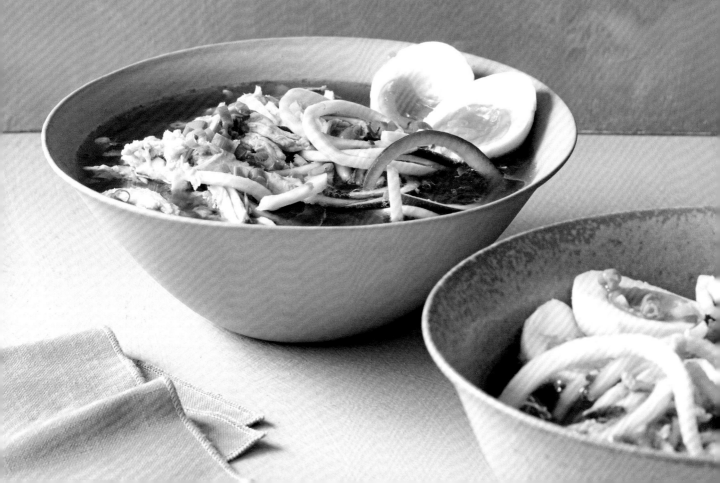

PART 4

THE ORIGINAL WHOLE30

The Original Whole30 is the version I completed and documented in 2009. During the elimination phase, you eat meat, seafood, and eggs; lots of vegetables and fruit; natural animal- and plant-based fats; and herbs, spices, and seasonings. You don't count or restrict calories, track your intake, or limit your portions. You eat real, whole foods to satiety, inspired by the delicious, satisfying, and diverse recipes starting on page 107.

The following is a summary of the rules. For a detailed description of the Original Whole30 Program Rules, return to page 36.

ORIGINAL WHOLE30 PROGRAM RULES (QUICK REFERENCE)

Original Whole30 elimination—30 days

- Added sugar (real or artificial)
- Alcohol (wine, beer, cider, liquor, etc.)
- Grains (wheat, oats, rice, corn, quinoa, etc.)
- Legumes (beans, lentils, soy, and peanuts)
- Dairy (milk, cheese, sour cream, yogurt, etc.)
- The Pancake Rule (baked goods, pasta, cereal, chips, and fries)
- The Scale Rule (weighing yourself or taking measurements)

The Fine Print (exceptions)

These foods *are* allowed during the Original Whole30 elimination phase:

- Green beans
- Most peas (sugar snap, snow, green, yellow, and split peas)
- Ghee and other forms of clarified butter
- Cooking oils (regardless of their source)
- Coconut aminos
- Alcohol-based botanical extracts (such as vanilla, lemon, or lavender)

- Cane, Champagne, red wine, rice, sherry, and white wine vinegar
- Iodized salt (which contains dextrose as a stabilizer)

Original Whole30 reintroduction—10+ days

- Added sugar (optional)
- Return to the Original Whole30 elimination phase for 2 to 3 days
- Legumes
- Return to the Original Whole30 elimination phase for 2 to 3 days
- Non-gluten grains
- Return to the Original Whole30 elimination phase for 2 to 3 days
- Dairy
- Return to the Original Whole30 elimination phase for 2 to 3 days
- Gluten-containing grains
- Return to the Original Whole30 elimination phase for 2 to 3 days
- Alcohol (optional)
- Return to the Original Whole30 elimination phase for 2 to 3 days

opposite: Zoodle Bowl with Chicken, Soft-Boiled Egg, and Green Onions, page 150

ORIGINAL WHOLE30 MEAL TEMPLATE

One of the benefits of the Whole30 is that the program gets you back in touch with your body's natural "hungry" and "full" signals. Most participants find by the second week of their Whole30, they're able to tune into their body for cues, and use their energy, focus, hunger, and mood to help them build a plate that suits their needs, activity levels, and schedule.

Until then, here is a general meal template for the Original Whole30. Use this as a starting place if you're not sure how much to eat. Treat this template as a *minimum,* so you're not eating less than the quantities recommended here.

Meal recommendations

Eat 3 to 4 meals a day, depending on your schedule, appetite, and activity levels. Base each meal on 1 to 2 palm-sized servings of protein. Fill the rest of your plate with vegetables. Add a serving of fruit, if you choose. Add fat in the recommended minimum amounts per meal. If using more than one fat source, like cooking oil and avocado, you can use the smaller end of the range for one or both.

- Oils and cooking fats (avocado oil, duck fat, etc.): 1 to 2 thumb-sized portions
- Butters (ghee, nut butter, coconut butter, etc.): 1 to 2 thumb-sized portions
- Coconut (shredded or flaked): 1 to 2 open (heaping) handfuls
- Olives: 1 to 2 open (heaping) handfuls
- Nuts and seeds: 1 small handful
- Avocado: ½ to 1 avocado
- Coconut milk: Between ¼ and ½ of one (13.5-ounce) full-fat can

Your schedule, hunger levels, or activity levels may require a snack between meals. For each snack, include at least two of the three macronutrients (protein, fat, and carbs) for satiety. Make your snack as big as you need to tide you over, but not so big that you're too full to eat your next scheduled meal. (See page 104 for snack ideas.)

If your activity levels necessitate a pre-workout or post-workout meal, follow the general guidelines on page 76, and work with your athletic trainer or sports nutritionist to ensure you are fueling your activities appropriately.

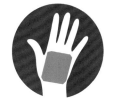
PROTEIN

VEGETABLES

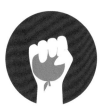
FRUIT

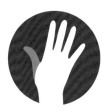
OILS & BUTTER

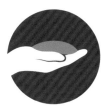
COCONUT & OLIVES

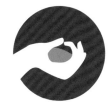
NUTS & SEEDS

ORIGINAL WHOLE30 SHOPPING LIST

PROTEINS

If you're purchasing processed meats (like chicken sausage, bacon, jerky, pre-made burgers), or canned meat or fish (like chicken, salmon, or tuna) read your labels to ensure compatibility.

- ☐ Anchovies
- ☐ Bacon
- ☐ Beef
- ☐ Bison
- ☐ Carne seca (dried beef)
- ☐ Catfish
- ☐ Chicken
- ☐ Clams
- ☐ Cod
- ☐ Crab
- ☐ Deli meat
- ☐ Duck
- ☐ Eggs
- ☐ Fish (other types)
- ☐ Flounder
- ☐ Halibut
- ☐ Hot dogs
- ☐ Jerky
- ☐ Lamb
- ☐ Liver
- ☐ Lobster
- ☐ Mackerel
- ☐ Mahi-mahi
- ☐ Meat sticks
- ☐ Mussels
- ☐ Mutton
- ☐ Octopus
- ☐ Organ meats (all types)
- ☐ Oysters
- ☐ Pollock
- ☐ Pork
- ☐ Prosciutto
- ☐ Sablefish
- ☐ Salami
- ☐ Salmon
- ☐ Sardines
- ☐ Sausage
- ☐ Scallops
- ☐ Seafood (other types)
- ☐ Shrimp
- ☐ Snapper
- ☐ Squid
- ☐ Trout
- ☐ Tuna
- ☐ Turkey
- ☐ Venison
- ☐ Whitefish

VEGETABLES

All vegetables but corn and lima beans are compatible with the Original Whole30 elimination phase. Use fresh, frozen, or canned vegetables.

- ☐ Artichokes
- ☐ Arugula
- ☐ Asparagus
- ☐ Beets
- ☐ Bok choy
- ☐ Broccoli/broccolini
- ☐ Broccoli rabe
- ☐ Brussels sprouts
- ☐ Cabbage
- ☐ Calabaza
- ☐ Callaloo
- ☐ Carrots
- ☐ Cassava
- ☐ Cauliflower
- ☐ Celery
- ☐ Chard
- ☐ Chayote
- ☐ Chile peppers (jalapeño, poblano, serrano, etc.)
- ☐ Cucumber
- ☐ Eggplant
- ☐ Endive
- ☐ Fennel (anise)
- ☐ Frisee (curly endive)
- ☐ Garlic
- ☐ Green beans
- ☐ Green onion
- ☐ Greens (beet, collard, dandelion, mustard, Swiss chard, turnip, etc.)
- ☐ Hearts of palm
- ☐ Jicama
- ☐ Kale
- ☐ Leeks
- ☐ Lettuce (all types, including Bibb, butter, romaine)
- ☐ Microgreens
- ☐ Mushrooms (all types)
- ☐ Nopal (prickly pear)
- ☐ Nori
- ☐ Okra
- ☐ Onions
- ☐ Parsnips
- ☐ Peas (English, garden, green, snow, split, sugar snap, yellow)
- ☐ Peppers, bell
- ☐ Peppers, dried (all types)
- ☐ Potatoes (all types)
- ☐ Pumpkin
- ☐ Radishes
- ☐ Rhubarb
- ☐ Romanesco
- ☐ Rutabaga
- ☐ Shallots
- ☐ Spinach
- ☐ Sprouts
- ☐ Squash (acorn, butternut, delicata, kabocha, spaghetti, summer, etc.)
- ☐ Sweet potato/yams
- ☐ Tomatillos
- ☐ Tomatoes
- ☐ Turnips
- ☐ Zucchini

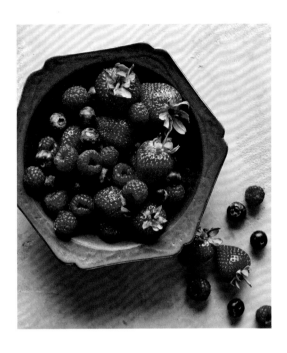

FATS

All cooking oils (regardless of their source) are compatible with the Whole30 elimination phase.

FOR COOKING

- ☐ Avocado oil
- ☐ Canola oil
- ☐ Clarified butter
- ☐ Coconut oil
- ☐ Corn oil
- ☐ Cultured oil (fermented)
- ☐ Duck fat
- ☐ Ghee
- ☐ Grapeseed oil
- ☐ Lard (pork fat)
- ☐ Olive oil (light, extra-virgin)
- ☐ Palm oil
- ☐ Safflower oil
- ☐ Sesame oil (toasted/ untoasted)
- ☐ Soybean oil
- ☐ Sunflower oil
- ☐ Tallow (beef fat)

FOR EATING

- ☐ Avocado
- ☐ Coconut butter
- ☐ Coconut (flakes, shredded)
- ☐ Coconut milk (canned)
- ☐ Olives (all types)

NUTS AND SEEDS

- ☐ Almonds/almond butter
- ☐ Brazil nuts
- ☐ Cashews/cashew butter
- ☐ Chia seeds
- ☐ Flax seeds
- ☐ Hazelnuts/hazelnut butter
- ☐ Hemp seeds (hearts)
- ☐ Macadamia/macadamia butter
- ☐ Pecans/pecan butter
- ☐ Pine nuts
- ☐ Pistachios
- ☐ Pumpkin seeds/ pepitas
- ☐ Sesame seeds/tahini
- ☐ Sunflower seeds/sunflower butter
- ☐ Walnuts

FRUITS

All fruit is compatible with the Whole30 elimination phase. Use fresh, frozen, or canned fruit (if canned in its own juice, without added sugar).

- ☐ Apples (all types)
- ☐ Apricots
- ☐ Bananas
- ☐ Blackberries
- ☐ Blueberries
- ☐ Cherries
- ☐ Cranberries
- ☐ Currants (all types)
- ☐ Dates
- ☐ Dried fruit (all types)
- ☐ Elderberries
- ☐ Figs
- ☐ Gooseberries (Cape gooseberries)
- ☐ Grapefruit
- ☐ Grapes (all types)
- ☐ Kiwifruit
- ☐ Kumquats
- ☐ Lemons
- ☐ Limes
- ☐ Mango
- ☐ Melon (all types)
- ☐ Nectarines
- ☐ Oranges (all types)
- ☐ Papaya
- ☐ Pawpaw
- ☐ Peaches
- ☐ Pears (all types)
- ☐ Persimmons
- ☐ Pineapple
- ☐ Plantains
- ☐ Plums
- ☐ Pomegranates
- ☐ Raisins
- ☐ Raspberries
- ☐ Salmonberries
- ☐ Strawberries
- ☐ Tangerines
- ☐ Xoconostle (cactus)
- ☐ Yuzu (citrus)

BEVERAGES

Avoid beverages with added sugar. Non-dairy milk should be made from coconut, nuts, or seeds.

- ☐ Apple cider
- ☐ Club soda
- ☐ Coconut water
- ☐ Coffee
- ☐ Coffee creamer (non-dairy)
- ☐ Fruit juice (all types)
- ☐ Kombucha
- ☐ Milk (non-dairy)
- ☐ Sparkling tea
- ☐ Tea (brewed)
- ☐ Tomato juice
- ☐ Vegetable juice (all types)
- ☐ Water (mineral/sparkling/seltzer)

HERBS, SPICES, SEASONINGS

Make sure your spices and spice blends are free from cornstarch, rice bran, added sugar, or other incompatible ingredients.

- ☐ Aleppo pepper flakes
- ☐ Allspice (whole/ground)
- ☐ Ancho chile powder
- ☐ Anise seeds
- ☐ Baharat (spice blend)
- ☐ Basil (fresh/dried)
- ☐ Bay leaves (fresh/dried)
- ☐ Black pepper (ground)
- ☐ Cacao powder (100%)
- ☐ Caraway seeds
- ☐ Cardamom seeds
- ☐ Cayenne
- ☐ Celery seeds
- ☐ Chervil (French parsley)
- ☐ Chili powder
- ☐ Chinese five-spice powder
- ☐ Chipotle powder
- ☐ Chives (fresh/dried)
- ☐ Cilantro (fresh/dried)
- ☐ Cinnamon (stick/ground)
- ☐ Cloves (whole/ground)
- ☐ Coriander (seeds/ground)
- ☐ Creole seasoning (blend)
- ☐ Cumin (seeds/ground)
- ☐ Curry powder (blend)
- ☐ Dill (fresh/dried)
- ☐ Everything bagel seasoning
- ☐ Galangal
- ☐ Garam masala
- ☐ Garlic powder
- ☐ Ginger (fresh/ground)
- ☐ Harissa (paste/sauce)
- ☐ Hibiscus flowers (dried)
- ☐ Hing (asafetida)
- ☐ Horseradish (fresh/prepared)
- ☐ Italian seasoning
- ☐ Lemongrass (fresh/dried)
- ☐ Liquid smoke
- ☐ Matcha powder
- ☐ Mint (fresh/dried)
- ☐ Mustard (powder)
- ☐ Nutmeg
- ☐ Onion powder
- ☐ Oregano (fresh/dried)
- ☐ Paprika (sweet/smoked)
- ☐ Parsley (fresh/dried)
- ☐ Peppercorns (black, pink)
- ☐ Red pepper flakes
- ☐ Rosemary (fresh/dried)
- ☐ Sage (fresh/dried)
- ☐ Salt
- ☐ Sumac (ground)
- ☐ Tajin (chile blend)
- ☐ Tarragon (fresh/dried)
- ☐ Thai basil
- ☐ Thyme (fresh/dried)
- ☐ Truffle salt
- ☐ Turmeric (whole/ground)
- ☐ Urfa biber (chile flakes)
- ☐ Vanilla (bean/extract)
- ☐ Wasabi powder
- ☐ Za'atar (blend)

PANTRY AND FRIDGE

This is one category in which reading labels is paramount. (For example, there is only one brand of fish sauce compatible with the Whole30: Red Boat fish sauce.) Better yet, just look for Whole30 Approved® products, and skip the label reading!

- ☐ Almond flour
- ☐ Anchovy paste
- ☐ Arrowroot powder
- ☐ Beet kvass
- ☐ Broth (beef, chicken, fish, vegetable)
- ☐ Capers
- ☐ Chicken (canned)
- ☐ Coconut aminos
- ☐ Coconut flour
- ☐ Collagen powder
- ☐ Cream cheese (dairy-free)
- ☐ Fish sauce
- ☐ Gelatin
- ☐ Hot sauce
- ☐ Ketchup (no-sugar)
- ☐ Kimchi
- ☐ Mayonnaise
- ☐ Mustard (all types)
- ☐ Nutritional yeast
- ☐ Olives (canned)
- ☐ Peppers, roasted (jarred)
- ☐ Pickled vegetables (jalapeño, red onion, etc.)
- ☐ Pickles
- ☐ Preserved lemons
- ☐ Pumpkin (canned)
- ☐ Queso (dairy-free)
- ☐ Ricotta (dairy-free)
- ☐ Salad dressing
- ☐ Salmon (canned)
- ☐ Sardines
- ☐ Sauerkraut
- ☐ Squash, butternut (canned)
- ☐ Sun-dried tomatoes
- ☐ Sweet potato (canned)
- ☐ Tapioca, instant
- ☐ Tapioca starch
- ☐ Tomato paste
- ☐ Tomato sauce
- ☐ Tomatoes (canned, crushed, diced, stewed)
- ☐ Tuna (canned/pouch)
- ☐ Vegetable broth
- ☐ Vinegar (apple cider, balsamic, cane, Champagne, red wine, rice, sherry, white, white wine)
- ☐ Yogurt (dairy-free)

ORIGINAL WHOLE30 FAQ

Why does the Original Whole30 eliminate _____?

The first question many people have after reading the rules is, "Wait, I thought whole grains/low-fat dairy/beans were *healthy*?" To which I respond, "Healthy for whom, and in what context?" There are no universally healthy foods. Not even broccoli! (Just ask my dad, who gets terrible gas and bloating every time he tries to eat it raw.)

Please visit our website (whole30.com) for detailed articles and references supporting these elimination groups.

Our bodies are unique, and we all respond to foods and ingredients differently. If you're sensitive to the gluten in bread, the lactose in dairy, or the fermentable carbohydrates in beans, it won't feel health-promoting when *you* consume them.

On the flip side, there are no universally *unhealthy* foods. Remember, Whole30 doesn't eliminate foods because they're "bad," and we certainly don't believe everyone needs to avoid them. These food groups have been shown in both the scientific literature and our fifteen-plus years of clinical experience to be commonly problematic—to varying degrees. I don't know if or how they're problematic for you, and neither do you until you eliminate them, reintroduce them, and compare your experience. What you choose to do with those learnings is completely up to you.

In summary:

- **Added sugar, real and artificial:** In the right context, added sugar can have health-promoting properties, making foods taste delicious and fueling your activities, mood, and energy levels. However, research overwhelmingly demonstrates that excess sugar consumption has a negative impact on cravings, blood sugar regulation and metabolism, digestion and gut health, systemic inflammation, and risk for chronic disease. While artificial sweeteners aren't believed to promote blood sugar dysregulation in the same way as natural forms of sugar, they can contribute to headaches, migraines, irritability, increased sugar cravings, gas, and bloating. Avoiding all forms of added sugar during your Whole30 elimination will help you become more aware of added sugar in your diet and help you identify which forms of sugar, in what amounts, and in what context work best for your body.

- **Alcohol:** Recent studies show that even small amounts of alcohol can have a negative effect on health—everything from cravings to blood sugar regulation and hormonal balance (particularly sex hormones), gut health, and systemic inflammation, particularly impacting the nervous system and brain. In addition, alcohol inhibits your judgment concerning all kinds of decisions, including food choices. Reintroduction will help you identify when, how often, in what amounts, and in what form alcohol may be "worth it" for you going forward.

- **Grains:** Whole grains provide fiber, vitamins, minerals, and other nutrients. Whole-grain foods can also help maintain healthy cholesterol levels and blood pressure, and assist in lowering the risk of diabetes, heart disease and other conditions. (In many studies, replacing refined grains with whole grains has been found to reduce inflammation, perhaps owing to their high fiber content.) However, there are different protein structures in grains that are particularly resistant to digestion and can improperly cross the gut barrier. This can trigger not only digestive issues but also an immune response that promotes systemic inflammation. You may be familiar with *gluten,* a protein component of wheat, rye, or barley that can be especially problematic. However, non-gluten grains like corn or pseudo-cereals like quinoa contain other proteins to which people can be similarly sensitive. Inflammation can also be the result of impaired metabolic health or blood sugar control. When grains (especially refined versions) are consumed in excess, it can be difficult to keep blood sugar within a healthy range. We replace all grains with fiber-rich, nutrient-dense vegetables and fruit during the Whole30 elimination to help you identify if or how grains may be impacting your health and how you feel.

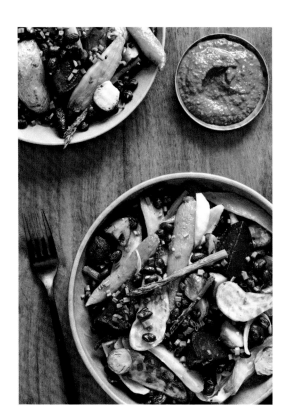

- **Legumes:** Beans and lentils can be a nourishing food for the gut and overall health. This is especially true when they're prepared in ways that make them easier to digest, such as soaking and sprouting. But for some, specific carbohydrates in beans and lentils can cause gastrointestinal symptoms like gas, bloating, and indigestion. The legume family also includes soy and peanuts. Both are commonly allergenic foods, and, if you are sensitive, can also promote gut disruption, systemic inflammation, and other negative health symptoms. As you'll be eating plenty of protein from animal sources on the Original Whole30, the program replaces legumes with vegetables and fruit during elimination to help you in later evaluating the impact of beans, lentils, soy, and peanuts in your body.

- **Dairy:** Dairy can offer a host of benefits, including bone health and heart health.

Dairy products are also a good source of protein, calcium, B vitamins, and vitamin D. However, not everyone tolerates dairy well. You may already know if you're one of the 60 to 70 percent of the global population with lactose intolerance, but lactose isn't the only potentially problematic component of dairy. In some people, milk proteins (casein and whey) may also contribute to digestive issues like gas, bloating, or stool changes; skin issues like eczema, hives, and acne; seasonal allergies and congestion; and asthma. For these reasons, we eliminate all forms of dairy on the Whole30, except clarified butter or various forms of ghee (which contains no lactose *or* milk proteins).

Roasted Veggies and Black Beans with Muhammara, page 304

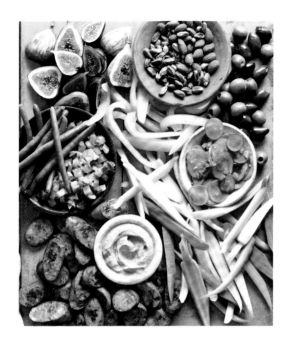

You can also serve a small leftover portion of last night's dinner as a snack! Snacks don't have to be grab-and-go options; a small bowl of chili, an egg muffin, or a few spoonfuls of Shepherd's Pie (page 171) would work just as well.

What are some on-the-go ideas for the Original Whole30?

Here are some easy on-the-go ideas for your Original Whole30. Not every option will be a good fit for your situation—please don't open canned tuna on an airplane—but you can certainly leave a can at the office to build a quick mini-meal between Zoom calls. Just make sure your on-the-go items fit the rules of the Original Whole30 elimination phase.

- Protein: Meat sticks or jerky, hard-boiled eggs, deli turkey, canned tuna/salmon/chicken, chicken or beef bone broth, smoothie
- Carbs: Fruit, sliced veggies, baby food pouches, applesauce, dried fruit, fruit-and-nut bars
- Fat: Avocado or guacamole, coconut flakes, olives, nuts and seeds, nut butter, coconut butter, salad dressing, nut "cheese" or dips

Smoothies (see page 105) generally contain protein, carbs from fruit and veggies, and healthy fats from coconut milk or nut butters, making them well-balanced on-the-go meals or snacks. In fact, many of these ideas (like eggs or dried fruit-and-nut bars) are good sources of at least two macronutrients.

What are some snack ideas for the Original Whole30?

Here are some ideas for snacks or mini-meals for your Original Whole30. Some require a bit of planning and preparation (like hard-cooking a dozen eggs). Others are more grab-and-go, like veggie sticks and guacamole. All contain at least two macronutrients to keep you satiated and energized.

- Meat sticks + carrots + nut-based cream cheese
- Deli turkey + berries + pistachios
- Hard-boiled eggs + apple slices + ranch dressing
- Banana + unsweetened nut butter
- Canned tuna + mayo + veggies
- Smoothie (see page 105)

Power Charcuterie Platter, page 141

How do I make an Original Whole30 smoothie?

Smoothies are a great way to add more protein to your day, and they can be an easy, portable source of energy when you're on the go. You can use fresh or frozen ingredients here. Be sure all the ingredients in your smoothie are compatible with the Original Whole30 elimination phase! Here is a general template:

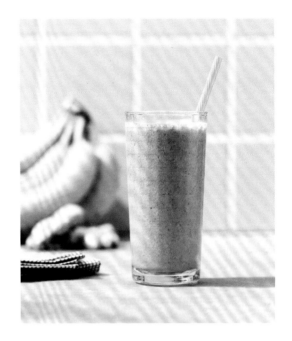

Liquids: 8 to 12 fluid ounces (1 to 1½ cups)

- Full-fat canned coconut milk (also counts as added fat)
- Unsweetened nut milk
- Brewed unsweetened tea
- Bone broth (chicken, beef, or vegetable)
- Water/ice

Protein: 15 to 20 grams

- Plant-based protein powder
- Collagen protein powder
- 100% egg white protein powder
- Cooked egg whites

Fat: 1 serving, minimum

- Avocado
- Seeds (chia, hemp, pumpkin, ground flaxseed, etc.)
- Nut butter, seed butter, or coconut butter
- Coconut flakes

Fruit: ½ to 1 cup

- Berries (up to 1 cup)
- Apple, pear, or peach (up to 1 cup)
- Pineapple or mango (up to ½ cup)
- Unsweetened acai puree (up to ½ cup)
- Banana (up to 1 small)

Veggies: 1 cup, minimum

- Leafy greens
- Mashed pumpkin
- Mashed butternut squash
- Mashed sweet potato
- Cauliflower rice
- Zucchini

Boosts: optional or to taste

- Cinnamon
- Chai seasoning
- Turmeric
- 100% cacao powder
- Sea salt
- Fresh herbs (mint, basil)

Golden Milk Green Tea Smoothie, page 220

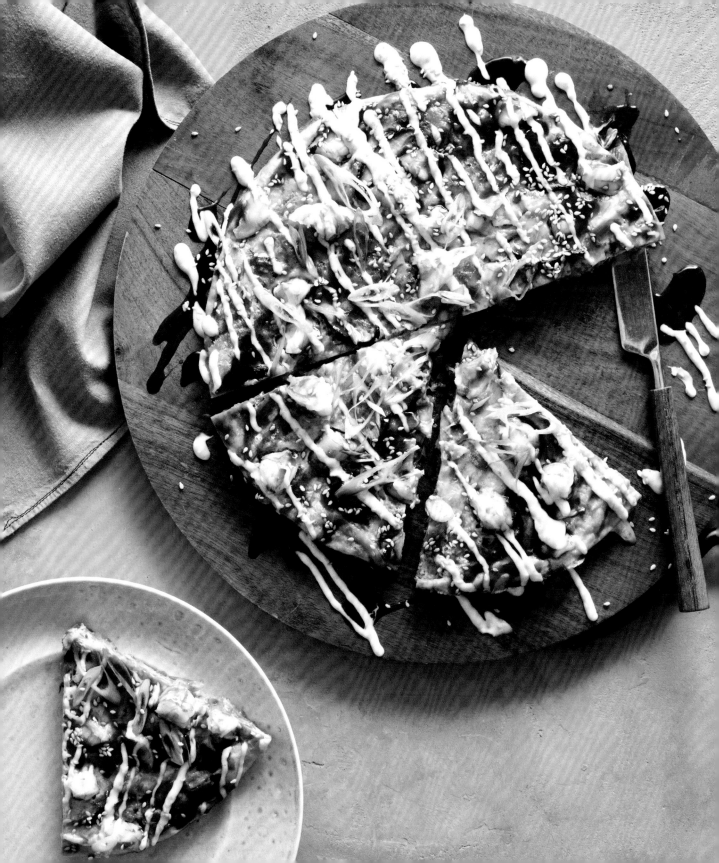

ORIGINAL WHOLE30 RECIPES

BREAKFASTS

Okonomiyaki-Style Omelet with Gingery Mayo and Teriyaki Sauce, page 128

MELISSA'S (NEW) CHICKEN HASH

SERVES 2 TO 3 • PREP: 30 MINUTES • COOK: 15 MINUTES • TOTAL: 45 MINUTES

FOR THE RAITA

⅔ cup Whole30-compatible dairy-free plain yogurt

1 small Persian cucumber, grated

¼ teaspoon salt

¼ teaspoon ground cumin

1 tablespoon chopped fresh mint or cilantro

2 teaspoons minced jalapeño or serrano chile

FOR THE HASH

1 tablespoon ghee or Clarified Butter (page 229)

1 pound boneless, skinless chicken thighs, cut into 1-inch dice

½ teaspoon salt

¼ teaspoon black pepper

¼ cup coarsely chopped roasted unsalted pistachios

1 large sweet potato, peeled and grated

1 Granny Smith apple, cored, peeled, and diced

¼ teaspoon red pepper flakes

1 teaspoon curry powder

¼ cup apple cider or juice

4 cups baby spinach

1 tablespoon apple cider vinegar

This is an update of the fan-favorite hash from the first Whole30 book, and it's one of my favorite breakfast dishes. This version swaps pistachios for walnuts and bumps up the overall flavor with curry powder and a splash of cider vinegar. The star of the show is a cooling raita made with dairy-free yogurt.

MAKE THE RAITA: In a small bowl, stir together the yogurt, cucumber, salt, cumin, mint, and jalapeño. Cover and refrigerate until serving time.

MAKE THE HASH: In a large skillet, heat the ghee over medium-high heat, swirling to coat the bottom of the pan. Add the chicken, being sure not to crowd the pieces. Season the chicken with salt and pepper. Cook until browned, 2 to 3 minutes. Turn the chicken to brown the other sides. Add the pistachios and cook 1 to 2 minutes, stirring occasionally.

Add the sweet potato, apple, red pepper flakes, and curry powder. Cook, stirring often, until the chicken is fully cooked and the sweet potato is tender, 2 to 3 minutes.

Add the apple cider and mix all the ingredients, scraping the bottom of the pan with a wooden spoon to bring up any tasty bits. Add the spinach and cook, stirring constantly, just until wilted, about 30 seconds. Stir in the vinegar.

Serve: Serve the hash immediately, topped with the raita.

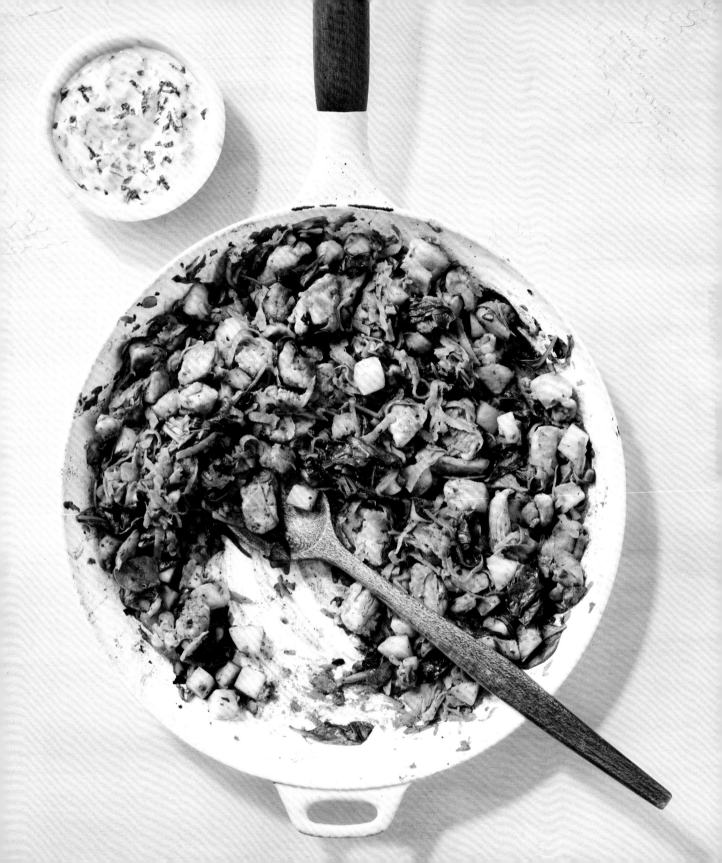

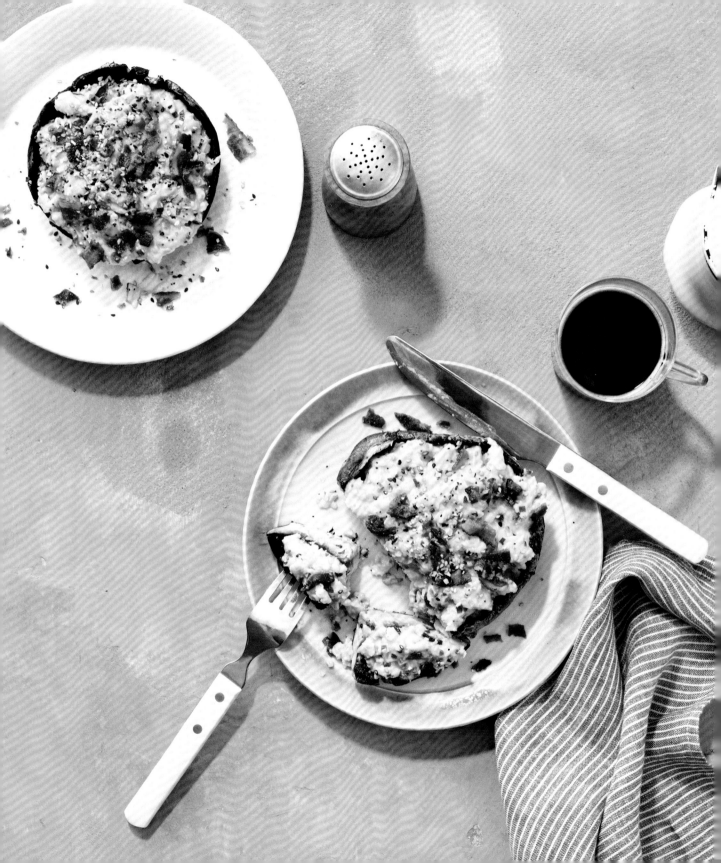

PORTOBELLO MUSHROOMS STUFFED WITH SCRAMBLED GREEN EGGS

SERVES 2 • PREP: 10 MINUTES • BAKE/COOK: 15 MINUTES • TOTAL: 25 MINUTES

2 large portobello mushrooms (about 5 inches in diameter)

2 teaspoons extra-virgin olive oil

Salt and black pepper

6 large eggs

3 tablespoons full-fat canned coconut milk or bone broth

¼ teaspoon salt

1 teaspoon ghee, Clarified Butter (page 229), or coconut oil

1 tablespoon chopped fresh chives, tarragon, chervil, basil, or parsley (see Tip)

2 slices Whole30-compatible bacon, cooked and crumbled

1 teaspoon everything bagel seasoning or black pepper

Juicy, meaty mushrooms are the vehicle for rich and fluffy eggs scrambled with a generous dose of fresh herbs. Bacon adds a touch of smokiness, and everything bagel seasoning brings some fun flavor and crunch.

Preheat the oven to 425°F.

Twist the mushroom stems to remove them from the caps (or use a paring knife). Use a spoon to scrape out and remove the dark brown gills. Wipe the mushroom caps clean with a damp paper towel. Brush lightly on all sides with the olive oil and sprinkle the undersides with salt and pepper. Place on a baking sheet, stem side up. Bake 15 minutes or until tender, turning over halfway through.

Meanwhile, crack the eggs into a medium bowl and whisk with a fork to combine. Whisk in the coconut milk and salt.

In a medium skillet, heat the ghee over medium heat, swirling to cover the bottom of the pan. Add the egg mixture. Cook without stirring until the eggs start to set on the bottom and edges. With a spatula, lift and fold the eggs. Add the herbs and continue to cook 1 to 2 minutes more, or until eggs are just cooked through but still glossy and moist, folding and lifting the eggs as needed to cook evenly.

Place the mushroom caps stem-side up on plates and spoon the eggs into them. Sprinkle with the bacon and the bagel seasoning or black pepper.

TIP: Scrambled eggs are a great place to get creative with what's in your refrigerator and spice cabinet. Try adding cooked chopped green onions, sweet bell pepper, baby spinach, or kale to your cooked eggs, or sprinkle the eggs with finely chopped olives.

To substitute dried herbs instead of fresh, use 1 teaspoon dried chives plus 1 teaspoon dried tarragon, chervil, basil, or parsley (for a total of 2 teaspoons).

PUMPKIN AND SAUSAGE BREAKFAST CUSTARD

SERVES 2 TO 3 • PREP: 15 MINUTES • COOK/BAKE: 45 MINUTES • TOTAL: 60 MINUTES

8 ounces Whole30-compatible bulk breakfast sausage (see Tip)

6 large eggs, lightly beaten

⅔ cup canned pumpkin

¾ cup full-fat canned coconut milk

3 tablespoons unsweetened applesauce

2 tablespoons dark or golden raisins (optional)

1 teaspoon vanilla extract

½ teaspoon Whole30-compatible pumpkin pie spice

½ teaspoon grated orange zest

Caramelized Onion Topper (optional; recipe follows)

TIP: If you can't find Whole30-compatible prepared breakfast sausage, use the recipe from the Sausage-Apple Stacks (page 114).

If you don't have pumpkin pie spice, mix ½ teaspoon ground cinnamon, ¼ teaspoon ground ginger, ⅛ teaspoon ground nutmeg, and ⅛ teaspoon ground allspice.

If you wake up one morning and find you just can't eat another fried or scrambled egg, try this popular breakfast ingredient in custard form. It's whipped with applesauce, pumpkin puree, vanilla, and warming spices, and baked with savory sausage. A caramelized onion topper adds buttery sweetness to the dish.

Preheat the oven to 325°F.

In a medium skillet, brown the sausage over medium-high heat, using a spatula to crumble it into small pieces. Cook until browned, about 6 minutes. Drain and discard any fat in pan. Set sauce aside to cool.

Place a 1½-quart baking dish or oven-safe bowl into a 3-quart baking dish. In a bowl, stir together the eggs, pumpkin, coconut milk, applesauce, raisins (if using), vanilla, pumpkin pie spice, and orange zest. Spoon the cooked sausage into the 1½-quart dish. Ladle the egg mixture over the sausage. Place the pan on the oven rack. Gently pour boiling water into the 3-quart baking dish, so it is around the smaller dish to a depth of 1 inch.

Bake for 40 to 45 minutes, or until a knife inserted near the center of the custard comes out clean. Remove the custard from the water. Cool on a wire rack. Top with the Caramelized Onion Topper (if using). Serve at room temperature, or cover and refrigerate up to 2 days. If refrigerated, serve cold or let stand at room temperature about 20 minutes before serving.

CARAMELIZED ONION TOPPER

Halve and thinly slice 1 small sweet onion (such as WallaWalla or Vidalia). In a large skillet, heat 1 tablespoon ghee (or Clarified Butter, page 229) or coconut oil over medium-low heat. Add the onion to the skillet and cook until tender and a rich brown color, 8 to 10 minutes, stirring occasionally. Season with salt and pepper.

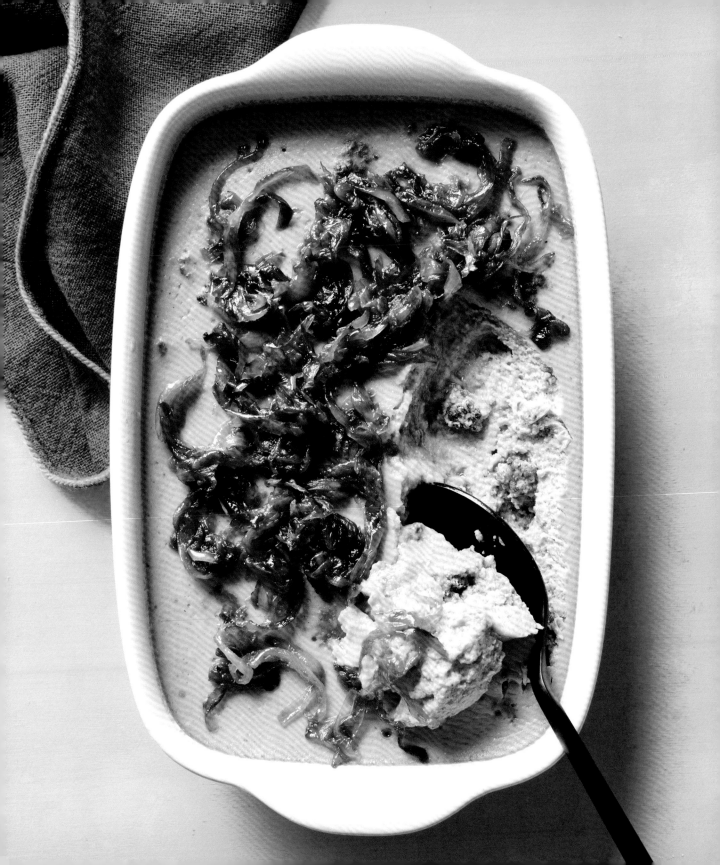

OPEN-FACED SCANDINAVIAN-STYLE BREAKFAST STACKS

SERVES 2 • PREP: SMOKED SALMON STACKS: 20 MINUTES • SAUSAGE-APPLE
STACKS: 30 MINUTES • COOK: 10 MINUTES (SAUSAGE-APPLE STACKS) • TOTAL: 30 TO 40 MINUTES

FOR THE SMOKED SALMON STACKS

¼ cup Whole30 Mayo (page 230) or Whole30-compatible mayonnaise

1 tablespoon capers, drained, rinsed, and coarsely chopped

1 teaspoon chopped fresh dill

8 large Bibb lettuce leaves

4 hard-cooked large eggs, sliced

4 ounces thinly sliced Whole30-compatible smoked salmon

½ Persian cucumber, sliced

2 radishes, sliced

Salt and black pepper

In Scandinavia, open-faced knife-and-fork sandwiches are popular fare for lunch and light dinners. These two Whole30 takes on these artfully arranged sandwiches offer a delicious, protein-packed way to start your day.

FOR THE SMOKED SALMON STACKS: In a small bowl, stir together the mayonnaise, capers, and ½ teaspoon of the dill. Set aside.

On each of 2 plates, arrange 4 Bibb lettuce leaves in stacks of 2. Top each stack with some of the sliced eggs, salmon, cucumber, and radish. Season lightly with salt and pepper.

Top each stack with about 1 tablespoon of the mayonnaise mixture. Sprinkle with the remaining ½ teaspoon dill.

FOR THE SAUSAGE-APPLE STACKS: In a small bowl, stir together the mayonnaise, mustard, and chives. On each of 2 plates, arrange 4 Bibb lettuce leaves in stacks of 2. Set aside.

In a medium bowl, combine the meat, sage, salt, pepper, onion powder, garlic powder, and red pepper flakes. Using your hands, combine well.

In a large skillet, heat the olive oil over medium-high heat. Add the seasoned meat to the skillet; cook, stirring occasionally, until meat is browned and cooked through, 6 to 8 minutes.

Divide the meat among the 4 lettuce stacks. Top with the diced apple. Top each stack with about 1 tablespoon each of the mayonnaise mixture and the microgreens. Sprinkle with almonds.

TIP: If you're using ground chicken or turkey, opt for ground thigh meat, not breast. Breast meat is very lean, so your sausage may taste dry. The fat in thigh meat will help you get a nice browning on the sausage.

FOR THE SAUSAGE-APPLE STACKS

- 2 tablespoons Whole30 Mayo (page 230) or Whole30-compatible mayonnaise
- 2 tablespoons Whole30-compatible Dijon mustard
- 1 tablespoon chopped fresh chives
- 8 large Bibb lettuce leaves
- 12 ounces ground meat (pork, chicken, or turkey) (see Tip)
- 2 teaspoons dried sage leaves, crushed
- ½ teaspoon salt
- ¼ teaspoon black pepper
- ½ teaspoon onion powder
- ½ teaspoon garlic powder
- ⅛ to ¼ teaspoon red pepper flakes
- 1 tablespoon extra-virgin olive oil
- 1 apple, cored, seeded, and diced
- ¼ cup microgreens or sprouts (such as pea, radish, or broccoli)
- 1 tablespoon sliced or slivered almonds, toasted

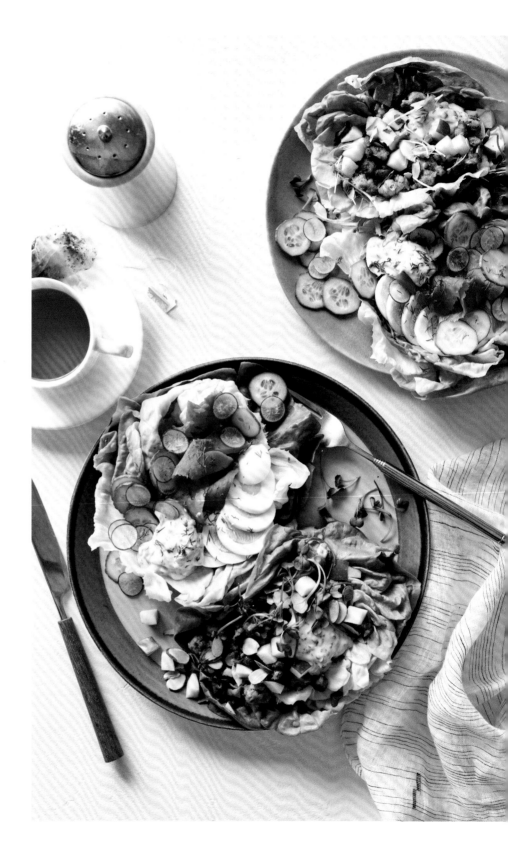

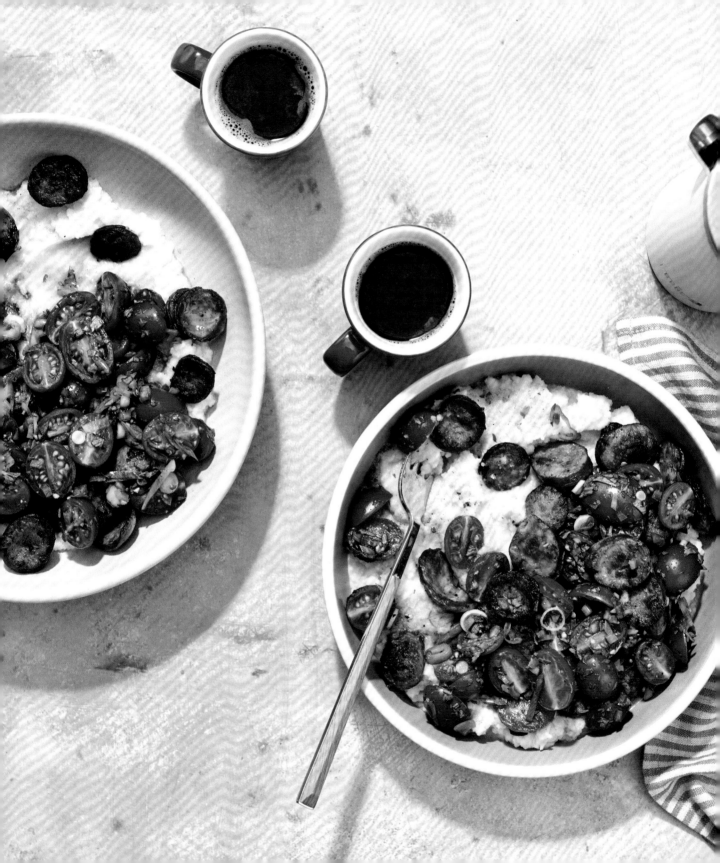

SAUSAGE AND CAULIFLOWER GRITS WITH TOMATO SALAD

SERVES 2 • PREP: 30 MINUTES • COOK: 15 MINUTES • TOTAL: 45 MINUTES

FOR THE TOMATO SALAD

1½ cups grape tomatoes, halved

1 small jalapeño or serrano chile, seeded and minced

1 green onion, sliced (green and white parts)

2 tablespoons chopped fresh cilantro or parsley

1 tablespoon extra-virgin olive oil

2 teaspoons white wine vinegar

¼ teaspoon salt

¼ teaspoon black pepper

FOR THE GRITS AND SAUSAGE

1 (12-ounce) bag frozen cauliflower rice

2 tablespoons ghee or Clarified Butter (page 229)

1 garlic clove, minced

¼ teaspoon salt

¼ teaspoon black pepper

¼ cup Whole30-compatible almond milk

1 tablespoon extra-virgin olive oil

4 links Whole30-compatible chicken sausage (preferably andouille style, fire-roasted red pepper, or Italian), sliced ¼ inch thick on the diagonal

You don't *have* to eat eggs for breakfast! In this anytime-dish, creamy cauliflower grits are the perfect complement to slices of spicy andouille-style chicken sausage. A juicy tomato salad topping adds a touch of freshness.

MAKE THE TOMATO SALAD: In a medium bowl, combine the tomatoes, jalapeño, green onion, and cilantro. Drizzle with the olive oil and vinegar, and sprinkle with the salt and pepper. Toss to combine. Set aside.

MAKE THE CAULIFLOWER GRITS: Break up any clumps of cauliflower while it's still in the bag, then place the frozen cauliflower rice in a medium microwave-safe bowl. Cover and cook on high for 4 minutes. Add the ghee, garlic, salt, pepper, and almond milk. Stir to combine. Cover and cook an additional 4 minutes. Using an immersion blender, blend until fairly smooth (see Tip). Cover and keep warm while cooking the sausage.

In a large skillet, heat the olive oil over medium heat. Cook the sausage, stirring occasionally, until browned and crisp around the edges, 4 to 5 minutes.

Serve: Divide the grits between 2 shallow bowls. Top with the sausage, then with the tomato salad.

> **TIP:** If you don't have an immersion blender, use a food processor or a potato masher to create a creamy texture. Don't try to use a traditional blender here! There isn't enough liquid for the ingredients to blend easily.
>
> To cook frozen cauliflower rice on the stove, drizzle olive oil into a large skillet to coat the bottom, and heat over medium heat. Add your frozen cauliflower rice. Cook 6 to 8 minutes, until the water evaporates and the cauliflower rice is tender. Add the ghee, garlic, salt, pepper, and almond milk. Stir to combine. Cover and cook an additional 3 to 4 minutes. Transfer the cauliflower grits to a bowl and blend with an immersion blender until fairly smooth.

SAUSAGE EGG CASSEROLE

SERVES 4 • PREP: 20 MINUTES • BAKE: 35 MINUTES • TOTAL: 55 MINUTES

Extra-virgin olive oil or avocado oil cooking spray

8 ounces Whole30-compatible bulk breakfast sausage (see Tip)

½ cup chopped red bell pepper

½ cup chopped green onions (green and white parts)

½ jalapeño, seeded and minced

1 teaspoon chili powder

Pinch of red pepper flakes

6 large eggs

1 teaspoon salt

½ teaspoon garlic powder

2 cups frozen hash-brown potatoes (see Tip)

Sausage, eggs, and frozen hash-brown potatoes all make an appearance in this hearty breakfast casserole. Kick up the heat by serving with salsa or hot sauce.

Preheat the oven to 350°F.

Coat a 9 × 13-inch baking dish with olive oil spray.

In a large skillet, cook the sausage with the bell pepper, green onions, and jalapeño over medium-high heat, breaking up the meat with a spoon. When the sausage is no longer pink, add the chili powder and red pepper flakes and cook a few minutes more.

In a large bowl, whisk the eggs together with the salt and garlic powder. Fold the hash browns and eggs into the sausage mixture, then transfer to the baking dish. Bake until set, 35 to 40 minutes.

Cut into squares and serve.

TIP: If you can't find Whole30-compatible prepared breakfast sausage, use the recipe from the Sausage-Apple Stacks (page 114).

You don't need to thaw the frozen hash-brown potatoes for this dish. If using freshly grated potato or refrigerated hash-brown potatoes, squeeze the water out into a clean kitchen towel before using.

To get a jump start, you can make the sausage and veggie mixture a day ahead and store it in the refrigerator. Then just mix with remaining ingredients and bake.

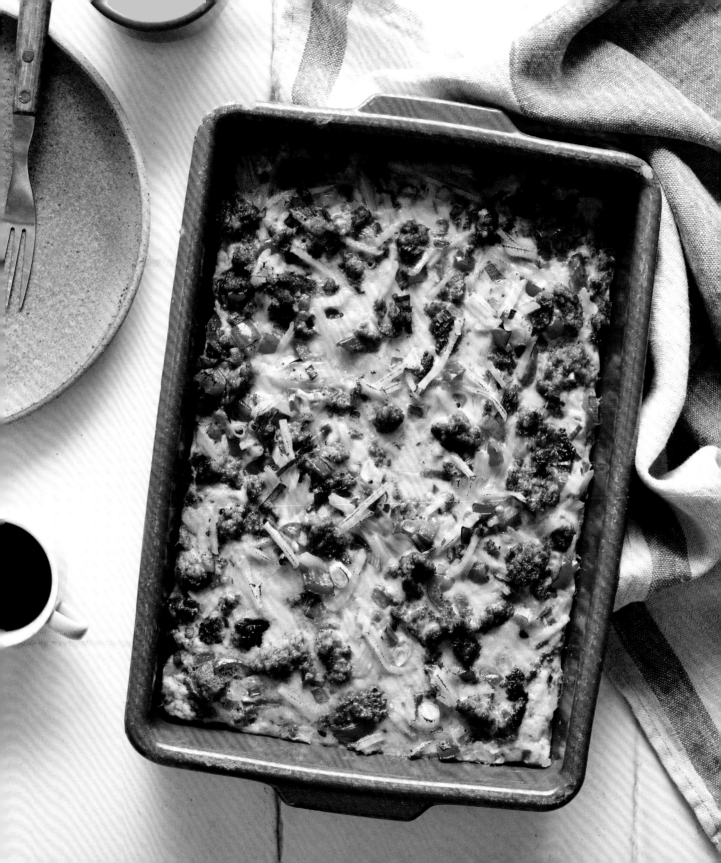

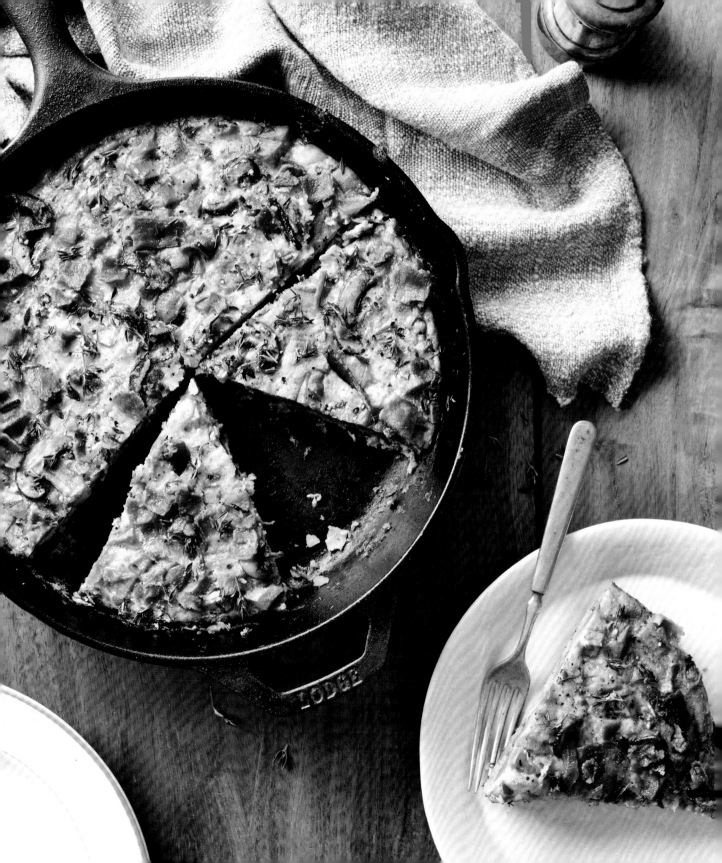

SEASONAL FRITTATA

SERVES 3 TO 4 • PREP: 20 MINUTES • COOK: 30 MINUTES • TOTAL: 50 MINUTES

FOR THE FRITTATA BASE

8 large eggs

½ teaspoon salt

¼ teaspoon black pepper

2 tablespoons extra-virgin olive oil, ghee, or Clarified Butter (page 229)

The frittata is a truly versatile dish. Follow our recipes, or use our frittata base and add whatever you have in the fridge. This is the perfect dish to double for leftovers! Slices are easily reheated in the microwave, but equally tasty eaten cold.

SPRING FRITTATA

1 tablespoon chopped fresh chives (or 2 teaspoons fresh dill), plus more for serving

2 green onions, chopped (green and white parts)

1 cup trimmed asparagus, diagonally sliced ¼ inch thick

1 cup sugar snap peas, diagonally sliced ¼ inch thick (strings removed, if present)

½ cup sliced fresh button mushrooms

1 ounce Whole30-compatible thin-sliced prosciutto

Preheat the oven to 350°F. Beat together the eggs, ¼ teaspoon salt, ⅛ teaspoon pepper, and 1 tablespoon of the chives; set aside.

In an 8-inch oven-safe skillet, heat the olive oil over medium heat, brushing the sides of the pan with some oil to prevent the eggs from sticking. Add the green onions, asparagus, sugar snap peas, and mushrooms to the pan. Cook and stir just until asparagus and snap peas start to turn bright green, 2 to 3 minutes.

Spread the vegetables in an even layer. Pour the egg mixture into the pan. Roughly tear the prosciutto over the top. Sprinkle with the remaining ¼ teaspoon salt and ⅛ teaspoon pepper. Bake until the center of the frittata is set and the prosciutto is lightly crisped, 20 to 25 minutes. Let stand 5 minutes before cutting. Garnish with additional chopped chives, if desired.

(continued)

SUMMER FRITTATA

2 tablespoons chopped fresh basil, plus more for serving

¾ cup chopped red onion

1 yellow bell pepper, chopped

1 small zucchini, halved lengthwise and sliced into half-moons

¾ cup cherry tomatoes, halved

Preheat the oven to 350°F. Beat together the eggs, ¼ teaspoon salt, ⅛ teaspoon black pepper, and 2 tablespoons chopped fresh basil; set aside.

In an 8-inch oven-safe skillet, heat the olive oil over medium heat, brushing the sides of the pan with some oil to prevent the eggs from sticking. Add the red onion and bell pepper to the pan. Cook, stirring frequently, until the vegetables are slightly softened, 2 to 3 minutes. Add the zucchini and cook, stirring frequently, until slightly softened and some of the liquid has evaporated, 3 to 4 minutes.

Spread the vegetables in an even layer. Pour the egg mixture into the pan. Scatter the cherry tomatoes over the top. Season with the remaining ¼ teaspoon salt and ⅛ teaspoon pepper. Bake until the center of the frittata is set, 20 to 25 minutes. Let stand 5 minutes before cutting. Garnish with torn fresh basil leaves, if desired.

FALL FRITTATA

1 teaspoon fresh thyme, plus more for serving

½ small yellow onion, chopped

1¼ cups sliced fresh button or cremini mushrooms

2 cups thinly sliced Brussels sprouts

1 cup diced cooked sweet potato

1 teaspoon extra-virgin olive oil or avocado oil

4 strips Whole30-compatible bacon, cooked until crisp and crumbled

Preheat the oven to 350°F. Beat together the eggs, ¼ teaspoon salt, ⅛ teaspoon pepper, and the 1 teaspoon fresh thyme; set aside.

In an 8-inch oven-safe skillet, heat the olive oil over medium heat, brushing the sides of the pan with some oil to prevent the eggs from sticking. Add the onion to the pan. Cook, stirring frequently, until onion is softened, 3 to 4 minutes. Add the mushrooms and cook, stirring frequently, until slightly softened, 2 to 3 minutes. Add the Brussels sprouts and cook, stirring frequently, until softened, 3 to 4 minutes.

Spread the vegetables in an even layer. Pour the egg mixture into the pan. Toss the sweet potato with the olive oil, then scatter over the eggs and add the crumbled bacon. Season with the remaining ¼ teaspoon salt and ⅛ teaspoon pepper. Bake until the center of the frittata is set, 20 to 25 minutes. Let stand 5 minutes before cutting. Garnish with additional thyme, if desired.

WINTER FRITTATA

1 tablespoon fresh oregano, chopped, plus more for serving

½ small yellow onion, chopped

1 garlic clove, minced

2 cups chopped fresh kale

4 ounces Whole30-compatible hot Italian bulk sausage, cooked (see Tip)

1 cup diced cooked Yukon Gold potato

1 teaspoon extra-virgin olive oil or avocado oil

¼ cup Kalamata olives, pitted and halved

Preheat the oven to 350°F. Beat together the eggs, ¼ teaspoon salt, ⅛ teaspoon pepper, and the 1 tablespoon chopped fresh oregano; set aside.

In an 8-inch oven-safe skillet, heat the olive oil over medium heat, brushing the sides of the pan with some oil to prevent the eggs from sticking. Add the onion to the pan. Cook, stirring frequently, until onion is softened, 3 to 4 minutes. Add the garlic and cook, stirring, until fragrant, about 1 minute. Add the kale and cook, stirring frequently, until wilted, 1 to 2 minutes. Stir the sausage into the egg mixture.

Spread the vegetables in an even layer. Pour the egg mixture into the pan. Toss the potatoes with the olive oil, then scatter them and the olives over the top. Season with the remaining ¼ teaspoon salt and ⅛ teaspoon pepper. Bake until the center of the frittata is set, 20 to 25 minutes. Let stand 5 minutes before cutting. Garnish with additional fresh oregano, if desired.

TIP: If you can't find Whole30-compatible hot Italian bulk sausage for the Winter Frittata, make your own. In a small bowl, stir together ½ to 1 teaspoon red pepper flakes, 2 teaspoons fennel seeds, 1 teaspoon garlic powder, 1 teaspoon dried oregano, ½ teaspoon paprika, ¾ teaspoon salt, and ½ teaspoon black pepper. Add the mixture to 1 pound ground meat of choice (pork, chicken thigh, or turkey thigh). Uncooked sausage can be refrigerated for 3 days or frozen for up to 3 months.

VEGGIE AND SHREDDED PORK BREAKFAST HASH

SERVES 4 • PREP: 20 MINUTES • ROAST: 20 MINUTES • TOTAL: 40 MINUTES

1 sweet potato, peeled and cut into 1-inch cubes

1 medium onion, cut into thin wedges

2 tablespoons extra-virgin olive oil, plus some for brushing

Salt and black pepper

8 ounces Brussels sprouts, trimmed and halved or quartered

½ red bell pepper, seeded and cut into bite-sized pieces

1 tablespoon chopped fresh thyme, or 1 teaspoon dried thyme

1 tablespoon apple cider vinegar or white vinegar

4 large eggs, poached (see Tip) or fried

2 cups Big-Batch Shredded Mexican-Style Pork Shoulder (page 133), warmed

Whole30-compatible salsa (optional)

TIP: The secret to successfully poaching eggs is to add vinegar to the water. This helps the eggs hold their shape as they cook. Cracking the eggs into a small bowl or ramekin first makes sure your yolks stay intact, and you won't get any shell fragments in the water. However, inexpensive egg poaching cups or an egg poaching pan will also make beautiful eggs.

This colorful dish is packed with a confetti of vegetables—sweet potato, onion, Brussels sprouts, and red bell pepper. The flavorful pork comes from the Big-Batch Shredded Mexican-Style Pork Shoulder on page 133. Top it off with a poached or fried egg.

Preheat the oven to 425°F. Line a large rimmed baking sheet with parchment or brush with a little olive oil.

In a large bowl, toss the sweet potato and onion with 1 tablespoon of the olive oil and season to taste with salt and pepper. Transfer to the baking sheet and roast for 5 minutes.

In the same bowl, toss the Brussels sprouts, bell pepper, and thyme with the remaining tablespoon oil. Season to taste with salt and pepper, and add to sweet potato mixture in the baking pan. Continue to roast until the Brussels sprouts are crisp-tender and browned on the edges and the sweet potato and onion are tender, 10 to 15 minutes more.

Near the end of the roasting time, poach the eggs. Add about 4 cups of water to a large skillet. Add the vinegar and bring to a boil. Reduce heat to a simmer (small bubbles will come to the surface), then break an egg into a small bowl. Lower the bowl very close to the water, and slip the egg into the water, being careful not to break the yolk. Quickly repeat with the remaining 3 eggs. Simmer the eggs, uncovered, for 3 minutes, or until whites are completely set and the yolks begin to thicken but are not hard.

Divide the vegetable mixture among 4 plates. Top each with some of the warm pork. With a slotted spoon, place an egg atop the pork mixture on each plate. Season to taste with salt and pepper. Serve with the salsa (if using).

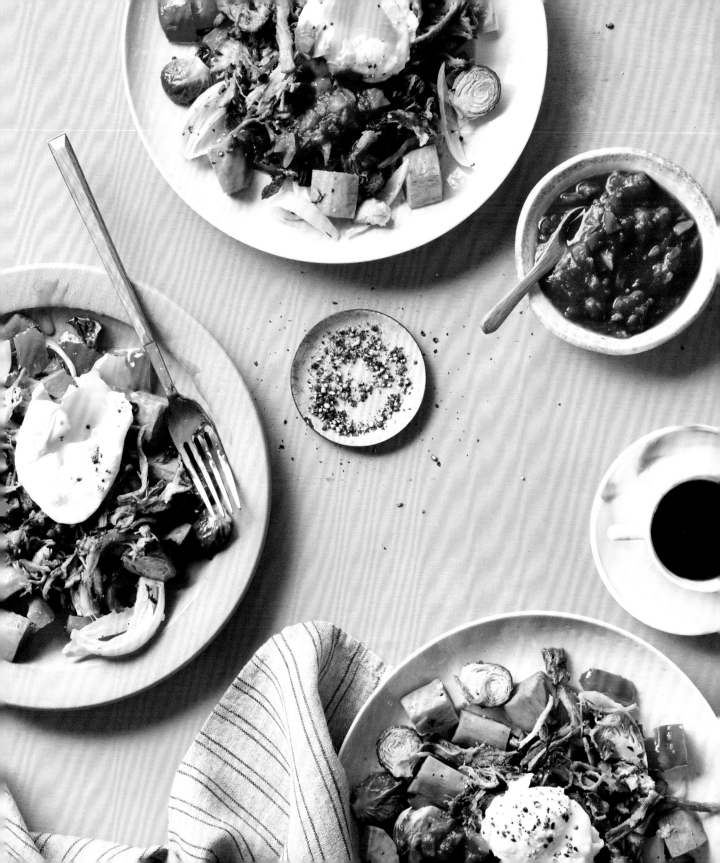

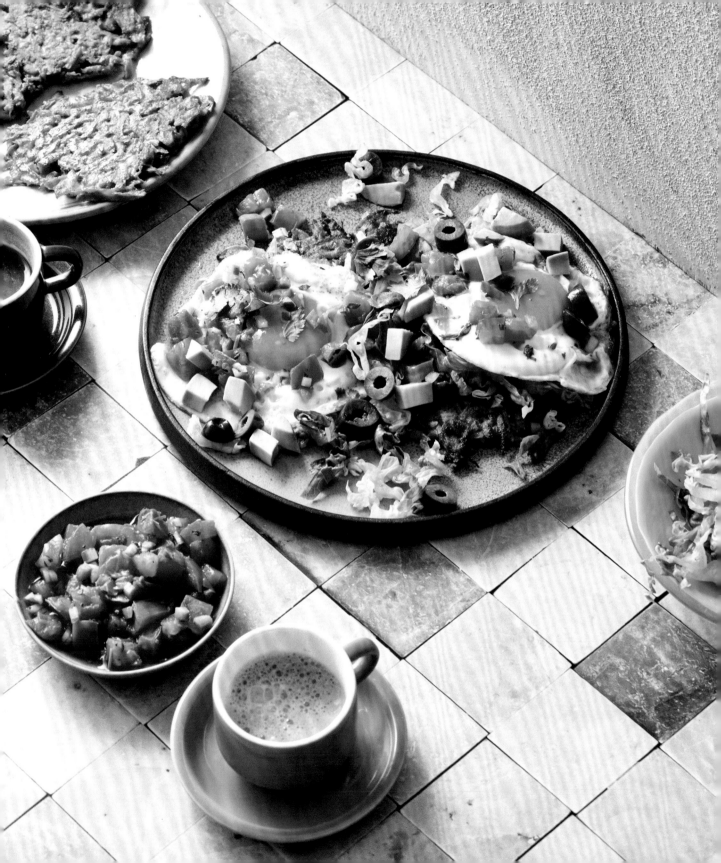

HUEVOS RANCHEROS WITH
SWEET POTATO–BACON HASH BROWNS

SERVES 2 • PREP: 30 MINUTES • COOK: 35 MINUTES • TOTAL: 1 HOUR 5 MINUTES

FOR THE SALSA

2 cups chopped fresh
   tomatoes, or drained
   canned diced tomatoes

¼ cup minced red onion

¼ cup chopped fresh cilantro

2 tablespoons white wine
   vinegar

1 teaspoon dried oregano

1 teaspoon salt

1 jalapeño, seeded and
   minced

FOR THE HASH BROWNS

1 large (10- to 12-ounce)
   sweet potato, peeled and
   coarsely grated

1½ tablespoons arrowroot
   powder

4 slices Whole30-compatible
   bacon, cooked and
   crumbled

2 large eggs

½ teaspoon garlic powder

½ teaspoon onion powder

½ teaspoon chili powder

Salt and black pepper

Extra-virgin olive oil or
   avocado oil

FOR THE HUEVOS
RANCHEROS

4 large eggs

Salt and black pepper

Shredded lettuce, diced
   avocado, sliced black
   olives, and chopped fresh
   cilantro, for serving

When we tested this recipe, one of our tasters pronounced it "really good—like, REALLY good." With fresh homemade salsa, cool and buttery avocado, *and* bacon, how could it be anything but?

MAKE THE SALSA: In a medium bowl, combine the tomatoes, onion, cilantro, vinegar, oregano, salt, and jalapeño. (Salsa can be made up to a day in advance and refrigerated.)

MAKE THE HASH BROWNS: Using a clean kitchen towel, squeeze the grated sweet potato to remove as much excess moisture as possible. In a large bowl, combine the sweet potato, arrowroot, and bacon; toss to combine. In another small bowl, whisk together the eggs, garlic powder, onion powder, chili powder, and salt and pepper to taste. Add to the potato mixture and stir together until everything is well combined.

Heat 2 tablespoons of the oil in a large nonstick skillet over medium-high heat. When hot, drop ⅓ cup of the shredded potato mixture into the skillet. Flatten with a spatula to a 3-inch round. Repeat for 3 other patties, maintaining some space between the patties. Cook until patties are browned and easily peel away from the bottom of the pan, about 6 minutes. Flip and continue cooking another 6 minutes, or until browned on the other side.

MAKE THE HUEVOS RANCHEROS: In a large saucepan or deep skillet, heat the salsa over medium heat. Crack the eggs into separate small dishes or cups. When the salsa comes to a simmer, gently add the eggs to the salsa. Season to taste with salt and pepper. Reduce the heat to medium-low, and cover the pan. Cook the eggs to desired doneness, 3 to 4 minutes for runny yolks. (Alternatively, fry the eggs in extra-virgin olive oil to desired doneness in a nonstick skillet; warm the salsa in a saucepan.)

Place 2 warm hash-brown patties on each serving plate. Top each with shredded lettuce, then place 2 eggs on top. Add the avocado and olives. Spoon some of the warm salsa on top of the eggs and around the hash browns. Sprinkle with cilantro before serving.

OKONOMIYAKI-STYLE OMELET WITH GINGERY MAYO AND TERIYAKI SAUCE

SERVES 2 TO 3 • PREP: 25 MINUTES • COOK/BAKE: 20 MINUTES • TOTAL: 45 MINUTES

FOR THE MAYO

½ cup Whole30 Mayo (page 230) or Whole30-compatible mayonnaise

1 tablespoon peeled and grated fresh ginger (see Tip)

1 tablespoon Whole30-compatible rice vinegar

1½ teaspoons toasted sesame oil or ¾ teaspoon hot sesame oil

FOR THE TERIYAKI SAUCE

½ cup coconut aminos

½ cup 100% pineapple juice

¼ cup Whole30-compatible rice vinegar

2 garlic cloves, minced

1 teaspoon peeled and grated fresh ginger

Pinch of red pepper flakes

1 tablespoon arrowroot powder

1 tablespoon water

Okonomiyaki is a crispy cabbage and egg pancake doused in savory sauces and mayo, traditionally cooked on a hot iron griddle called a teppan. It's a popular Japanese street food originating in the city of Osaka. *Okonomi* translates to "as you like," so it's a highly variable dish that can include all kinds of vegetables and proteins. Our version has carrot, shiitake mushroom, sweet potato, green onion, and shrimp.

MAKE THE MAYO: In a small bowl, whisk together the mayonnaise, ginger, vinegar, and sesame oil until well combined. Cover and refrigerate until serving time.

MAKE THE TERIYAKI SAUCE: In a small saucepan, combine the coconut aminos, pineapple juice, vinegar, garlic, ginger, and red pepper flakes. Bring to a simmer over medium-high heat and cook until reduced slightly, about 5 minutes. Meanwhile, combine the arrowroot powder and water in a small dish. Whisk the arrowroot mixture into the juice mixture and simmer until sauce is thickened, 1 to 2 minutes. Set aside to cool. (See Tip.)

MAKE THE OMELET: Preheat the oven to 400°F. In a large, oven-safe nonstick skillet, heat 2 tablespoons of the oil over medium-high heat. Add the cabbage, carrot, mushrooms, sweet potato, green onion, and ginger. Cook, stirring occasionally, until cabbage is crisp-tender, about 5 minutes.

Meanwhile, in a medium bowl, whisk the eggs. Add the remaining tablespoon oil to the pan. Pour the eggs over the vegetables and sprinkle the shrimp over the top. Cook until set on the bottom, using a rubber spatula to lift underneath the omelet to prevent sticking, 3 to 4 minutes.

Transfer the pan to the oven and finish cooking until the top is no longer wet, about 10 minutes more. Remove from the oven and let stand 5 minutes before cutting into wedges and serving.

(continued)

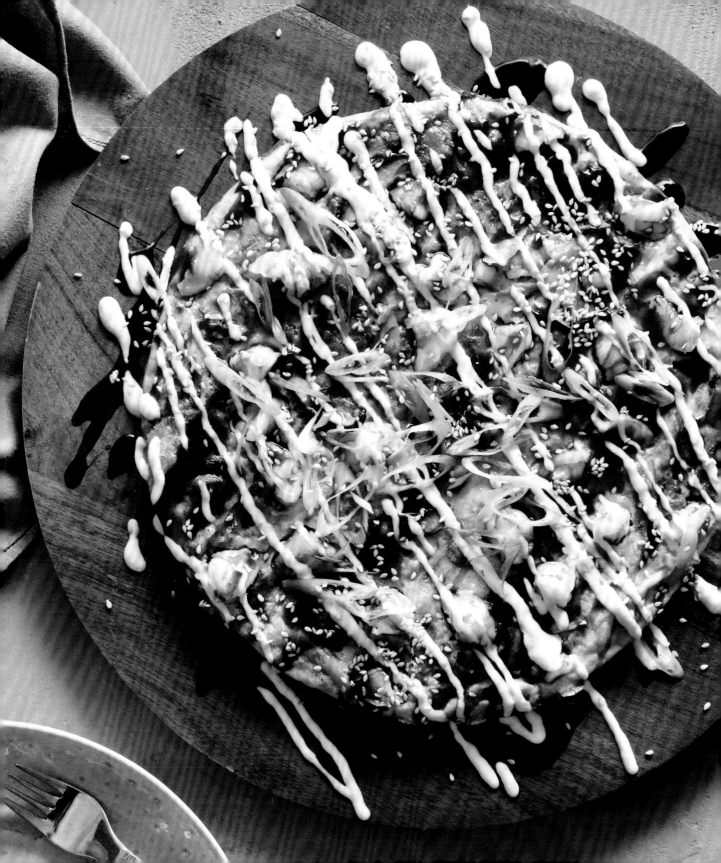

FOR THE OMELET

3 tablespoons avocado oil

2 cups coarsely chopped
   green cabbage

½ cup grated carrot

½ cup thinly sliced fresh
   shiitake mushrooms

⅓ cup grated sweet potato

¼ cup thinly sliced green
   onion (green and white
   parts), plus more for serving

2 teaspoons peeled and
   grated fresh ginger

6 large eggs

1 cup chopped peeled and
   deveined shrimp

Sesame seeds, toasted, for
   serving

Serve: Drizzle the omelet with the teriyaki sauce and a generous amount of mayo. If desired, sprinkle with additional sliced green onion and the sesame seeds.

TIP: The teriyaki sauce and mayo can be made a day ahead and stored in the refrigerator.

Here are two tips for grating ginger: First, use a microplane (not a cheese grater), as it's less likely the ginger will get stuck in the holes. Second, keep a piece of fresh ginger in your freezer! Frozen ginger is much easier to grate, and it thaws in seconds in the pan. You can also buy minced ginger in a jar or tube, which makes it easy to add to any recipe. A 1-inch piece of fresh ginger equates to 1 tablespoon of minced ginger.

ORIGINAL WHOLE30 LUNCHES

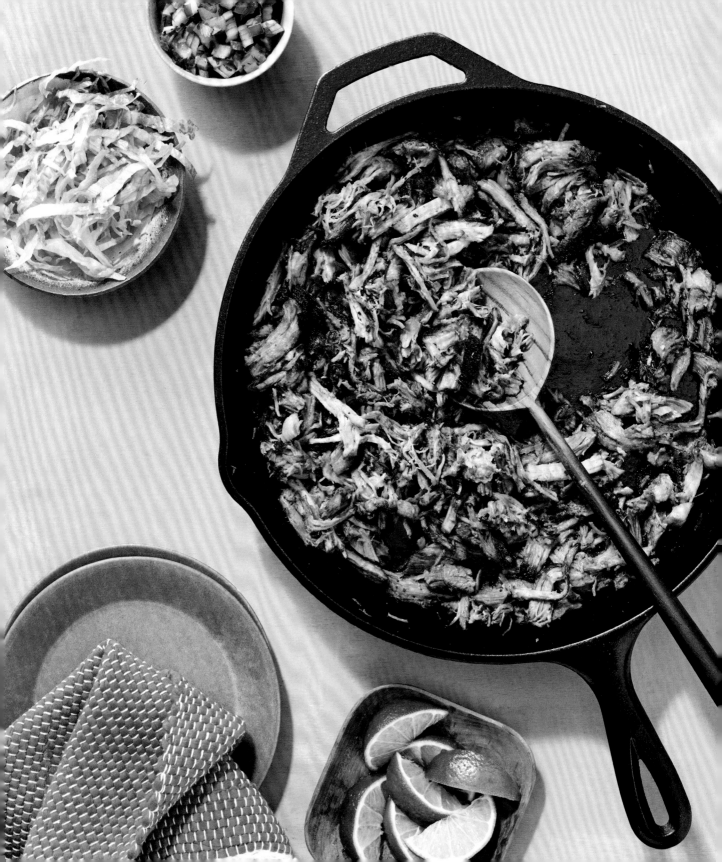

BIG-BATCH SHREDDED MEXICAN-STYLE PORK SHOULDER

MAKES 6 CUPS (8 TO 12 SERVINGS) • PREP: 20 MINUTES • SLOW COOK: 4 TO 5 HOURS •
TOTAL: 4 HOURS, 20 MINUTES

3 pounds boneless pork shoulder roast, trimmed and cut into 3 equal pieces

1 small onion, chopped

4 garlic cloves, minced

1 tablespoon apple cider vinegar

1 tablespoon ground cumin

2 teaspoons salt

2 teaspoons chipotle powder or 1 jalapeño, seeded and finely chopped

2 teaspoons dried Mexican or Italian oregano

1 small orange, cut into wedges

4 teaspoons avocado oil

This easy-to-prep pork shoulder comes together in the slow cooker and is extremely versatile to use in meals throughout the day. It comes out pull-apart tender, then the edges get crisped in a skillet to become that Whole30 fan favorite—carnitas. (See Tip.)

In a 3½- to 4-quart slow cooker, combine the pork, onion, and garlic. Drizzle with the vinegar. Sprinkle with the cumin, salt, chipotle powder, and oregano. Squeeze the orange wedges over the mixture, then drop the wedges into the cooker. Cover and cook on low heat for 8 to 10 hours or on high heat for 4 to 5 hours, or until pork is tender.

Remove the pork from the cooker and transfer to a cutting board, reserving the cooking juices, if desired, but discarding orange wedges. Shred the pork with 2 forks.

In a large skillet, heat 2 teaspoons of the oil over medium-high heat. Spoon half the pork into the skillet in an even layer. Cook 1 to 2 minutes or until crispy on the edges, flipping it halfway through with a spatula. Transfer to a bowl and repeat with the remaining 2 teaspoons oil and remaining pork.

Divide the pork into 3 (2-cup) portions. If using one portion immediately, cover to keep warm. Cool the remaining portions, reserving for later, and place in storage containers. If desired, strain the cooking liquid and place in a separate storage container. Refrigerate the pork and cooking liquid for up to 3 days or freeze for up to 3 months. If frozen, thaw overnight in the refrigerator and heat through before using.

TIP: This pork is endlessly versatile! Use warm shredded pork in Veggie and Shredded Pork Breakfast Hash (page 124); pile on top of spaghetti squash or zucchini noodles; serve over thinly sliced jicama topped with fresh salsa, green onion, and shredded lettuce; or spoon over grilled pepper and onion strips with guacamole and lime wedges. Use a small amount of the reserved cooking liquid to add moisture when reheating leftovers.

CRUNCHY CHICKEN SALAD WITH LEMON AND TARRAGON

SERVES 2 TO 3 • PREP: 20 MINUTES • TOTAL: 20 MINUTES

½ cup Whole30 Mayo (page 230) or Whole30-compatible mayonnaise

2 tablespoons fresh lemon juice

1 tablespoon chopped fresh tarragon or basil

½ teaspoon salt

¼ teaspoon black pepper

2 cups shredded cooked chicken breast

1½ cups shredded coleslaw mix

1 green onion, sliced (green and white parts)

¼ cup slivered almonds, toasted

4 to 6 romaine lettuce leaves

This protein- and veggie-packed chicken salad is perfect for a quick midday meal. Use a cooked rotisserie chicken to make your prep even easier. We give you three variations, so you can mix up your flavor profiles and ingredients using the base recipe as your blueprint.

In a medium bowl, whisk together the mayonnaise, lemon juice, tarragon, salt, and pepper. Add the chicken, coleslaw mix, green onion, and almonds. Stir well to combine.

Place 2 romaine lettuce leaves on each plate. Divide the chicken salad among the leaves and serve. Chicken salad can also be served in a hollowed-out bell pepper, on sweet potato "toast," or simply in a bowl.

GREEK-STYLE CHICKEN SALAD: Substitute 2 teaspoons chopped fresh dill for the tarragon. Substitute 2 tablespoons finely diced red onion for the green onion. Omit the coleslaw mix. Stir in 1 diced small Persian cucumber, ¼ cup halved Kalamata olives, and 1 seeded and diced Roma (plum) tomato.

SUMMER CHICKEN SALAD: Substitute 1 tablespoon chopped fresh basil for the tarragon. Omit the coleslaw mix. Stir in ⅓ cup diced celery and 1 pitted and diced ripe peach. Serve topped with diced fresh strawberries and additional fresh basil.

CURRIED CHICKEN SALAD: Substitute 3 tablespoons chopped fresh cilantro for the tarragon. Whisk 1 teaspoon curry powder into the mayonnaise mixture before adding the other ingredients. Omit the coleslaw mix. Stir in 1 cored, peeled, and diced small Granny Smith apple, 1 cup coarsely chopped baby spinach leaves, and 1 seeded and minced small jalapeño. Substitute ¼ cup chopped roasted cashews for the almonds.

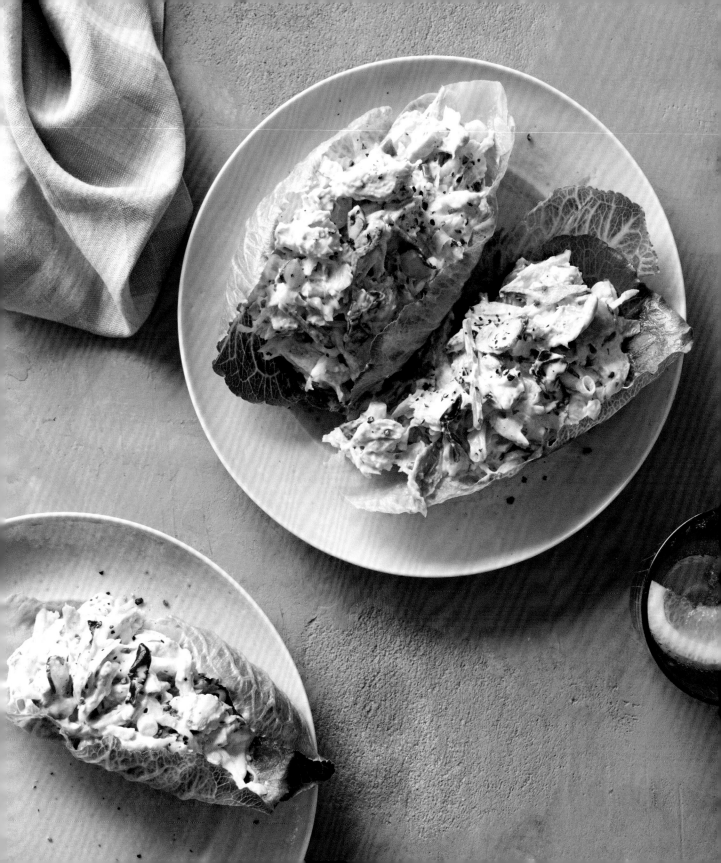

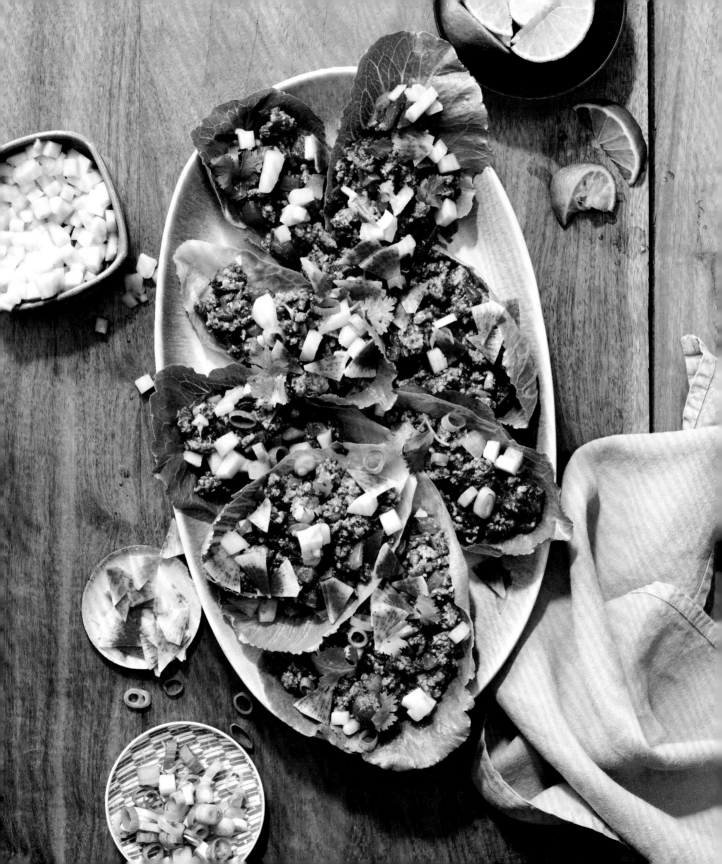

JAMAICAN JERK TURKEY SLOPPY JOES IN LETTUCE WRAPS

SERVES 4 • PREP: 15 MINUTES • COOK: 15 MINUTES • TOTAL: 30 MINUTES

2 teaspoons coconut oil or avocado oil

1 small onion, chopped

1 pound ground turkey breast or thigh

1 green or red bell pepper, cored, seeded, and chopped

½ to 1 jalapeño, seeded and finely chopped

1 tablespoon Whole30-compatible Jamaican jerk seasoning (or homemade; see Tip)

1 teaspoon salt

½ teaspoon sweet or smoked paprika

1 (14-ounce) can diced fire-roasted tomatoes

2 tablespoons coconut aminos

12 to 16 large romaine or Bibb lettuce leaves

1 cup chopped ripe mango or fresh pineapple

Lime wedges, sliced green onion, and cilantro leaves for serving

Nicely spicy and perfectly seasoned, these saucy wraps are big on flavor and freshness. Diced mango offers a touch of sweetness, and the heat is easily adjusted by using less (or more) jalapeño and a mild sweet or smoked paprika.

In a large skillet, heat the oil over medium heat. When hot, add the onion and cook for 2 minutes. Add the turkey, bell pepper, jalapeño, jerk seasoning, salt, and paprika. Cook until the onion is tender and the turkey is lightly browned, 6 to 8 minutes, stirring occasionally and breaking up the turkey. Stir in the tomatoes. Bring to a boil, reduce the heat to low, and simmer, uncovered, for 7 minutes, stirring occasionally. Stir in the coconut aminos.

Arrange the lettuce leaves on a platter. Fill with the turkey mixture and add the mango. Squeeze the lime wedges over the top to taste, then sprinkle with the green onion and cilantro. Serve with additional lime wedges.

TIP: To make Whole30 jerk seasoning, stir together 1 tablespoon dried onion flakes, 1 tablespoon garlic powder, 1 tablespoon dried parsley, 2 teaspoons smoked or sweet paprika, 2 teaspoons salt, 2 teaspoons ground allspice, 2 teaspoons dried thyme, 1 teaspoon black pepper, 1 teaspoon ground cumin, ½ teaspoon cayenne, ½ teaspoon ground cinnamon, and ½ teaspoon ground nutmeg. Transfer to a jar with a lid, and store at room temperature for up to 6 months. Makes about ⅓ cup.

LEMON-MUSTARD SALMON WITH A KALE AND APPLE SALAD

SERVES 2 • PREP: 25 MINUTES • BROIL: 10 MINUTES • TOTAL: 35 MINUTES

FOR THE SALMON

2 (6- to 8-ounce) salmon fillets, about 1 inch thick, skin removed

2 tablespoons extra-virgin olive oil

1 tablespoon Whole30-compatible Dijon mustard

¼ teaspoon salt

Black pepper

FOR THE SALAD

3 cups very finely chopped or slivered fresh kale

2 tablespoons extra-virgin olive oil, plus additional for massaging kale

¼ teaspoon salt, plus a pinch for massaging kale

1 tablespoon fresh lemon juice

½ small garlic clove, minced

1 small apple, cored and cut into ¼-inch dice

1 tablespoon sliced or slivered almonds, toasted

Lemony, mustardy broiled salmon, served with a sprightly kale and apple salad, makes for a hearty and high-fiber lunch. Look for crisp apples that won't brown too quickly when chopped, like Honeycrisp, Fuji, Pink Lady, or Jazz. Add roasted sweet potatoes or beets to the salad to bump up the carbs.

MAKE THE SALMON: Line a large rimmed baking sheet with parchment. Position the top oven rack 6 inches from the broiler. Preheat the broiler to high. Place the salmon on the baking sheet.

In a small bowl, whisk together the olive oil and mustard. Brush the tops and sides of the salmon fillets with the mixture. Season with the salt and add pepper to taste. Broil until the salmon is cooked through and has a deep brown crust on top, 7 to 8 minutes.

MAKE THE SALAD: While the salmon is cooking, place the kale in a medium bowl. Drizzle with a little olive oil and sprinkle with a pinch of salt. Massage with your hands until the kale is softened, about 1 minute.

In a small jar with a lid, combine the 2 tablespoons olive oil, the ¼ teaspoon salt, the lemon juice, and the minced garlic. Shake until emulsified. Pour over kale and toss to coat.

Serve: Divide the kale between 2 plates. Top each with diced apple, then sprinkle with the toasted almonds. Serve the salmon with the salad.

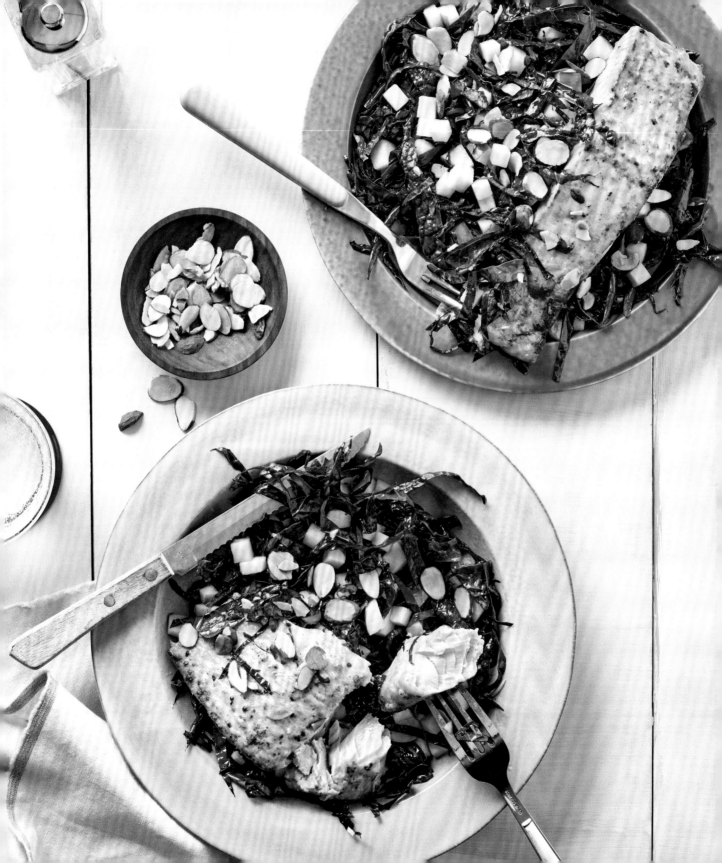

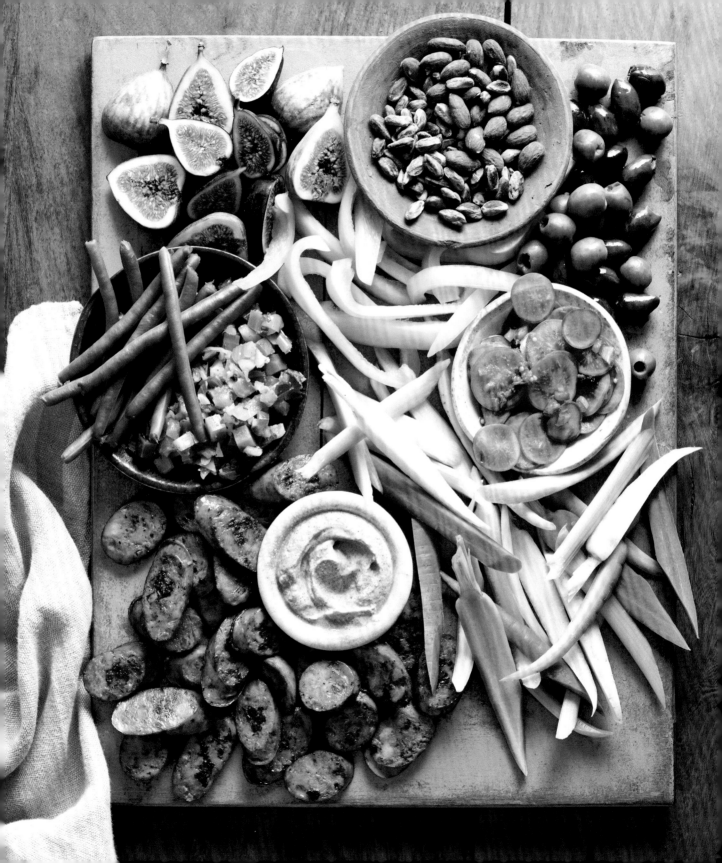

POWER CHARCUTERIE PLATTER

SERVES 2 • PREP: 20 MINUTES • TOTAL: 20 MINUTES

FOR THE RADISH PICKLES

4 radishes

½ cup apple cider vinegar

½ cup water

2 pitted dates, chopped

1 teaspoon salt

1 teaspoon mustard seeds, coriander seeds, and/or peppercorns

FOR THE CHARCUTERIE PLATTER

2 cooked Whole30-compatible chicken sausage links (apple or roasted red pepper works well)

1 tablespoon Whole30-compatible brown mustard

1 cup Whole30-compatible pickled vegetables (cauliflower, giardiniera, green beans, or cucumbers) (see Tip)

1 medium carrot and/or celery stalk, peeled, trimmed, and cut into sticks

½ yellow bell pepper, seeded and cut into strips

4 fresh figs, halved, or 1 sliced pear, and/or ¼ cup Whole30-compatible dried fruit

8 green or Kalamata olives

3 tablespoons shelled pistachios or almonds, toasted

This power platter for two is very accommodating. Use any sliced, dried, or bite-sized fruits, plus raw vegetables, olives, and/or nuts. If you fancy a dipping sauce, try guacamole, the Revamped Ranch Dressing (page 212), or Avocado Green Goddess Dressing (page 201).

MAKE THE RADISH PICKLES: Trim and very thinly slice the radishes with a mandoline slicer or sharp knife. Place the radishes in a bowl or jar.

In a small saucepan, stir together the vinegar, water, dates, salt, and mustard seeds. Bring to a boil over medium-high heat. Pour the vinegar mixture over the radishes and cool to room temperature. If using immediately, set aside half the pickles for the charcuterie plate and cover and refrigerate the remainder for up to 1 week.

MAKE THE CHARCUTERIE PLATTER: Slice the sausages into ½-inch pieces and heat in a skillet until browned around the edges. If the slices start to stick, add a little water to the skillet.

On a platter large enough for 2 servings, arrange the sausage slices. Place the reserved radishes and the mustard into separate small dishes. Place the mustard dish and the radish dish next to the sausages on the platter. Arrange the pickled vegetables, carrot, bell pepper, figs, olives, and pistachios on the platter and serve.

> **TIP:** You can quickly pickle many vegetables (such as green beans, cauliflower, cucumber, beets, red onion, carrots, asparagus, or jalapeños) at home. Slice your veggies into strips or chunks and pack them into a large jar. Add 3 or 4 cloves of garlic, peeled, and other herbs or spices as desired (such as peppercorns, dill, hot pepper flakes, or mustard seed). In a small sauce pot, add 1 cup of water, 1 cup of white or apple cider vinegar, and 1 tablespoon of salt. Bring to a boil. Once all the salt has dissolved, pour the liquid carefully over the vegetables. Allow to cool, then cover the jar tightly and place it in the fridge. You can eat them in a few hours or the next day, but the longer they sit, the better they'll taste. Pickled vegetables will last for up to 2 months in a closed container in the fridge.

SPANISH-STYLE BEEF SOUP TO GO

SERVES 1 • PREP: 20 MINUTES • COOK: 5 MINUTES • TOTAL: 25 MINUTES

1½ cups baby spinach

¾ cup diced cooked sweet potato

1 Roma (plum) tomato, seeded and diced

¾ cup cooked shredded or ground beef

¼ cup Whole30-compatible red pepper–stuffed Spanish olives, sliced

¼ teaspoon smoked paprika

¼ teaspoon garlic powder

¼ teaspoon onion powder

¼ teaspoon salt

¼ teaspoon black pepper

1 (16-ounce) package Whole30-compatible beef bone broth

This perfect single-serving office recipe layers cooked beef, veggies, olives, and seasonings in a glass jar with a lid. Then just add bone broth and heat it in the microwave.

In a 1-quart wide-mouth glass jar with a lid, combine the spinach, sweet potato, tomato, beef, olives, paprika, garlic powder, onion powder, salt, and pepper. Store, covered, in the refrigerator until ready to use, up to 4 days. Remove the jar from the refrigerator 15 minutes before you plan to eat it to allow the glass to come to room temperature.

When ready to eat, pour the broth into the jar and place the jar in the microwave. (See Tip.) Cook on high heat, uncovered, for 2 minutes. Using oven mitts, carefully remove the jar from the microwave and stir. Cook for an additional 2 to 3 minutes, or until simmering.

Carefully remove the hot jar from the microwave and pour into a bowl.

TIP: For the freshest flavors and textures, don't pour the broth over the ingredients until just before serving. Otherwise, the broth starts to break down the spinach and tomato.

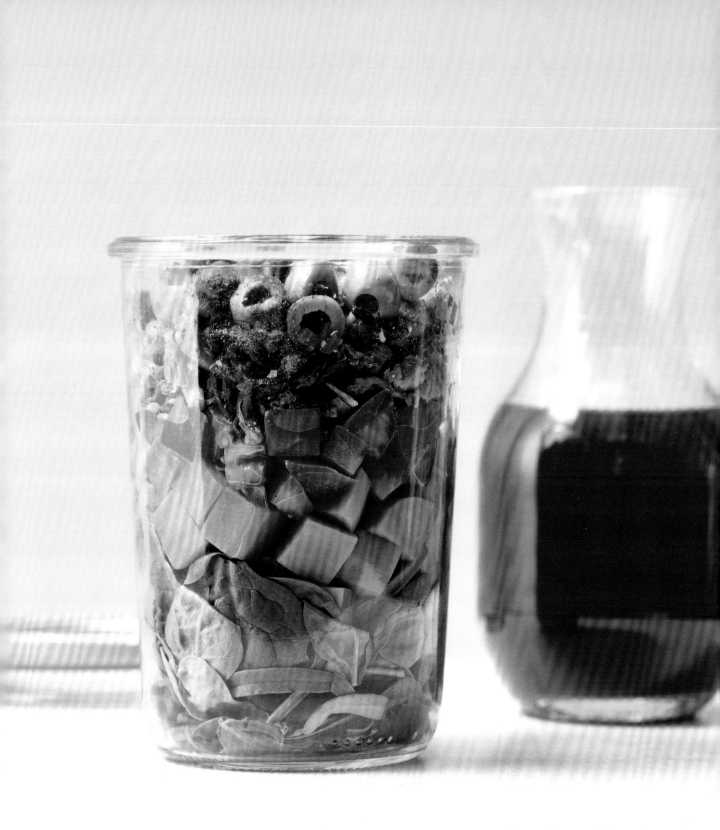

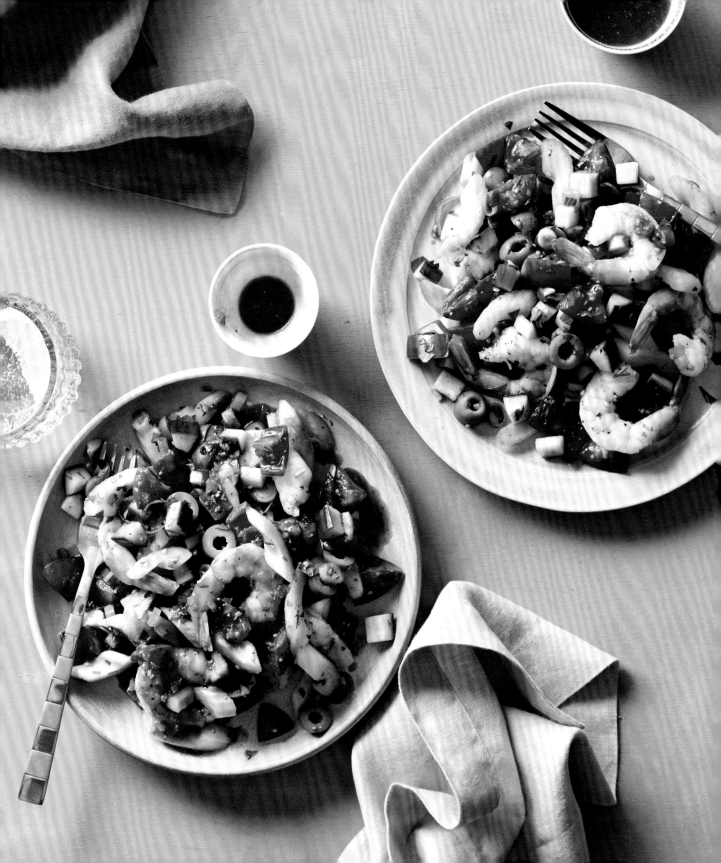

BLOODY MARY CHOPPED SALAD

SERVES 2 • PREP: 20 MINUTES • COOK: 10 MINUTES • TOTAL: 30 MINUTES

FOR THE DRESSING

1 tablespoon extra-virgin olive oil

1 tablespoon minced shallot

¼ cup Chicken Bone Broth (page 231) or Whole30-compatible chicken broth

⅔ cup Whole30-compatible spicy tomato juice

2 tablespoons red wine vinegar

1 tablespoon coconut aminos

2 teaspoons Whole30-compatible fish sauce

1 teaspoon Whole30-compatible Dijon mustard

1 teaspoon prepared horseradish

½ teaspoon celery seeds

Juice of ½ lemon

Black pepper

FOR THE SALAD

8 ounces cooked large shrimp, thawed if frozen

2 cups chopped ripe tomatoes

1 cup sliced celery

½ cup diced cucumber

⅓ cup sliced pitted Whole30-compatible green olives

¼ cup sliced green onion (green and white parts)

¼ cup chopped fresh parsley

Black pepper

This fresh salad features all the flavors of the famous brunch cocktail—tomato, horseradish, lemon, celery seed, and black pepper—and includes all the "fixings." A "shot" of the dressing is served alongside so diners can dress the salad to taste.

MAKE THE DRESSING: In a small saucepan, heat the olive oil over medium-high heat. Add the shallot and cook until soft, about 3 minutes. Deglaze the pan with the chicken broth and simmer until nearly evaporated. Add the tomato juice, vinegar, coconut aminos, fish sauce, mustard, horseradish, celery seed, and lemon juice. Simmer 3 minutes, then season to taste with pepper. Remove from the heat and chill. (Dressing may be made up to 2 days ahead.)

MAKE THE SALAD: In a large bowl, combine the shrimp, tomatoes, celery, cucumber, olives, green onion, parsley, and pepper to taste. Toss to combine.

Serve: Divide the salad between 2 serving plates and serve with shot glasses of the dressing on the side.

LARB-INSPIRED BUTTERNUT SQUASH SOUP

SERVES 3 TO 4 • PREP: 30 MINUTES • COOK: 20 MINUTES • TOTAL: 50 MINUTES

FOR THE SOUP

1 tablespoon coconut oil

½ cup diced onion

1 tablespoon peeled and minced fresh ginger

2 garlic cloves, minced

1 jalapeño, seeded and minced

3 cups peeled and cubed butternut squash

1½ tablespoons mild curry powder

Pinch of red pepper flakes

4 cups Chicken Bone Broth (page 231) or Whole30-compatible chicken broth

1 (13.5-ounce) can full-fat coconut milk

FOR THE LARB

2 cups chopped cooked chicken (see Tip)

1 apple (any variety), peeled, cored, and diced

⅓ cup chopped fresh mint

⅓ cup chopped fresh cilantro

¼ cup unsweetened coconut flakes

¼ cup roasted salted cashews

1 tablespoon Whole30-compatible fish sauce

Juice of 1 lime

Larb is a delicious Thai and Laotian meat salad, seasoned with fish sauce, red pepper flakes, lime juice, and fresh herbs. In our version, we turn the delicious flavors of larb into a hearty soup, with a spice profile you can easily adjust to your liking.

MAKE THE SOUP: In a Dutch oven or large saucepan, melt the coconut oil over medium-high heat. Add the onion, ginger, garlic, jalapeño, squash, curry powder, and red pepper flakes. Cover and cook, stirring frequently, until the onion is translucent, about 10 minutes. Add the broth. Cover and simmer until the squash is very tender, about 15 minutes.

Blend the soup with an immersion blender (or use an upright blender for a smoother consistency). Stir in the coconut milk. Keep warm.

MAKE THE LARB: In a medium bowl, combine the chicken, apple, mint, cilantro, coconut, cashews, fish sauce, and lime juice. Toss until well blended.

Serve: Place one serving of larb in the bottom of each bowl, then ladle the soup over the top.

> **TIP:** As larb is typically made with *ground* meat, you could use ground chicken or turkey in this dish, too. In a large skillet or Dutch oven, heat 1 tablespoon of extra-virgin olive oil over medium heat. Add the ground meat. Cook, stirring often, until the meat is browned, 7 to 10 minutes.
>
> In a pinch you can substitute two 12-ounce packages of frozen butternut squash; no need to thaw before adding to the pan.

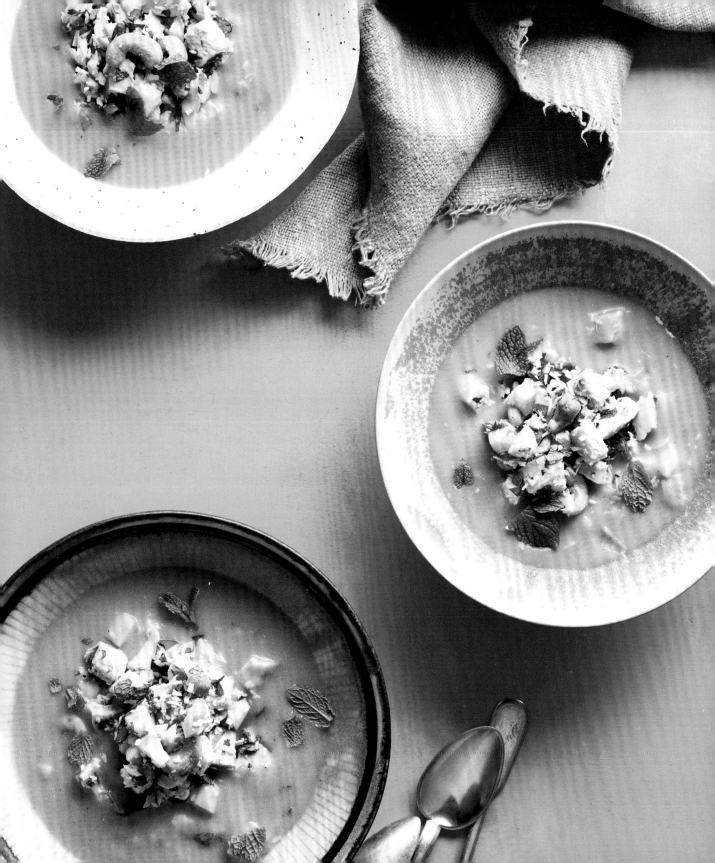

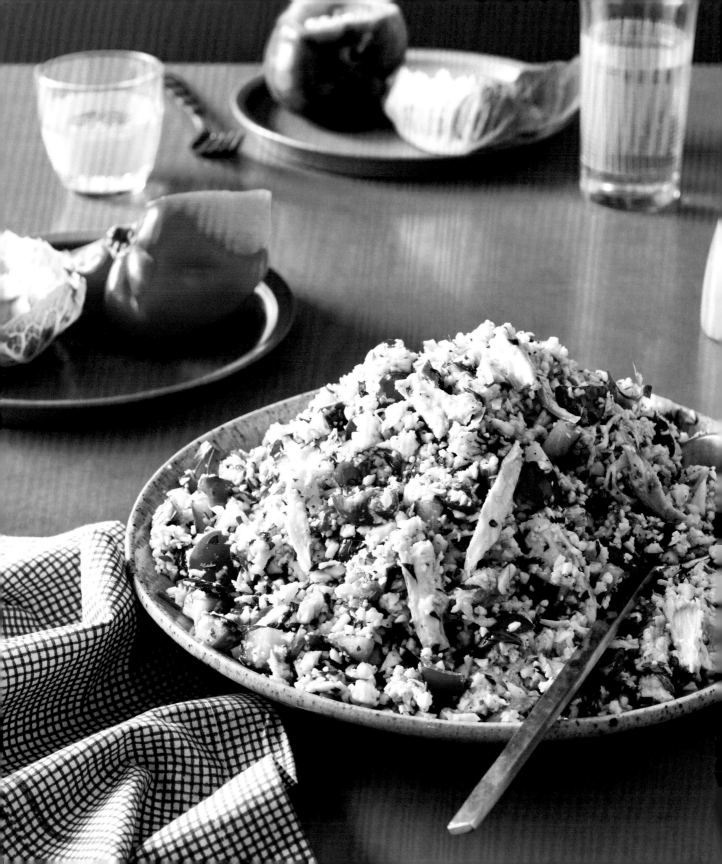

ZA'ATAR "TABBOULEH" WITH PULLED CHICKEN

SERVES 4 • PREP: 25 MINUTES • TOTAL: 25 MINUTES

1 small head Romanesco, broccoli, or cauliflower, trimmed and cut into florets

2 green onions, chopped (green and white parts)

¼ cup chopped fresh mint

¼ cup chopped fresh parsley

3 tablespoons fresh lemon juice

3 tablespoons extra-virgin olive oil or avocado oil

1 tablespoon za'atar

1 teaspoon salt

1 teaspoon black pepper

3 cups shredded cooked chicken breast (see Tip)

1 cup diced hothouse cucumber

1½ cups quartered grape tomatoes

Za'atar is an herby, flavorful spice with ancient roots in the Middle East and the eastern Mediterranean. It gives big flavor to this riff on the classic grain-and-herb salad normally served as one dish in a mezze (an offering of small plates). Riced Romanesco or cauliflower steps in here for the traditional bulgur or cracked wheat.

Place half the Romanesco in a food processor and pulse until it reaches a rice-like consistency, 15 to 20 pulses. (Don't overcrowd it in the food processor, and don't over-pulse or it will get mushy.) Transfer to a large bowl and repeat with the remaining Romanesco.

Add the green onions, mint, parsley, lemon juice, olive oil, za'atar, salt, and pepper to the bowl and mix well. Gently fold in the chicken, cucumber, and grape tomatoes. If the chicken is warm, cover and refrigerate for 2 hours, or up to 3 days.

This dish can be served in a hollowed-out bell pepper, on lettuce leaves, or in a bowl. If you're eating this salad as leftovers, add an extra drizzle of olive oil and a squeeze of lemon before serving.

TIP: To cook and shred a chicken breast, place 2 boneless, skinless chicken breast halves in a saucepan, side by side. Cover with at least 1 inch of water. Bring the water to a boil, then reduce the heat to low and simmer, covered, for about 8 minutes, or just until cooked through and no longer pink (160°F). Transfer the chicken to a cutting board or plate and let stand until cool enough to handle. Use 2 forks to pull the chicken apart into bite-sized shreds.

ZOODLE BOWL WITH CHICKEN, SOFT-BOILED EGG, AND GREEN ONIONS

SERVES 2 • PREP: 20 MINUTES • COOK: 5 MINUTES • TOTAL: 25 MINUTES

2 large eggs

2 cups Chicken Bone Broth (page 231) or Whole30-compatible chicken broth

2 tablespoons coconut aminos

1 tablespoon Whole30-compatible rice vinegar

¼ teaspoon salt

1 (10-ounce) package refrigerated zucchini spirals (see Tip)

½ cup shredded carrots

1 cup shredded cooked chicken breast (see Tip, page 149)

Black pepper

1 large green onion, finely chopped (green and white parts)

2 teaspoons toasted sesame oil

Flaky sea salt

This fragrant bowl of broth, chicken, soft-boiled egg, and veggies is delicious on a chilly day, or anytime you're in the mood for a comforting light meal.

Fill a small saucepan with water, then bring to a boil over high heat. Gently lower the eggs into the water and cook for 7 minutes. Use a slotted spoon to transfer the eggs to a bowl of ice water. Let cool 5 minutes. Drain and peel the eggs; set aside.

In a medium saucepan, combine the broth, coconut aminos, vinegar, and salt, then bring to a boil. Meanwhile, divide the zucchini spirals, shredded carrots, and chicken between 2 large microwave-safe bowls. Microwave each on high heat for 45 seconds to 1 minute, or until heated through.

Pour the boiling broth over the vegetables and chicken. Cut the eggs in half lengthwise and add 2 halves to each bowl. Season the bowl to taste with pepper. Sprinkle with the green onion and drizzle with the sesame oil. Sprinkle with flaky salt.

TIP: Be sure to use refrigerated, not frozen, zucchini spirals. Frozen zucchini spirals break down too quickly in the hot broth and become mushy; refrigerated spirals retain a toothsome bite. You can also spiralize your own zoodles for this soup, using 1 large or 2 small zucchini.

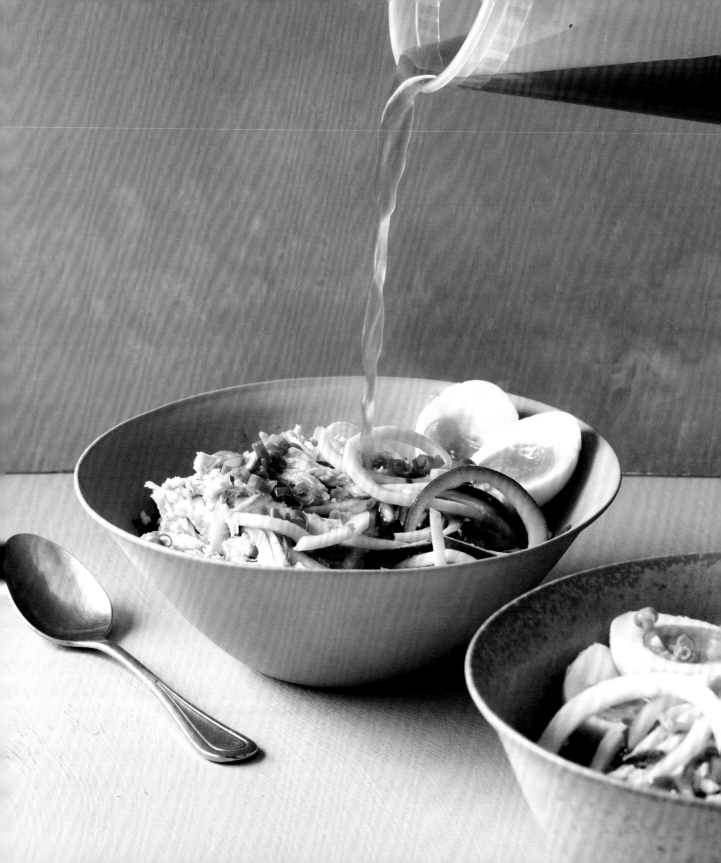

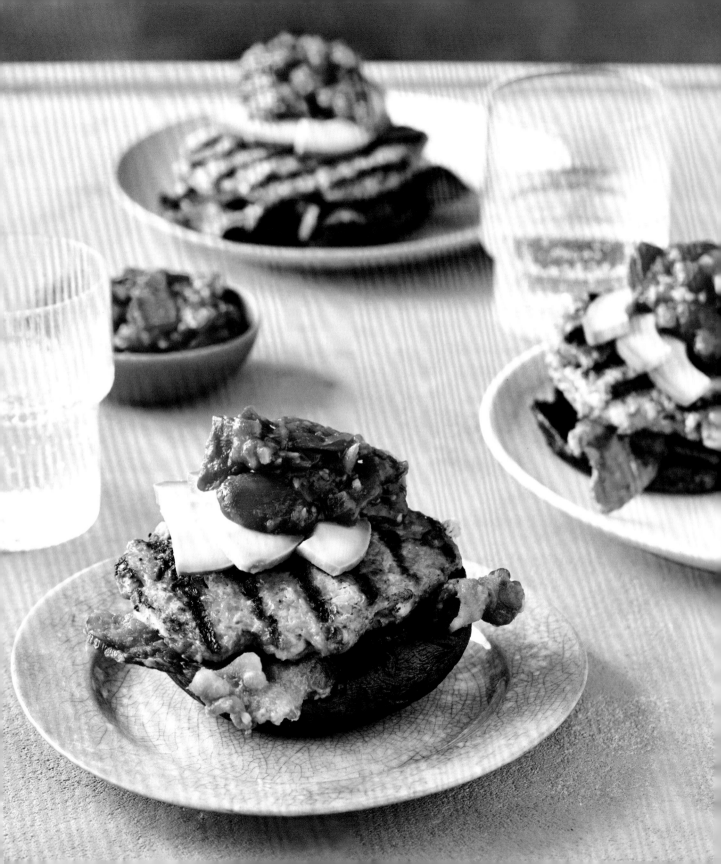

TURKEY BURGERS WITH BACON, TOMATO JAM, AND PORTOBELLO "BUNS"

SERVES 4 • PREP: 35 MINUTES • COOK: 15 MINUTES • GRILL: 10 MINUTES • TOTAL: 1 HOUR

FOR THE TOMATO JAM

1½ cups cherry or grape tomatoes, halved

¼ cup diced red onion

5 Medjool dates, pitted and chopped

2 tablespoons white wine vinegar

2 tablespoons peeled and minced fresh ginger

1 teaspoon minced garlic

1 teaspoon ground coriander

3 tablespoons fresh lime juice

2 teaspoons tomato paste

1 teaspoon minced seeded jalapeño

Salt

FOR THE BURGERS

8 ounces ground turkey breast

8 ounces ground turkey thigh

1 Granny Smith apple, cored and grated

1 teaspoon salt, plus more to taste

½ teaspoon black pepper, plus more to taste

4 portobello mushroom caps, stems removed and gills scraped

Extra-virgin olive oil

4 Whole30-compatible bacon strips, cooked

Sliced avocado

If you make the tomato jam ahead and cook your bacon ahead of time, these tasty burgers come together in a snap. The portobello "buns" make for a very hearty lunch; serve the burgers over crisp lettuce leaves if you want a lighter meal.

MAKE THE TOMATO JAM: In a medium saucepan, combine 1 cup of the tomatoes, the onion, dates, vinegar, ginger, garlic, and coriander. Bring to a simmer over medium-high heat. Cover and cook, stirring often, until the tomatoes break down and release their juices, about 10 minutes. Add the remaining ½ cup tomatoes, the lime juice, and tomato paste. Return the mixture to a boil, and simmer until thickened to a jammy consistency, about 3 minutes. Stir in the jalapeño and salt to taste. (See Tip.)

MAKE THE BURGERS: Preheat the grill to medium-high. In a large bowl, combine the ground turkey breast and thigh, the apple, 1 teaspoon salt, and ½ teaspoon pepper. Mix gently to combine ingredients. (Don't overwork or meat could become tough.) Shape the mixture into 4 burgers. Brush both sides of the burgers and the mushroom caps with olive oil. Season the mushroom caps on both sides with salt and pepper to taste.

Arrange the burgers on the grill. Cover and cook for 5 to 6 minutes. Flip the burgers, then arrange the mushroom caps on the grill, stem side down. Cover and cook until the burgers reach an internal temperature of 160°F on an instant-read thermometer, 5 to 6 more minutes. Flip the mushrooms after 4 minutes, then cook for 2 to 3 minutes on the other side. Remove the mushrooms from the grill when they are lightly charred and tender but not overcooked.

Serve: Place a burger on each mushroom cap. Top each burger with a bacon strip, then spoon on the tomato jam and arrange the avocado slices on top.

TIP: The jam can be made up to a week ahead and stored in the fridge in an airtight container.

ORIGINAL WHOLE30 DINNERS

CATALAN-STYLE STEW

SERVES 4 • PREP: 15 MINUTES • COOK: 40 MINUTES + 15 MINUTES SLOW-RELEASE TIME •
TOTAL: 1 HOUR 10 MINUTES

2 slices Whole30-compatible bacon, cut into bite-sized pieces

1½ pounds boneless beef or lamb stew meat, cubed

1 medium onion, chopped

1 large parsnip (see Tip, page 157) or 2 medium carrots, chopped

3 garlic cloves, minced

1 (14.5-ounce) can diced fire-roasted tomatoes

1¾ cups Whole30-compatible beef broth

2 tablespoons red wine vinegar

1 tablespoon tomato paste

1 ounce 100% cacao (see Tip, page 157)

1 tablespoon chopped fresh thyme

1 tablespoon chopped fresh rosemary

2 strips orange peel (2 inches long and 1 inch wide)

1 teaspoon smoked paprika

1 cinnamon stick (about 2 inches)

½ teaspoon black pepper, plus more to taste

1 tablespoon Whole30-compatible instant tapioca (small balls), crushed

Salt

Chopped fresh Italian parsley

Chopped or sliced almonds, toasted

Estofado de Ternera a la Catalana is a hearty beef stew from the region of Catalonia, in northeastern Spain. Two distinctive ingredients—cinnamon and orange—infuse it with flavor. Serve as is or over Quick Cauliflower Rice (page 189).

In a 4- to 6-quart multifunction electric pressure cooker, cook the bacon on the sauté setting until crisp. Remove the bacon, leaving 1 tablespoon drippings in the cooker pot. Reserve any remaining drippings.

Pat the meat dry with a paper towel. Brown half the meat in the drippings in the cooker pot. Transfer to a bowl and repeat with the remaining meat, adding additional drippings if needed. Place the meat in the bowl.

Add any remaining drippings (or add extra-virgin olive oil to equal 1 teaspoon) to the cooker pot. Add the onion and sauté in the hot fat for 2 minutes. Add the parsnip and garlic and cook 3 minutes more, or until the onion is tender, stirring occasionally. Add the bacon and meat to the cooker pot, then add the tomatoes, broth, vinegar, tomato paste, cacao, thyme, rosemary, orange peel, paprika, cinnamon stick, and ½ teaspoon pepper. Set the pressure cooker to high pressure for 15 minutes.

Let the pressure cooker stand for 15 minutes to release the pressure naturally, then quick-release any remaining pressure. Open the lid and stir in the tapioca until mostly dissolved and stew is thickened slightly (some small pieces of tapioca may soften but not dissolve completely).

Season to taste with salt and additional pepper. Remove the orange peel and cinnamon stick. Ladle the stew into bowls and top with the parsley and almonds.

(continued)

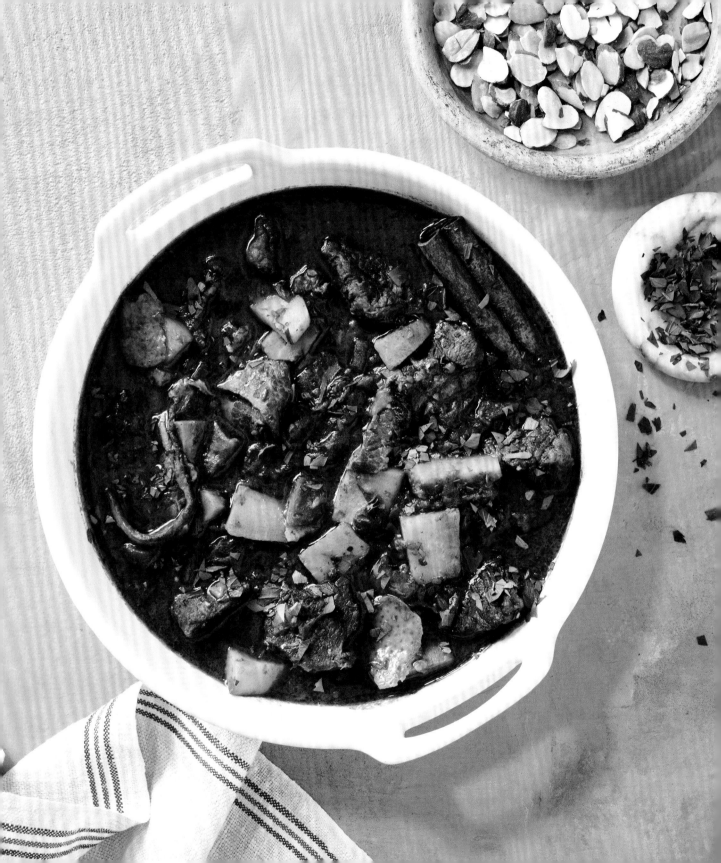

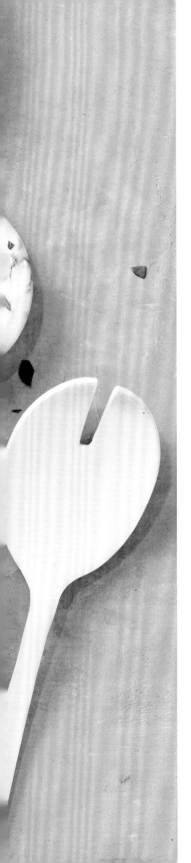

STOVETOP DIRECTIONS: Prepare as directed, using a Dutch oven on medium-high heat to cook the bacon, brown the meat, and cook the onion, parsnip, and garlic. Return the bacon and meat to the pot with the onion, parsnip, and garlic, then add the remaining stew ingredients. Bring the stew to a boil, then reduce the heat to low and simmer, covered, for 2 hours, or until the meat is very tender. Stir in the tapioca and continue as directed.

TIP: This stew is full of flavor right out of the pot, but you can also make it 24 hours ahead, then cool and refrigerate.

Larger parsnips can have a tough, woody core in the center, which should be removed before roasting. After peeling, trim the top and bottom of the parsnip, then cut it in half (crosswise, not lengthwise). Working with the largest piece, stand the chunk up on its base—you'll see the core running down the middle. Cut each chunk into quarters. Then, using a paring knife, trim the core sections away and discard.

This recipe calls for one ounce of a 100% cacao bar. You can find unsweetened 100% cacao from popular brands like Lindt, Alter Eco, and Ghirardelli. If you can't find an unsweetened cacao bar, you can substitute with 3 tablespoons of 100% cacao powder combined with 1 tablespoon of melted coconut oil.

CURRIED PINEAPPLE AND PORK FRIED "RICE"

SERVES 2 • PREP: 25 MINUTES • COOK: 10 MINUTES • TOTAL: 35 MINUTES

⅓ cup whole raw cashews

8 ounces boneless pork tenderloin, sliced into bite-sized strips

2 teaspoons curry powder

Salt

1 tablespoon ghee, Clarified Butter (page 229), or avocado oil

3 garlic cloves, minced

1 cup trimmed and halved snow peas or ½ cup thawed frozen green peas

½ cup chopped red bell pepper

3 green onions, thinly sliced (green and white parts)

1 (10- to 12-ounce) package frozen cauliflower rice

1 cup cubed fresh pineapple or drained canned pineapple chunks packed in juice, reserving 2 tablespoons juice

¼ cup chopped dried apricots, golden raisins, or pitted dates

2 tablespoons Whole30-compatible fish sauce

2 tablespoon coconut aminos

⅛ to ¼ teaspoon red pepper flakes

2 tablespoons chopped fresh cilantro, Thai basil, or sweet basil

Quick to fix, filling, and flavorful, this colorful dish gets hints of heat from the red pepper flakes, sweetness from the pineapple and apricots, and savory saltiness from the coconut aminos and fish sauce. Pan-roasted cashews and red bell pepper add a nice crunch.

In a large dry skillet or wok over medium-high heat, toast the cashews until lightly golden, about 2 minutes. Remove from the pan and set aside.

Sprinkle the pork with 1 teaspoon of the curry powder and salt to taste. In the skillet or wok, heat the ghee over medium-high heat. Add the pork and garlic and stir-fry for 2 minutes. Stir in the snow peas, bell pepper, and green onions. Cook 2 minutes more. Stir in the remaining teaspoon curry powder, the cauliflower rice, pineapple (and pineapple juice if using canned), apricots, fish sauce, coconut aminos, and red pepper flakes. Cook and stir 2 minutes, or until heated through. Stir in the cashews and cilantro and serve immediately.

TIP: Add a dash of toasted sesame oil and a squeeze of lemon or orange juice just before serving to boost the flavors even more.

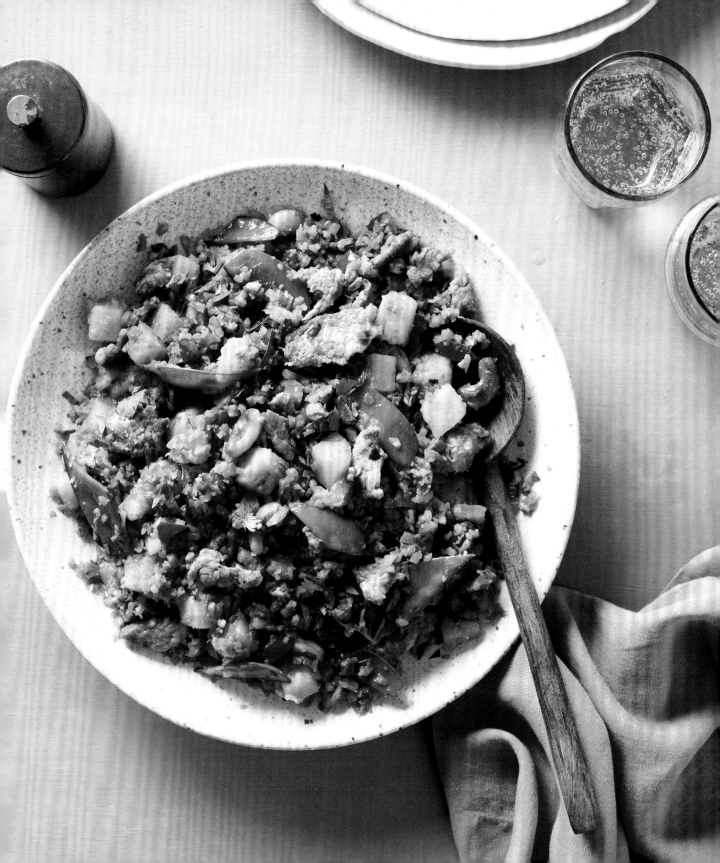

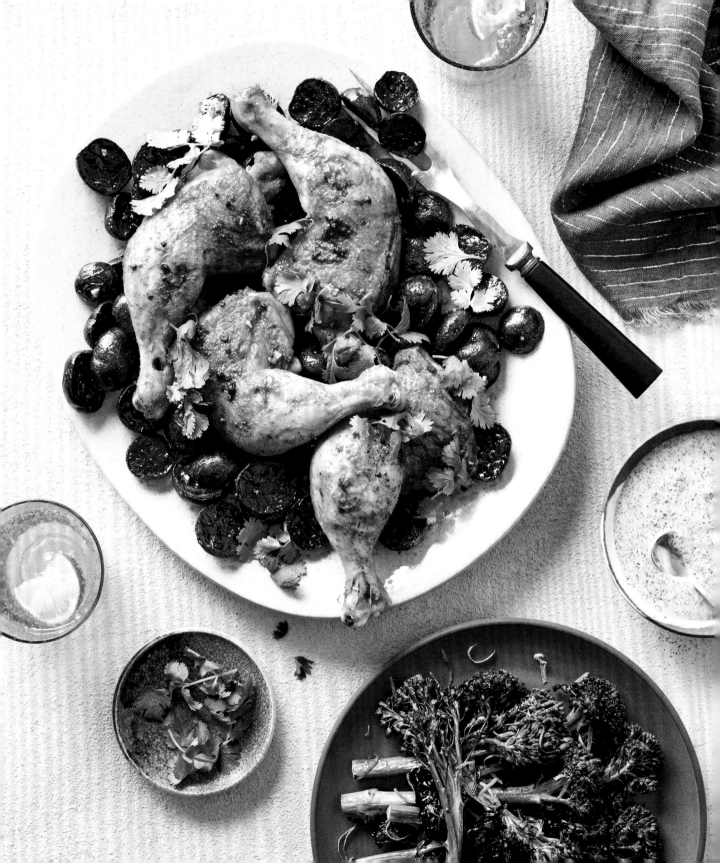

PERUVIAN-INSPIRED ROAST CHICKEN AND POTATOES WITH GREEN SAUCE AND BROCCOLINI

SERVES 4 • PREP: 20 MINUTES • ROAST: 35 MINUTES • TOTAL: 55 MINUTES

FOR THE CHICKEN AND POTATOES

Juice and grated zest of 1 lime

3 tablespoons extra-virgin olive oil

3 garlic cloves, minced

1 tablespoon ground cumin

1 teaspoon smoked paprika or sweet paprika

¾ teaspoon salt

4 chicken leg quarters (attached drumstick and thigh)

1½ pounds baby purple Peruvian potatoes (or baby potato medley), halved

1 teaspoon dried oregano, crushed

Black pepper

FOR THE BROCCOLINI

2 bunches fresh broccolini

1 teaspoon extra-virgin olive oil or avocado oil

Salt and black pepper

FOR THE GREEN SAUCE

1 cup packed fresh cilantro (leaves and stems)

¼ cup Whole30 Mayo (page 230) or Whole30-compatible mayonnaise

2 tablespoons extra-virgin olive oil

1 tablespoon fresh mint leaves

½ to 1 jalapeño, seeded and coarsely chopped

1 garlic clove, minced

¼ teaspoon salt

Rotisserie chicken and potatoes served with a zippy, herby green sauce is a classic dish in Peruvian cooking. Increase the heat in the green sauce by leaving the pith and seeds in the jalapeño, if desired.

MAKE THE CHICKEN AND POTATOES: Preheat the oven to 400°F. In a small bowl, combine 1 teaspoon of the lime zest, 1 tablespoon of the lime juice (reserve the remaining zest and juice for the green sauce and broccolini), 1 tablespoon of the olive oil, half the garlic, the cumin, paprika, and ½ teaspoon of the salt.

Line a large rimmed baking sheet with parchment. Place the chicken, skin side up, on one side of the pan. Carefully slide your fingertips between the meat and skin of each chicken piece to loosen the skin from the meat. Spoon some of the seasoning mixture under the skin of each piece. Brush any remaining mixture over the chicken.

In a medium bowl, toss the potatoes with the remaining 2 tablespoons olive oil, remaining half of garlic, remaining ¼ teaspoon salt, and the oregano. Season with pepper to taste and arrange skin side down on baking sheet opposite the chicken. Roast until the chicken is no longer pink (180°F on an instant-read thermometer), and the potatoes are browned and tender, about 35 minutes.

MAKE THE BROCCOLINI: Arrange the broccolini in a shallow baking pan lined with parchment. Brush with the olive oil and season with salt and pepper to taste. Roast in the 400°F oven along with the chicken and potatoes for the last 10 to 15 minutes, until just tender and starting to brown on the edges. Sprinkle with any remaining lime zest before serving.

MAKE THE GREEN SAUCE: In a blender, combine the cilantro, mayonnaise, olive oil, mint, 1 tablespoon of the reserved lime juice, the jalapeño, garlic, and salt. Cover and blend until mostly smooth. Transfer to a serving bowl.

Serve: Place the chicken and potatoes on a serving platter. Serve with the green sauce and broccolini.

ROASTED SALMON, ASPARAGUS, AND POTATOES WITH OLIVE-WALNUT VINAIGRETTE

SERVES 2 • PREP: 30 MINUTES • ROAST: 25 MINUTES • TOTAL: 55 MINUTES

FOR THE SALMON AND VEGETABLES

2 tablespoons extra-virgin olive oil

½ teaspoon smoked paprika

½ teaspoon ground coriander

1 teaspoon grated lemon zest

2 teaspoons fresh lemon juice

12 ounces fingerling potatoes, halved lengthwise, or baby Yukon Gold potatoes, quartered

¾ teaspoon salt

½ teaspoon black pepper

2 (6-ounce) salmon fillets, about 1 inch thick

10 to 12 asparagus spears, trimmed

FOR THE VINAIGRETTE

3 tablespoons extra-virgin olive oil

2 tablespoons white wine vinegar

2 tablespoons finely chopped fresh parsley

2 tablespoons finely chopped walnuts, toasted (see Tip)

2 tablespoons finely chopped pitted Kalamata olives

2 tablespoons finely chopped pitted firm green olives, such as Castelvetrano, Picholine, Cerignola, or Manzanilla olives

¼ teaspoon salt

¼ teaspoon black pepper

Buttery salmon, crispy potatoes, and tender asparagus form the center of this simple but company-worthy recipe. The vinaigrette is more like a thick sauce, which pairs beautifully with the rich salmon.

MAKE THE SALMON AND VEGETABLES: Preheat the oven to 425°F. Line a large rimmed baking sheet with parchment.

In a small bowl, stir together 1 tablespoon of the olive oil, the paprika, coriander, and lemon zest and juice; set aside.

In a medium bowl, toss the potatoes with 1½ teaspoons of the olive oil, ¼ teaspoon of the salt, and ⅛ teaspoon of the pepper. Arrange the potatoes on one side of the sheet pan, being careful not to crowd the pieces. Roast for 15 minutes.

In the same bowl, toss the asparagus with the remaining 1½ teaspoons olive oil, ¼ teaspoon of the salt, and ⅛ teaspoon of the pepper.

Remove the pan from the oven. Stir the potatoes. Place the salmon fillets opposite the potatoes. Brush the seasoned olive oil mixture over the tops and sides of the fillets. Season with the remaining ¼ teaspoon salt and ¼ teaspoon pepper. Add the asparagus to the pan between the salmon and the potatoes. Roast until the potatoes are browned and crisp, asparagus is tender, and the salmon is cooked through, 10 to 12 minutes.

MAKE THE VINAIGRETTE: While the salmon and vegetables finish cooking, in a small jar with a lid, combine the olive oil, vinegar, parsley, walnuts, olives, salt, and pepper. Shake until emulsified.

Serve: Divide the salmon fillets, asparagus, and potatoes between 2 plates. Spoon the vinaigrette over all.

> **TIP:** To toast walnuts, spread them on a rimmed baking sheet and bake in a 375°F oven for 6 to 8 minutes, or until lightly browned, stirring once.

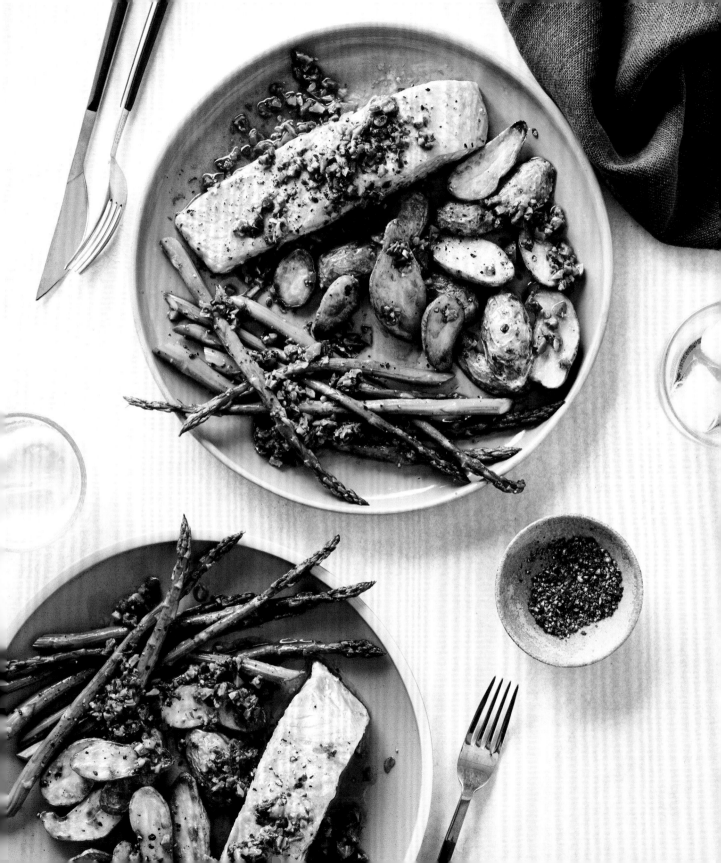

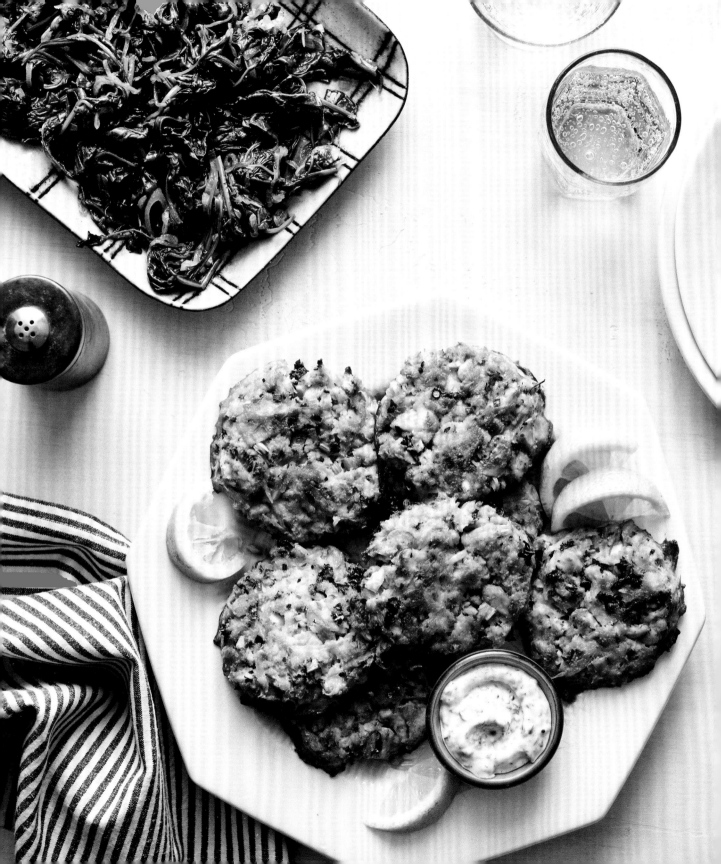

SALMON CAKES WITH LEMON-CAPER MAYO AND SHALLOT-SAUTÉED SPINACH

SERVES 2 • PREP: 30 MINUTES • BAKE/COOK: 30 MINUTES • TOTAL: 60 MINUTES

FOR THE MAYO

- ¼ cup Whole30 Mayo (page 230) or Whole30-compatible mayonnaise
- 1 tablespoon capers, drained, rinsed, and coarsely chopped
- 1½ teaspoons fresh lemon juice
- 1½ teaspoons lemon zest
- ⅛ teaspoon salt
- ⅛ teaspoon black pepper

FOR THE SALMON CAKES

- Extra-virgin olive oil spray
- 3 (6-ounce) cans boneless wild-caught salmon, drained
- 1 medium Yukon Gold potato, peeled and shredded (see Tip)
- 1 large egg, lightly beaten
- ⅓ cup finely diced celery
- ¼ cup finely diced red onion
- 1 teaspoon Whole30-compatible Dijon mustard
- ¼ cup superfine almond flour
- 2 teaspoons grated lemon zest
- 1 tablespoon chopped fresh chives
- 2 tablespoons chopped fresh parsley
- ½ teaspoon salt
- ¼ teaspoon black pepper

It's no secret that lemon and salmon are fast friends, so there's lemon in the mayonnaise, lemon in the salmon-cake mix, and a squeeze of fresh lemon right before serving. Lightly spraying or glazing the salmon cakes with oil before baking gives them a lightly crisp crust. Consider making a double batch, as these cakes make a quick and delicious lunch the next day.

MAKE THE MAYO: In a small bowl, stir together the mayonnaise, capers, lemon juice and zest, salt, and pepper. Cover and refrigerate until serving time.

MAKE THE SALMON CAKES: Preheat the oven to 425°F. Line a large rimmed baking sheet with parchment or foil. Spray with cooking spray.

Crumble the salmon into a large bowl. Add the potato, egg, celery, onion, mustard, almond flour, lemon zest, chives, parsley, salt, and pepper. Stir gently until all ingredients are well combined. Scoop portions of the mixture into a ⅓-cup measuring cup, pressing on the mixture to compact it slightly, then turn out onto the baking sheet. Flatten and shape the patty with your hands. Repeat with remaining mixture, flattening and shaping to get patties of the same size and thickness. Spray lightly with olive oil spray.

Bake for 20 minutes, then gently turn the patties with a spatula. Spray the tops lightly with olive oil spray and return to the oven. Bake until golden brown, about 10 more minutes.

(continued)

FOR THE SPINACH AND SERVING

1 tablespoon extra-virgin olive oil

1 large shallot, thinly sliced

2 (5-ounce) packages baby spinach

¼ teaspoon salt

¼ teaspoon black pepper

Lemon wedges, for serving

MAKE THE SPINACH: While the salmon cakes are baking, heat the olive oil in a very large skillet over medium heat until shimmering. Add the shallot and cook, stirring frequently, until softened and lightly browned, 3 to 4 minutes. Add the spinach in handfuls, tossing with tongs, and cook just until wilted, 4 to 5 minutes. Season with salt and pepper.

Serve: Place the salmon cakes on serving plates and add the mayonnaise and spinach; arrange the lemon wedges alongside.

TIP: To make quick work of your meal prep, use 1 cup of refrigerated shredded potatoes instead of shredding a whole potato.

If using frozen hash brown potatoes, thaw them and squeeze out as much water as possible using a clean kitchen towel.

SEA BASS WITH APPLE-POMEGRANATE SLAW AND BUTTERNUT SQUASH PUREE

SERVES 2 • PREP: 15 MINUTES • COOK: 10 MINUTES • GRILL: 10 MINUTES • TOTAL: 35 MINUTES

FOR THE SQUASH

4 cups cubed butternut squash

2 tablespoons ghee, Clarified Butter (page 229), or coconut oil

½ teaspoon salt

¼ teaspoon black pepper

FOR THE SLAW AND FISH

1 small crisp, tart apple (such as Granny Smith or Pink Lady), cored and cut into 2-inch julienne (matchstick) pieces

⅓ cup pomegranate arils (seeds, see Tip) or quartered red grapes

¼ cup Whole30-compatible ginger kombucha, or apple cider with a splash of apple cider vinegar

1 tablespoon chopped fresh mint or basil

¼ teaspoon Whole30-compatible wasabi powder or Aleppo pepper flakes

Salt and black pepper

2 (5- to 6-ounce) fillets sea bass, cod, or snapper, about 1 inch thick, skin left on

Extra-virgin olive oil

A crisp slaw dressed with ginger kombucha, mint, and wasabi makes a refreshing side for rich and buttery sea bass served on a bed of creamy pureed butternut squash. It's restaurant-level fancy, but the meal comes together in just 35 minutes.

MAKE THE SQUASH: Place the squash in a steamer basket and put into a large saucepan. Fill the saucepan with water to just below the bottom of the basket. Bring the water to a boil, reduce the heat, cover, and steam until the squash is tender, about 10 minutes.

Drain and return the squash to the pan. Add the ghee, salt, and pepper. Use an immersion blender to puree (or transfer to a food processor to puree). If the mixture is too thick to puree, stir in a little coconut milk or chicken broth until desired consistency. Cover and keep warm.

MAKE THE SLAW AND FISH: While the squash is cooking, toss the apple, pomegranate, kombucha, mint, and wasabi powder together in a medium bowl. Season to taste with salt and pepper. Cover and set aside.

Preheat a grill to medium. Measure the thickness of the fish. Brush the fish with olive oil on all sides. Season to taste with salt and pepper. Grill the fish on the rack of the uncovered grill directly over medium heat for 8 to 10 minutes, or until the fish begins to flake easily when tested with a fork, turning once (allow about 5 minutes per ½ inch thickness of fish).

Serve: Divide the squash puree between 2 dinner plates. Top each with a fish fillet. With a slotted spoon, place the apple-pomegranate slaw next to the fish and squash.

(continued)

BROILING DIRECTIONS: To broil the fish, prepare as directed, but place the fish fillets on a large foil-lined baking sheet and broil for 8 to 10 minutes, or until the fish just flakes when tested with a fork.

> **TIP:** There are two tricks for removing pomegranate seeds from the fruit's flesh. One is to cut the pomegranate into quarters, then submerge them in a big bowl of cool water. Rub the seeds with your thumbs underwater until they separate from the flesh. Most of the light membrane will float to the top, while the heavier seeds will sink to the bottom of the bowl. The other trick is to "spank" the pomegranate. Cut the fruit in half, then cup it in your hand seed side down over a bowl. Firmly whack the back of the fruit with a wooden spatula or spoon. Use the spoon over the entire surface of the fruit, until all the seeds have dropped out. Pick off any white membrane left on the seeds.

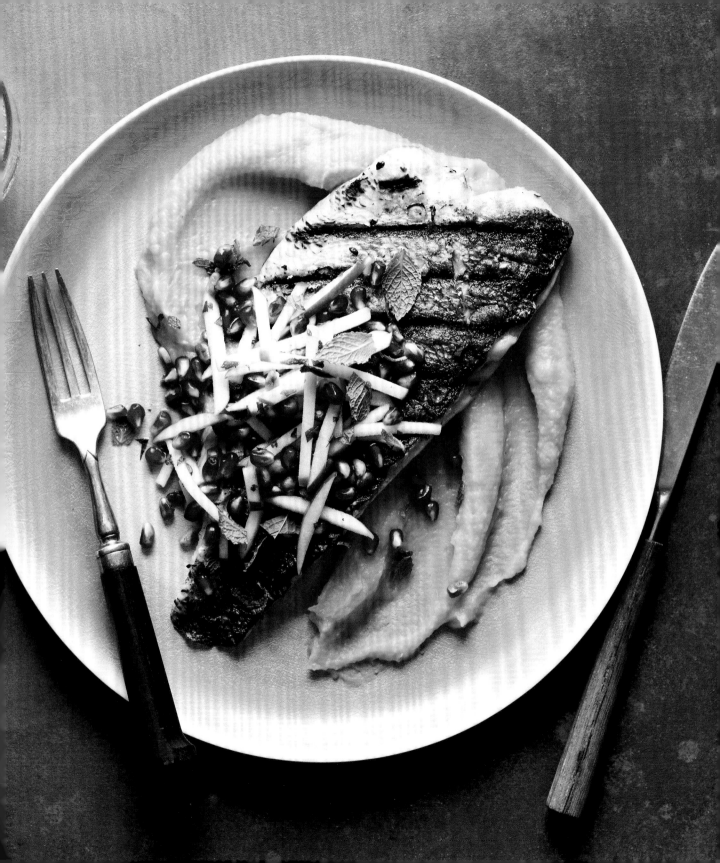

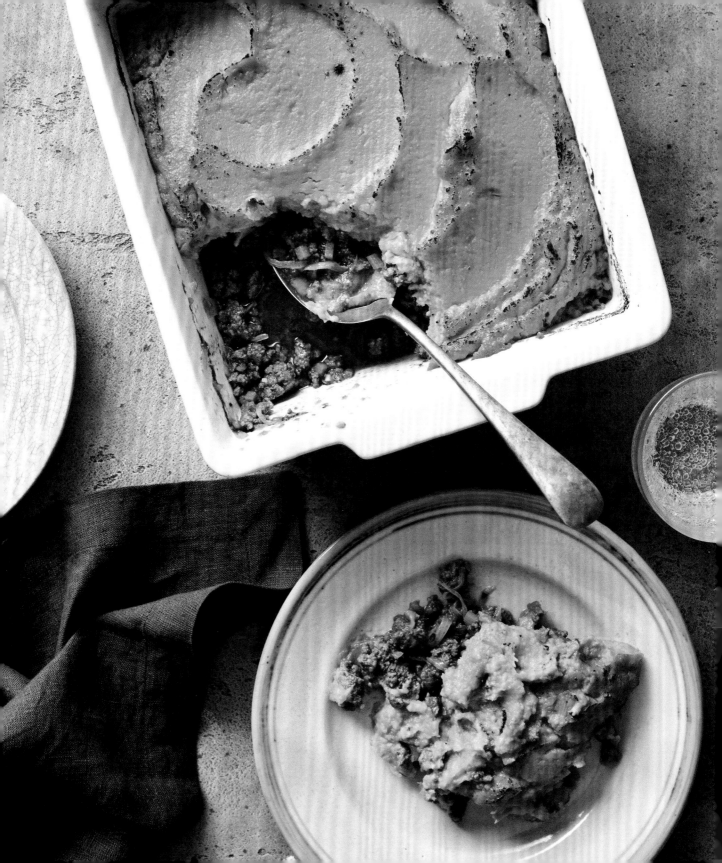

SHEPHERD'S PIE

SERVES 3 TO 4 • PREP: 20 MINUTES • COOK: 25 MINUTES • BAKE: 25 MINUTES
+ 10 MINUTES RESTING • TOTAL: 1 HOUR 20 MINUTES

2 medium sweet potatoes, peeled and cut into large chunks

2 tablespoons ghee or Clarified Butter (page 229)

½ cup full-fat canned coconut milk

1½ teaspoons salt

¾ teaspoon black pepper

1 tablespoon extra-virgin olive oil

2 shallots, sliced

2 celery stalks, finely chopped

1 medium carrot, peeled and finely chopped

1 pound ground beef, lamb, or bison

2 garlic cloves, minced

2 teaspoons chopped fresh thyme, or ½ teaspoon dried thyme

1 tablespoon tomato paste

1 cup Whole30-compatible beef broth

1 tablespoon potato starch (see Tip)

This modest update to the shepherd's pie in the first Whole30 book shakes things up in a delicious way. Shallots step in for the original onion, a little bit of tomato paste is added for flavor, and a slurry made with beef broth and potato starch helps create a bubbly gravy.

Preheat the oven to 375°F. Place the sweet potatoes in a large saucepan and cover with cold water. Bring to a boil over high heat, then reduce the heat and cook until the potatoes are fork-tender, 10 to 15 minutes.

Drain the potatoes and return them to the pan. Add the ghee, coconut milk, ½ teaspoon of the salt, and ¼ teaspoon of the pepper. Mash with a potato masher or blend with an immersion blender until creamy; set aside.

In a large skillet, heat the olive oil over medium heat. Add the shallots, celery, and carrot and cook, stirring frequently, until the vegetables are softened, about 5 minutes. Add the ground meat of choice and the garlic. Cook, stirring often, until meat is browned, 7 to 10 minutes. Season with the remaining 1 teaspoon salt, ½ teaspoon pepper, and the thyme. Add the tomato paste and cook, stirring constantly, until the tomato paste begins to darken, about 1 minute.

In a small bowl or measuring cup, stir together the beef broth and potato starch until smooth. Add to the meat mixture and cook, stirring constantly, until slightly thickened, 1 to 2 minutes.

Spoon the meat mixture evenly into a 2-quart casserole or 8-inch square glass baking dish. Carefully spread the mashed sweet potatoes over the top. Bake until bubbling, about 25 minutes. (See Tip.) Let stand 10 minutes before serving.

TIP: To get the sweet potato topping lightly browned and caramelized in a few places, place it under the broiler for just 1 to 2 minutes—and watch carefully to avoid burning. If you don't have potato starch, you can substitute 2 tablespoons of tapioca starch or ½ tablespoon of arrowroot powder.

BALSAMIC-GLAZED PORK TENDERLOIN WITH ROASTED GRAPES, BRUSSELS SPROUTS, AND WALNUTS

SERVES 3 • PREP: 20 MINUTES • ROAST: 30 MINUTES • TOTAL: 50 MINUTES

Avocado oil cooking spray

½ cup balsamic vinegar

1 tablespoon Whole30-compatible whole-grain or Dijon mustard

1 pound boneless pork tenderloin, trimmed

1 pound Brussels sprouts, trimmed and quartered

1 tablespoon extra-virgin olive oil

Salt and black pepper

8 ounces red grape clusters

½ cup coarsely chopped walnuts

Just a few ingredients add up to a dish that is so much greater than the sum of its parts. While it's a welcome end to the day any time of year, it seems especially right for a cool fall or winter night. With only 20 minutes of prep time, this might be your new weeknight staple.

Preheat the oven to 425°F. Lightly coat a large rimmed baking sheet with cooking spray.

Whisk together ¼ cup of the vinegar and the mustard in a shallow dish (such as a pie plate). Add the tenderloin, turn to coat, and marinate for 10 minutes.

Meanwhile, toss the Brussels sprouts with 2 teaspoons of the olive oil, and season to taste with salt and pepper. Gently coat the grape clusters with the remaining teaspoon oil and sprinkle with some salt and pepper.

Remove the pork from the marinade (reserve excess marinade for basting) and season to taste with salt and pepper. Roast the tenderloin and Brussels sprouts for 10 minutes. Remove the pan from the oven, brush the pork with some of the reserved marinade, then flip it over and brush the other side.

Add the grapes and walnuts to the baking sheet alongside the tenderloin and Brussels sprouts. Return the baking sheet to the oven and continue to roast until the pork reaches an internal temperature of 160°F on an instant-read thermometer, about 10 minutes more. The Brussels sprouts should be starting to brown and the grapes starting to shrivel.

Let the tenderloin rest for 5 minutes. While tenderloin rests, simmer the remaining ¼ cup balsamic vinegar in a small skillet over medium-high heat. Cook until glaze is syrupy, about 5 minutes. (Watch carefully—it can overreduce and quickly burn.)

Slice the pork and plate with the Brussels sprouts and grape clusters. Drizzle the balsamic glaze over all.

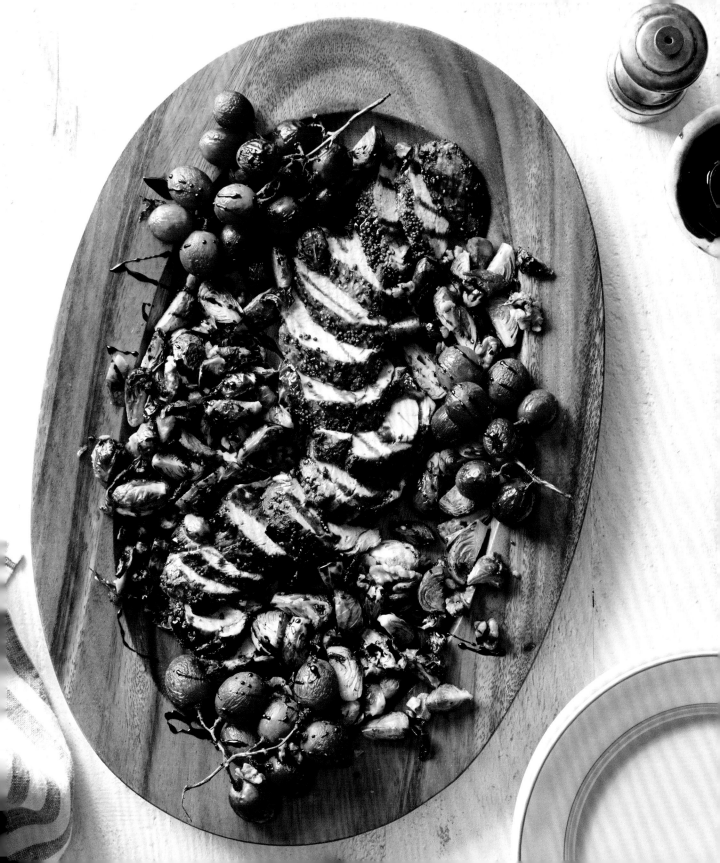

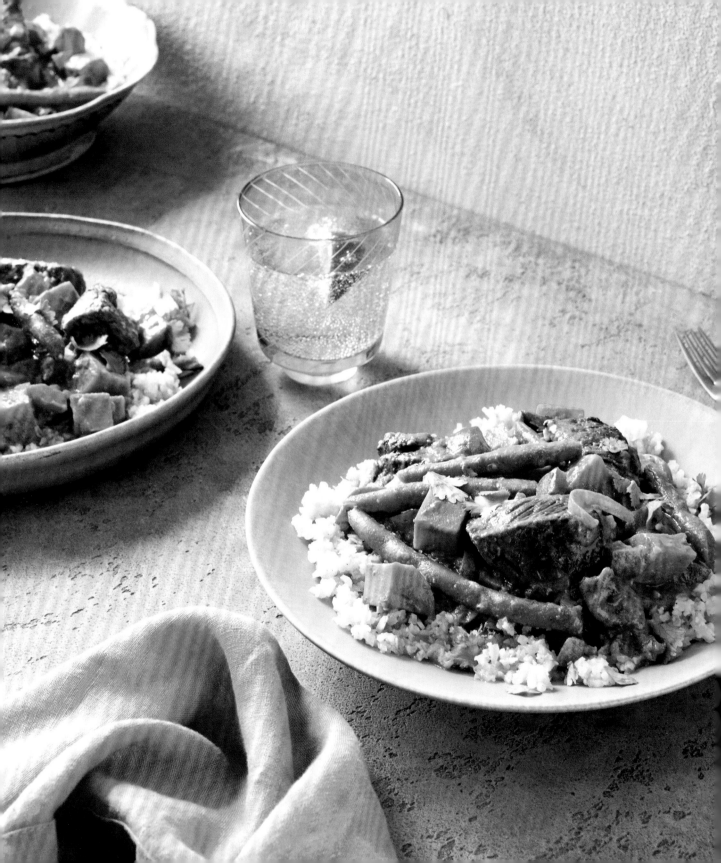

CURRIED BEEF WITH SWEET POTATOES

SERVES 2 TO 3 • PREP: 25 MINUTES • COOK: 30 MINUTES • TOTAL: 55 MINUTES

FOR THE CURRY

1 pound boneless ribeye steak, trimmed, cut into 2-inch cubes

Salt and black pepper

2 tablespoons coconut oil

1 cinnamon stick

8 whole cloves

1 small onion, thinly sliced

1 bay leaf

2 tablespoons peeled and minced fresh ginger

3 garlic cloves, minced

2 teaspoons curry powder

½ teaspoon red pepper flakes

2 cups peeled and cubed sweet potatoes

1 (13.5-ounce) can full-fat coconut milk

1 (14.5-ounce) can diced tomatoes

4 ounces fresh green beans, trimmed

½ cup diced red bell pepper

Juice of ½ lime

Chopped fresh cilantro

FOR THE CAULIFLOWER RICE

1 teaspoon coconut oil

2 teaspoons peeled and minced fresh ginger

⅛ teaspoon Chinese five-spice powder

1 (10- to 12-ounce) bag frozen cauliflower rice

Salt

Tender cubes of beef, sweet potatoes, tomatoes, green beans, and red bell peppers are simmered together with coconut milk and spices. Serve over a five-spice–infused cauliflower rice to create this colorful one-pot wonder.

MAKE THE CURRY: Season steak cubes to taste with salt and pepper. In a large skillet, heat the coconut oil over medium-high heat. Add the cinnamon stick and cloves and fry the spices, stirring frequently, until the cloves swell and the cinnamon unfurls, about 2 minutes. Remove the spices and discard.

Add the steak cubes to the skillet and sear on all sides (do not cook through), then transfer to a plate. Add the onion and bay leaf, and cook, stirring occasionally and scraping up any brown bits from the bottom of the pan, until the onion begins to brown, 6 to 8 minutes. Add the ginger, garlic, curry powder, and red pepper flakes. Cook until fragrant, 1 minute, then stir in the sweet potatoes, coconut milk, and tomatoes. Cover the pan, reduce the heat to medium, and simmer until the potatoes are tender, about 15 minutes.

MAKE THE CAULIFLOWER RICE: While the curry simmers, melt the coconut oil in a medium saucepan over medium heat, then add the ginger and five-spice powder. Cook 1 minute, then add the cauliflower. Cover and simmer until tender but not mushy, 5 to 6 minutes. Remove from the heat and keep warm.

Finish the curry and serve: Add the steak cubes and any accumulated juices, the green beans, and the red pepper to the curry. Cover and simmer until the vegetables are crisp tender, about 5 minutes.

Drizzle the curry with the lime juice and sprinkle with the cilantro. Serve the curry over the cauliflower rice.

ROASTED SPATCHCOCK CHICKEN WITH KABOCHA SQUASH SALAD

SERVES 4 • PREP: 20 MINUTES • ROAST: 50 MINUTES • TOTAL: 1 HOUR 10 MINUTES

1 whole (3- to 4-pound) chicken

¼ cup extra-virgin olive oil

2 teaspoons chopped fresh rosemary or sage

2 teaspoons chopped fresh thyme

Juice and grated zest of 1 lemon

1 teaspoon salt

1 teaspoon black pepper

1 kabocha squash, seeded and cut into wedges (see Tip)

3 tablespoons sherry vinegar

1 tablespoon minced shallot

1 teaspoon Whole30-compatible Dijon mustard

1 tablespoon walnut oil (optional)

4 cups baby kale or arugula

½ cup chopped walnuts, toasted (see Tip, page 162)

TIP: Kabocha squash—also called Japanese pumpkin—is a sweet, orange-fleshed winter squash. If you can't find it, you can substitute acorn or delicata squash.

When you're craving a cozy roast chicken but don't have time to cook a whole bird, spatchcock it! This simple technique of removing the backbone and flattening the bird helps the chicken cook faster and more evenly. Plus, it's just fun to say.

Preheat the oven to 400°F. Line a large rimmed baking sheet with parchment.

To spatchcock the chicken, remove any giblets from the cavity and pat the chicken dry with a paper towel. Place the chicken on your work surface breast side down, with the neck facing you. Using a pair of strong kitchen shears, cut down both sides of the backbone, close to the spine. Remove and discard the backbone. Flip the bird over and open it like a book. Then use your hands to press along the breastbone to flatten the chicken. Place the chicken on the baking sheet, breast side up.

In a bowl, stir together 1 tablespoon of the olive oil, the rosemary, thyme, lemon juice and zest, salt, and pepper. Rub the paste all over the chicken, then roast the chicken for 30 minutes.

Meanwhile, toss the squash with 1 tablespoon of the olive oil. Season to taste with salt and pepper.

After 30 minutes, remove the chicken from the oven and arrange the squash on the baking sheet. Return the pan to the oven and continue roasting until the squash is browned and tender and the chicken registers 170°F on an instant-read thermometer inserted in the thigh, 20 to 25 minutes. Let the chicken and squash rest for 10 minutes before carving the chicken and plating.

In a small bowl, whisk together the vinegar, shallot, and mustard, then drizzle in the remaining 2 tablespoons olive oil and the walnut oil (if using).

Once the chicken has been carved, arrange the kale on a large platter and top with the squash wedges; sprinkle on the walnuts. Place the chicken on top of the kale. Drizzle the vinaigrette over everything and serve.

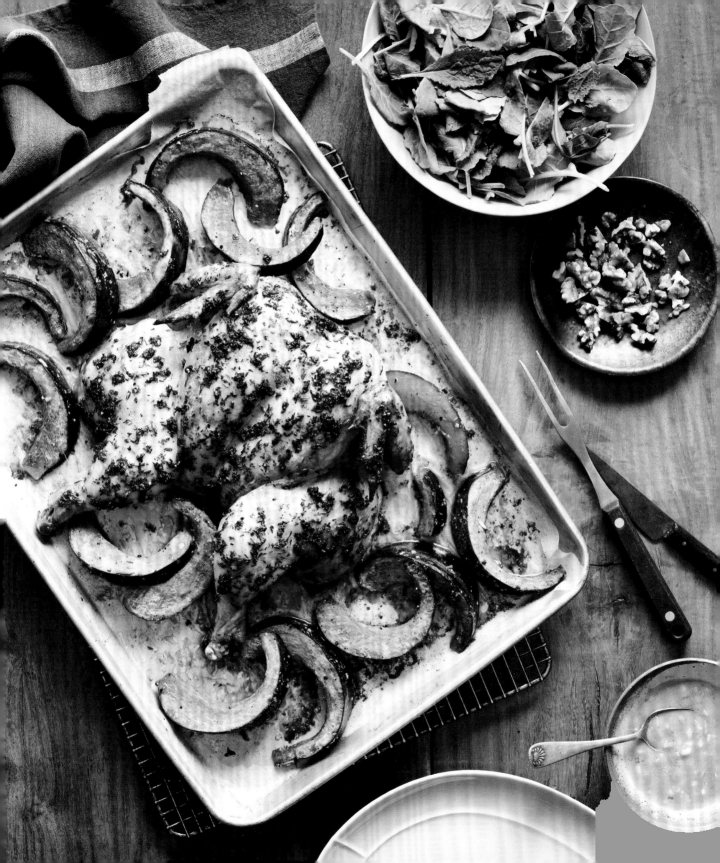

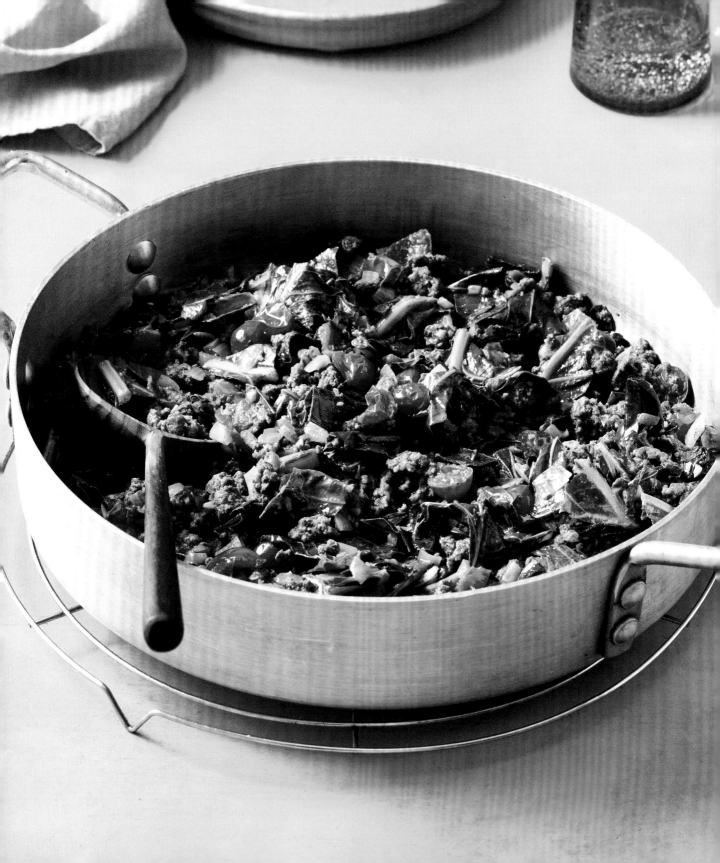

SOMALI-INSPIRED BEEF AND COLLARDS SAUTÉ

SERVES 3 TO 4 • PREP: 25 MINUTES • COOK: 20 MINUTES • TOTAL: 45 MINUTES

FOR THE SPICE BLEND

1 teaspoon ground cumin

1 teaspoon ground coriander

1 teaspoon salt

½ teaspoon ground ginger

½ teaspoon ground cinnamon

½ teaspoon black pepper

½ teaspoon ground turmeric

¼ teaspoon ground cloves

FOR THE SAUTÉ

1 tablespoon ghee, Clarified Butter (page 229), or extra-virgin olive oil

1 small yellow onion, chopped

2 garlic cloves, minced

1 jalapeño or serrano chile, minced (and seeded, if desired)

1 pound ground beef

1 bunch collard greens (about 8 leaves), center ribs removed, leaves cut into 1-inch ribbons (see Tip)

1 (10-ounce) package grape tomatoes, quartered

1 tablespoon fresh lemon juice

Salt and black pepper

The spice blend for this quick beef and collards dish is inspired by the popular Somali spice blend xawaash (pronounced ha-wash). The word xawaash is from the Arabic word *hawaij*, which simply means "mixture." Like garam masala, the exact blend varies from cook to cook, but most versions feature a combination of warmly flavored spices like cumin, coriander, cloves, ginger, and cinnamon. If desired, serve the sauté over Quick Cauliflower Rice (page 189).

MAKE THE SPICE BLEND: In a small bowl, stir together the cumin, coriander, salt, ginger, cinnamon, pepper, turmeric, and cloves; set aside.

MAKE THE SAUTÉ: In a large skillet, heat the ghee over medium heat until shimmering. Add the onion and cook, stirring frequently, until softened, 4 to 5 minutes. Add the garlic and jalapeño and cook, stirring constantly, until fragrant, about 1 minute.

Add the beef and spice blend, and cook, stirring frequently until browned, 6 to 8 minutes. Add the collard greens and tomatoes, and cook, stirring frequently, until collards are wilted, 3 to 4 minutes, being careful not to crush the tomatoes.

Stir in the lemon juice and season to taste with salt and pepper.

> **TIP:** If you can't find fresh collard greens, you can use frozen. Rinse them under cool water first to remove any ice particles. Watch the collards carefully as you cook—frozen veggies tend to cook faster than fresh.

TANDOORI-SPICED FISH WITH APPLE-COCONUT RAITA AND COCONUT-CAULIFLOWER RICE

SERVES 4 • PREP: 30 MINUTES + 1 HOUR MARINATING • COOK: 10 MINUTES •
BROIL: 10 MINUTES • TOTAL: 1 HOUR 50 MINUTES

FOR THE FISH

½ cup Whole30-compatible plain coconut yogurt

2 tablespoons peeled and grated fresh ginger (see Tip, page 130)

3 garlic cloves, minced

1 tablespoon fresh lime juice

1 tablespoon minced seeded jalapeño

2 teaspoons mild curry powder

1 teaspoon smoked paprika

½ teaspoon salt

4 (5- to 6-ounces each) mild fish fillets (cod, snapper, halibut, mahi-mahi), skin removed

Avocado oil cooking spray

FOR THE RAITA

½ cup unsweetened coconut flakes

1 Granny Smith apple, cored and diced

1 small jalapeño, seeded and chopped

1 bunch fresh cilantro

¼ teaspoon ground cumin

Juice of ½ lime

Pinch of salt

3 tablespoons Whole30-compatible plain coconut yogurt

The flavors in this dish are next level. The fish soaks up the goodness of the seasoned yogurt marinade. Once broiled, it's served on top of creamy coconut-cauliflower rice with a spicy, tart, cooling raita (a classic Indian side dish).

MARINATE THE FISH: In a shallow ceramic or wide glass dish (such as a pie plate), combine the yogurt, ginger, garlic, lime juice, jalapeño, curry powder, paprika, and salt. Add the fish fillets and coat both sides generously with the yogurt mixture. Cover and let marinate in the refrigerator for at least 1 hour and up to 4 hours. Prepare the raita and cauliflower rice while the fish marinates.

MAKE THE RAITA: In a food processor or blender, combine the coconut, apple, jalapeño, cilantro, cumin, lime juice, and salt. Process until finely minced. Transfer to a serving bowl. Stir in the yogurt. Cover and chill the raita until ready to serve. (Raita is best served within an hour or two of being made.)

MAKE THE CAULIFLOWER RICE: In a large saucepan, melt the coconut oil over medium-high heat. Add the cauliflower rice and salt. Cook, stirring occasionally, for about 5 minutes, then stir in the coconut milk. Simmer about 3 minutes, then finish with the lime juice and cilantro. Remove from the heat and cover to keep warm. If you plan to marinate your fish for longer than an hour, store cooked cauliflower rice in the refrigerator, then reheat just before serving.

(continued)

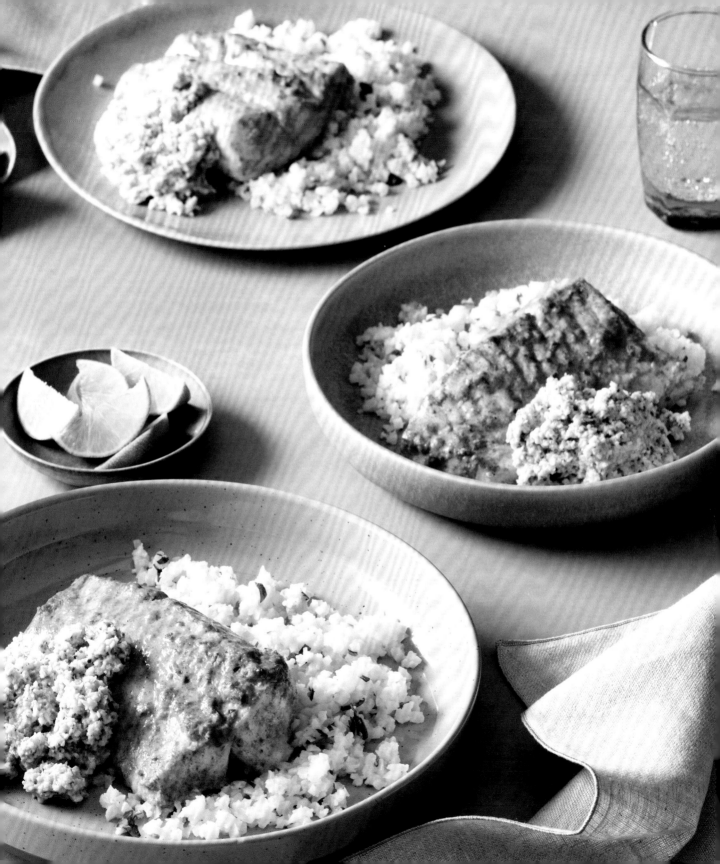

FOR THE CAULIFLOWER RICE

1 tablespoon coconut oil

1 (10- to 12-ounce) package frozen cauliflower rice

½ teaspoon salt

½ cup full-fat canned coconut milk

Juice of ½ lime

Chopped fresh cilantro

COOK THE FISH: Line a large rimmed baking sheet with foil. Spray with cooking spray. Preheat the broiler to high. Scrape off most (but not all) the marinade from the fish; discard any remaining marinade. (See Tip.) Arrange the fillets on the baking sheet and broil until cooked through, 8 to 12 minutes depending on the thickness of the fillets.

Serve: Spoon the coconut-cauliflower rice into shallow serving bowls and top each with a fish fillet. Serve with some raita on the side.

> **TIP:** It may be tempting to leave that delicious marinade on the fish when you pop it into the broiler, but it will start to brown (and then burn). If you do leave a little too much on and notice it starting to blacken the top of the fish, briefly remove fish from the broiler, carefully scrape it off to the side, and resume broiling.

ORIGINAL WHOLE30 SIDES

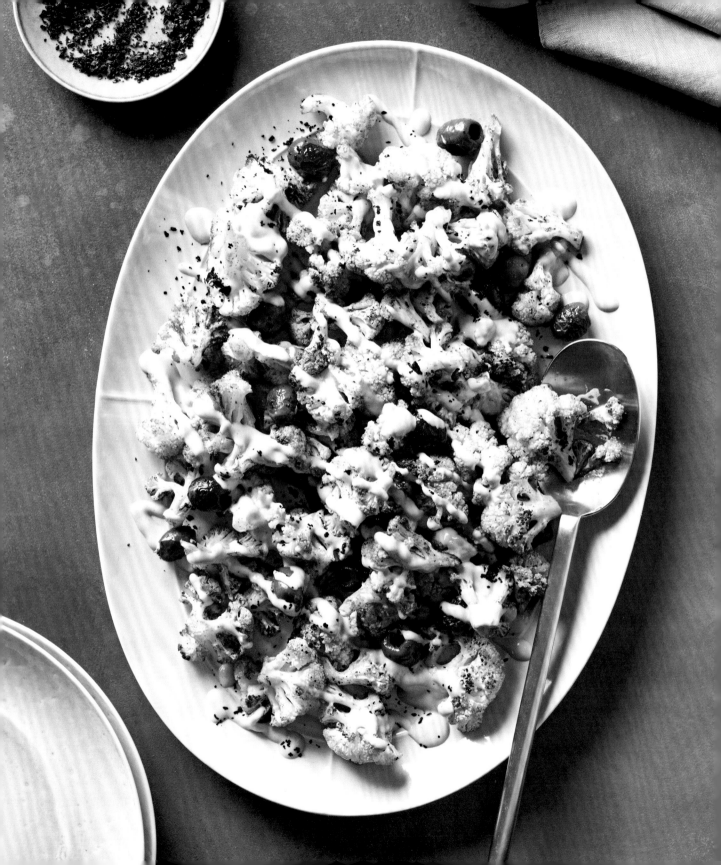

7-SPICE ROASTED CAULIFLOWER
WITH TAHINI SAUCE

SERVES 3 TO 4 • PREP: 20 MINUTES • ROAST: 20 MINUTES • TOTAL: 40 MINUTES

FOR THE CAULIFLOWER

1 head of cauliflower (about 2 pounds), trimmed, cored, and broken into bite-sized florets

2 tablespoons olive oil

1 teaspoon baharat (see Tip)

½ teaspoon salt

½ cup mixed pitted olives

FOR THE TAHINI SAUCE AND SERVING

2 large garlic cloves, crushed

2 tablespoons fresh lemon juice, or more to taste

¼ cup tahini, or more to taste

¼ teaspoon salt, or more to taste

⅛ teaspoon ground cumin, or more to taste

¼ cup ice water, or more as needed

Urfa chile flakes (see Tip) or Aleppo pepper flakes

This roasted cauliflower is seasoned with baharat (the Arabic word for "spices"), also known as "7 spice." Baharat is a warm spice blend widely used in Middle Eastern cuisine. The specific spices used vary by region and even household, but it often includes cumin, coriander, black pepper, cardamom, paprika, cloves, and nutmeg.

MAKE THE CAULIFLOWER: Preheat the oven to 450°F. Line a large rimmed baking sheet with parchment.

In a large bowl, toss together the cauliflower florets and the olive oil. Sprinkle with the baharat and salt. Toss again. Arrange the cauliflower on the baking sheet. Add the olives, then roast until the cauliflower is golden and tender and starting to get browned on the edges, about 20 minutes, stirring once.

MAKE THE TAHINI SAUCE: While the cauliflower roasts, combine the garlic and lemon juice in a medium bowl. Let stand 10 minutes. Remove the garlic and press through a small-mesh strainer to squeeze out as much of the flavorful liquid as possible. Discard the garlic.

Add the ¼ cup tahini, ¼ teaspoon salt, and ⅛ teaspoon cumin to the bowl. Whisk until blended. Add the ice water, 1 tablespoon at a time, whisking after each addition until smooth. If necessary, whisk in a little additional water to achieve a drizzling consistency. Taste and add more tahini, salt, cumin, or lemon juice, if desired.

Serve: Transfer the cauliflower and olives to a serving platter. Drizzle with the tahini sauce. Sprinkle with the Urfa chile flakes. Serve immediately.

> **TIP:** If you can't find baharat, use equal parts paprika, cumin, and cinnamon. Urfa (sometimes called urfa biber) is a Turkish chile that has a dark burgundy color and a wonderful smoky/sweet/sour/fruity flavor with a modest amount of heat. Aleppo pepper flakes add more of a fruity flavor, and a mild level of spice. If you have neither, red pepper flakes will work in a pinch but will add more heat to the dish.

POTATOES AND KALE
IN INDIAN-STYLE BUTTER SAUCE

SERVES 4 • PREP: 15 MINUTES • SLOW COOK: 2 HOURS 30 MINUTES •
TOTAL: 2 HOURS 45 MINUTES

½ (14.5-ounce) can diced tomatoes, undrained (1 cup)

3 garlic cloves, crushed

1½ teaspoons garam masala

1 teaspoon peeled and grated fresh ginger, or ½ teaspoon dried ginger (see Tip, page 130)

½ teaspoon ground turmeric

½ teaspoon salt

¼ teaspoon red pepper flakes

1½ pounds baby Yukon Gold or red potatoes, quartered

1 tablespoon water

4 cups coarsely chopped baby kale

¼ cup full-fat canned coconut milk

3 tablespoons ghee or Clarified Butter (page 229)

2 tablespoons chopped fresh cilantro and/or chopped green onions (green and white parts)

Whether you make this dish in a slow cooker, on the stovetop, or in a pressure cooker, it fills the kitchen with the aroma of Indian spices as it simmers.

In a 3½- to 4-quart slow cooker, stir together the tomatoes, garlic, garam masala, ginger, turmeric, salt, and red pepper flakes. Add the potatoes and drizzle in the water. Cover and cook on high for 2 hours 30 minutes, or until potatoes are tender. Turn off the cooker and stir in the kale. Cover and let stand for 5 minutes.

Stir the coconut milk and ghee into the slightly cooled potato mixture. Transfer to a serving dish and sprinkle with the cilantro.

STOVETOP DIRECTIONS: Prepare as directed, but use a large saucepan to stir together the tomatoes, garlic, garam masala, ginger, turmeric, salt, and red pepper flakes. Add the potatoes and water. Bring to a boil, then reduce the heat and simmer, covered, 10 to 15 minutes, or until potatoes are tender. Remove from the heat and continue as directed.

PRESSURE COOKER DIRECTIONS: In a 6-quart multifunction electric pressure cooker, stir together the tomatoes, garlic, garam masala, ginger, turmeric, salt, and red pepper flakes. Add the potatoes. Lock the lid in place. Set the pressure cooker to high pressure for 4 minutes. Quick-release the pressure, then open the lid carefully. Continue as directed.

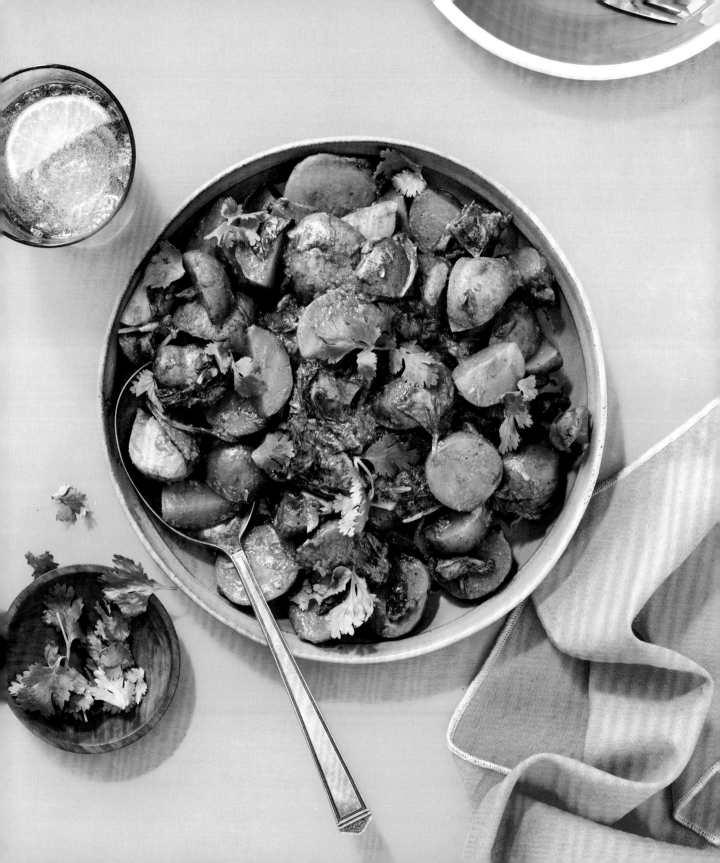

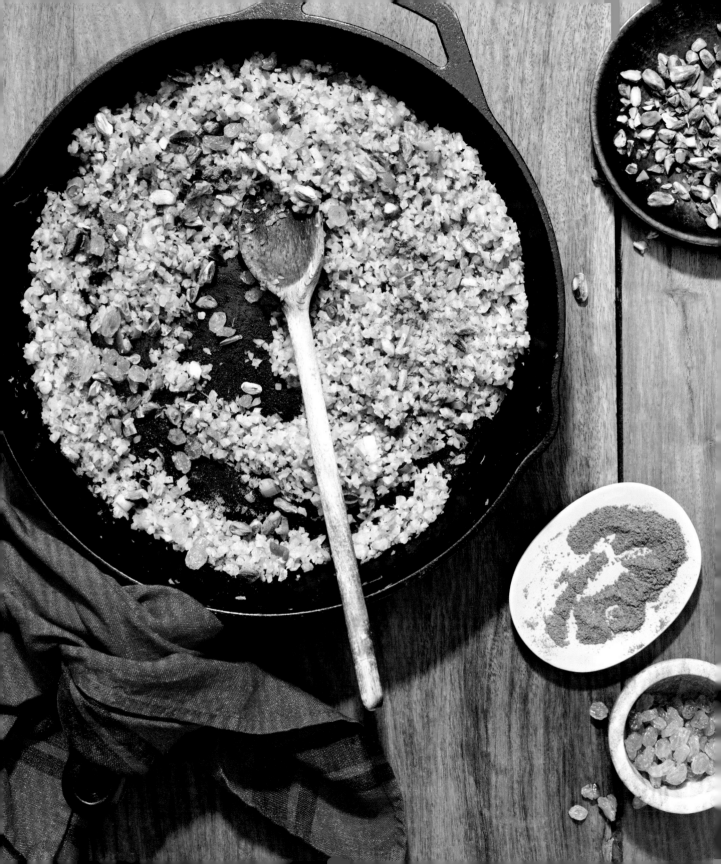

QUICK CAULIFLOWER RICE

SERVES 2 TO 3 • PREP: 5 MINUTES • COOK: 10 MINUTES • TOTAL: 15 MINUTES

2 tablespoons ghee, Clarified Butter (page 229), or extra-virgin olive oil

2 green onions, thinly sliced, green and white parts separated

1 garlic clove, minced

1 small carrot, finely shredded

1 (10- to 12-ounce) bag frozen cauliflower rice

½ teaspoon salt

¼ teaspoon black pepper

This is your go-to cauliflower rice, and it can form the perfect base for stir-fries or curries. Starting with frozen riced cauliflower greatly simplifies and shortens the prep time. We've included variations too, so you'll always have the right flavor profile to pair with any dish.

In a medium nonstick skillet, heat the ghee over medium heat. Add the green onion whites, the garlic, and carrot. Cook, stirring frequently, until the garlic is fragrant and the carrot and green onion whites are slightly softened, 2 to 3 minutes.

Break up any lumps of frozen cauliflower rice by gently whacking the sealed bag on the countertop. Add the cauliflower rice to the skillet and cook, stirring occasionally, until it is tender (but not mushy) and lightly browned, 6 to 8 minutes.

Stir in the green onion greens, salt, and pepper.

SAFFRON LEMON RICE: Add a pinch of saffron threads to ¼ cup hot Chicken Bone Broth (page 231) or Whole30-compatible chicken broth and let steep 5 minutes. Add when adding cauliflower rice to the pan. Stir in 1 tablespoon fresh lemon juice along with the green onion greens, salt, and pepper.

INDIAN-SPICED RICE: Stir in ½ teaspoon garam masala and 2 tablespoons golden raisins or finely diced apricots when adding the cauliflower rice to the pan. Stir in 2 tablespoons chopped roasted pistachios with the green onion greens, salt, and pepper.

MEXICAN-INSPIRED GREEN RICE: Add 1 finely chopped (seeded, if desired) jalapeño to the pan along with the green onion whites, garlic, and carrot. Stir in ½ teaspoon ground cumin when adding the cauliflower rice to the pan. Stir in 1 tablespoon each finely chopped fresh cilantro and parsley along with the green onion greens, salt, and pepper.

ROASTED BACON-WRAPPED ASPARAGUS AND TOMATOES

SERVES 4 • PREP: 20 MINUTES • ROAST: 15 MINUTES • TOTAL: 35 MINUTES

1 pound asparagus spears, trimmed

2 teaspoons avocado oil or extra-virgin olive oil

Black pepper

Garlic powder

4 thin-cut slices Whole30-compatible bacon, halved lengthwise

1 cup grape tomatoes, halved lengthwise

2 teaspoons chopped fresh thyme, or ½ teaspoon dried thyme

Salt

½ teaspoon grated lemon zest

Everything's better with bacon, right? As these asparagus bundles roast, the bacon infuses the asparagus with flavors of salt and smoke. Thyme-seasoned grape tomatoes roasted alongside the bundles turn beautifully soft and juicy, forming a textural balance with the crisp bacon.

Preheat the oven to 425°F. Line a large rimmed baking sheet with foil or parchment.

Lightly brush the asparagus with 1 teaspoon of the oil and sprinkle with pepper and garlic powder. Divide the asparagus into 8 equal bundles with spears facing the same direction. Wrap each bundle with one halved strip of bacon, starting just below the ferny tops and ending near the bases. Place the bundles on one side of the baking sheet. Roast for 7 minutes.

Brush the cut sides of the tomatoes with the remaining teaspoon oil. Carefully remove the baking sheet from the oven. Place the tomatoes, cut sides up, alongside the asparagus bundles. Sprinkle the tomatoes with the thyme and salt to taste. Roast until the asparagus is crisp-tender and the bacon is cooked (it may not be crispy, but should be cooked through), 8 to 10 minutes more (see Tip). Transfer the asparagus bundles and tomatoes to a serving platter or plates, and sprinkle with the lemon zest.

TIP: The cooking time will depend on how thick and how tender the asparagus is. Use a knife inserted into the thickest part of a spear to test for desired doneness.

Tomatoes are done when the cut sides begin to puff up and look juicy.

If the bacon is not as crisp as desired, remove the tomatoes from the baking sheet and broil the asparagus bundles on high for a few minutes before serving, watching them closely to prevent overcooking.

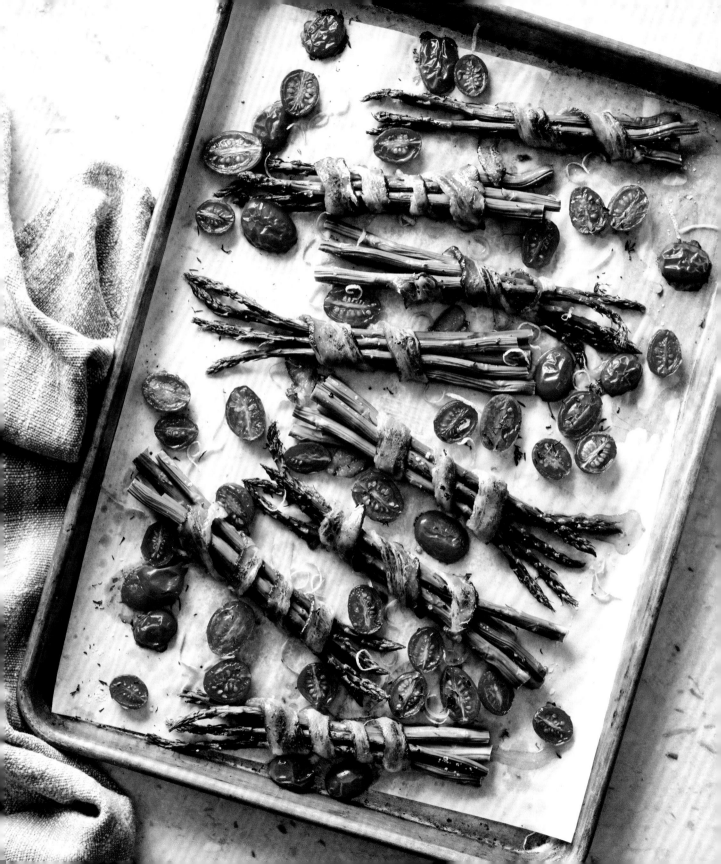

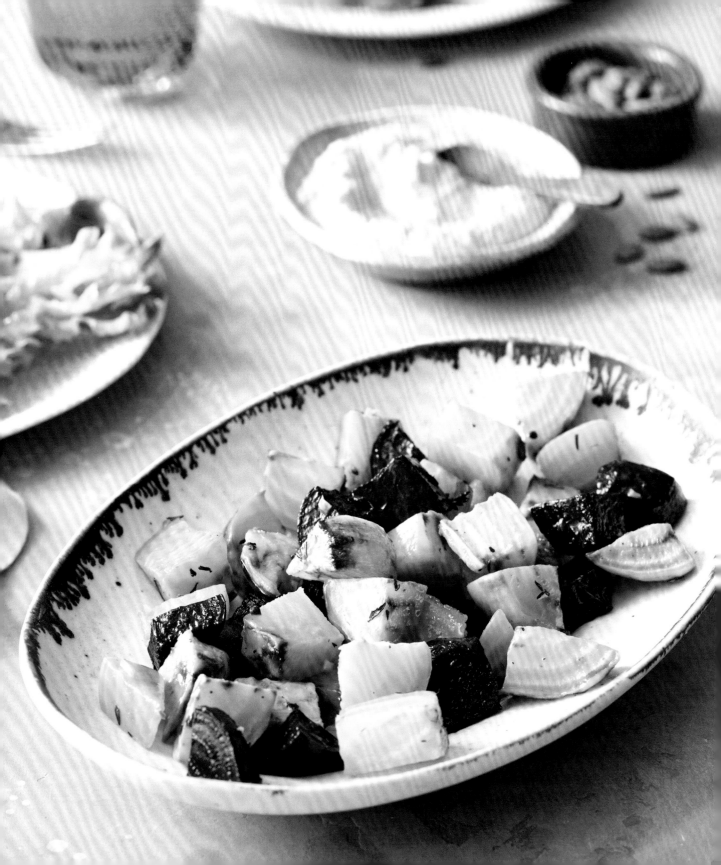

ROASTED BEET SALAD
WITH HORSERADISH CREAM

SERVES 2 • PREP: 15 MINUTES • ROAST: 30 MINUTES • TOTAL: 45 MINUTES

FOR THE BEETS

1 pound red and/or yellow beets, peeled and cut into ¾-inch cubes

1 tablespoon extra-virgin olive oil

2 large garlic cloves, minced

2 teaspoons chopped fresh thyme, or ½ teaspoon dried thyme

¼ teaspoon salt

⅛ teaspoon black pepper

FOR THE HORSERADISH CREAM

½ cup raw cashews, soaked in water at least 1 hour (and up to 12 hours)

3 tablespoons fresh lemon juice

3 tablespoons water

1 tablespoon Whole30-compatible prepared horseradish

1 tablespoon apple cider vinegar

2 teaspoons nutritional yeast

Pinch of salt

FOR SERVING

4 cups lightly packed mixed salad greens

2 tablespoons Lemony Shallot-Mustard Vinaigrette (page 216)

1 tablespoon dry-roasted pepitas (pumpkin seeds)

The heat of this horseradish cream offers an invigorating contrast to the sweetness of the roasted beets. If you love the nose-tingling effect of horseradish, bump up the amount by a teaspoon or two.

MAKE THE BEETS: Preheat the oven to 400°F. Line a large rimmed baking sheet with parchment.

In a medium bowl, combine the beets, olive oil, garlic, thyme, salt, and pepper. Toss to coat. Arrange the beets in a single layer on the baking sheet and roast until tender, turning once or twice, 30 to 35 minutes. Let cool while you make the horseradish cream.

MAKE THE HORSERADISH CREAM: Drain the cashews. In a blender, combine the cashews, lemon juice, water, horseradish, vinegar, nutritional yeast, and salt. Blend until smooth. (See Tip.)

SERVE: Dress the greens with the vinaigrette. Divide the salad greens between 2 plates. Top the greens with the beets. Top each plate with 1 tablespoon horseradish cream, then sprinkle with the pepitas and serve.

TIP: This recipe generates about ½ cup horseradish cream, which gives you leftovers to use in other dishes. Use this cream on top of a grilled steak or burger, stir it into mashed potatoes, or serve with scrambled eggs.

SWEET AND SPICY SAUTÉED SPINACH

SERVES 2 • PREP: 10 MINUTES • COOK: 5 MINUTES • TOTAL: 15 MINUTES

2 tablespoons golden raisins

1 tablespoon extra-virgin olive oil

2 teaspoons ghee or Clarified Butter (page 229)

1 large garlic clove, thinly sliced

2 (5-ounce) packages baby spinach

¼ teaspoon salt

¼ teaspoon red pepper flakes

1 tablespoon pine nuts or slivered almonds, toasted

This simple side is a flash in the pan—literally. It takes no time to make, but it delivers big on both freshness and flavor. It also pairs well with any protein—beef, bison, pork, lamb, chicken, or fish.

In a small bowl, cover the raisins with warm water and soak for 10 minutes.

Meanwhile, in a large skillet, heat the olive oil and ghee over medium heat. Add the garlic and cook, stirring constantly, until fragrant, about 1 minute. Add the spinach in handfuls, tossing with tongs, and cook just until wilted, 4 to 5 minutes.

Drain the raisins and add to the pan. Toss to combine. Season with salt and red pepper flakes.

Transfer the spinach to a serving platter and sprinkle with the pine nuts.

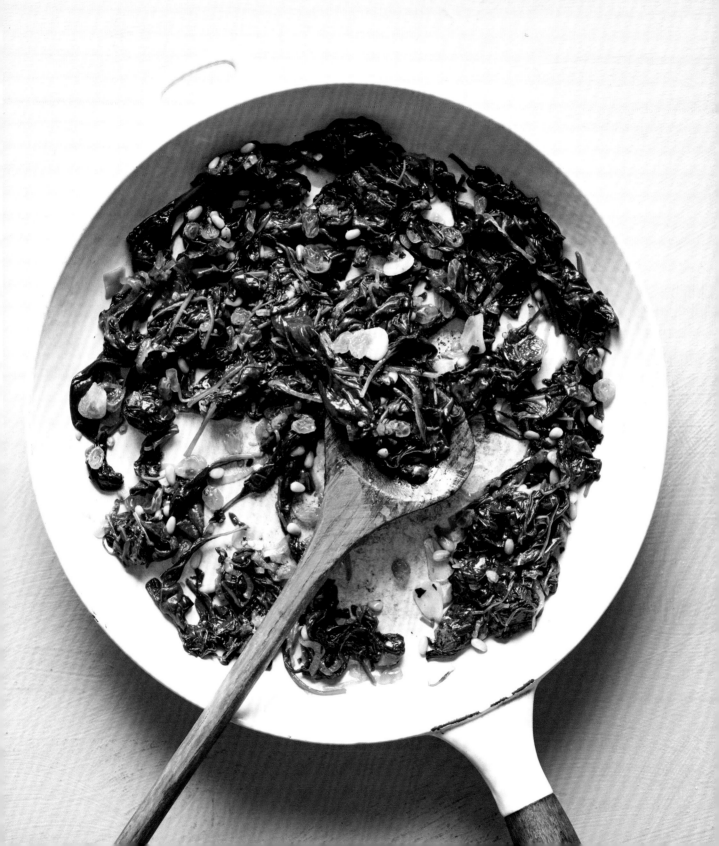

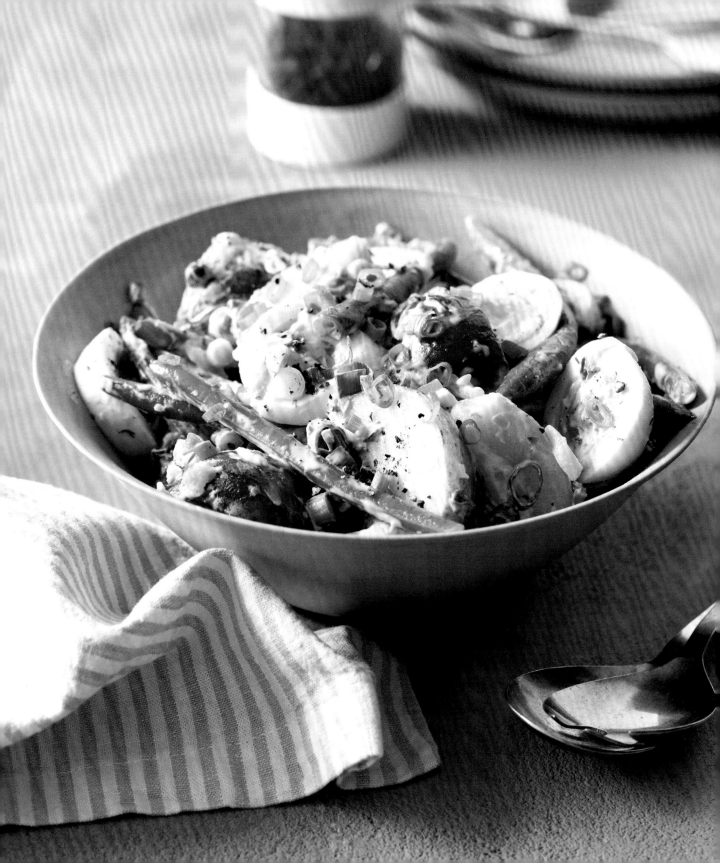

POTATO AND GREEN BEAN SALAD

SERVES 4 • PREP: 5 MINUTES • COOK: 10 MINUTES • TOTAL: 15 MINUTES

1 pound medium potatoes (red-skinned or Yukon Gold), quartered

2 large eggs

4 ounces fresh green beans, trimmed

1 tablespoon drained and rinsed capers, chopped

⅓ to ½ cup Creamy Cucumber-Dill Dressing (page 205)

Salt and black pepper

2 tablespoons chopped green onions, fresh chives, and/or fresh parsley

This picnic-perfect salad can be served slightly warm (immediately after making it), at room temperature, or chilled. The dressing is mayonnaise based, so if you do pack it for a picnic, keep it chilled in a cooler until serving time. (See Tip.)

Place the potatoes and eggs in a large saucepan with salted water and bring to a boil over high heat, then reduce the heat to medium and cook for 10 minutes, or until the potatoes are nearly tender. Add the beans and cook another 3 minutes; drain and cool completely.

Run the eggs under cold water until cool enough to handle, then peel and slice into rounds.

Remove the loose skins from the potatoes and rough-chop the potatoes into ½-inch chunks.

Toss the potatoes, eggs, beans, and capers in a large bowl with the desired amount of dressing. Season to taste with salt and pepper and sprinkle with the chopped green onions, chives, and/or parsley.

TIP: This salad can be made a day or two ahead; the flavors meld even more as it chills in the fridge. (Keep refrigerated in an airtight container for up to 5 days.)

ROASTED CARROTS AND PARSNIPS WITH CHAMOY AND PISTACHIOS

SERVES 2 • PREP: 15 MINUTES • ROAST: 15 MINUTES • TOTAL: 30 MINUTES

8 ounces carrots, peeled and cut into 2-inch chunks

8 ounces parsnips, peeled and cut into 2-inch chunks (see Tip, page 157)

1 tablespoon extra-virgin olive oil

Salt and black pepper

2 tablespoons Mexican Chamoy Sauce (page 209), thinned with 1 to 2 tablespoons water

1 tablespoon chopped fresh cilantro

1 tablespoon chopped fresh dill

Pinch of red pepper flakes

2 tablespoons chopped pistachios

Fresh lime juice

Chamoy sauce is a bold, stone fruit–based Mexican sauce that lends a salty, sweet, and sour flavor with a kick of heat from chiles. Top these parsnips and carrots with crunchy pistachios, fresh herbs, and a splash of lime juice.

Preheat the oven to 400°F. Line a large rimmed baking sheet with parchment.

In a medium bowl, toss the carrot and parsnip chunks in the olive oil. Season to taste with salt and pepper. Arrange in a single layer on the baking sheet. Roast until crisp-tender and lightly browned, about 15 minutes.

Transfer the vegetables to a serving bowl or platter, then drizzle with the sauce, and finish with the cilantro, dill, red pepper flakes, pistachios, and lime juice.

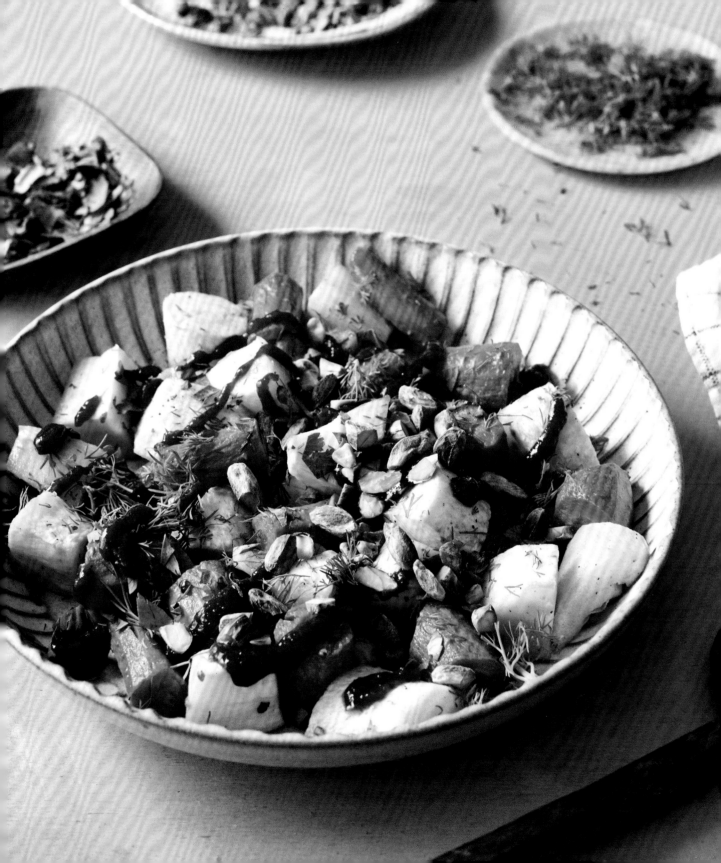

ORIGINAL WHOLE30 SAUCES AND DRESSINGS

AVOCADO GREEN GODDESS DRESSING

MAKES 1⅓ CUPS   •   PREP: 15 MINUTES   •   TOTAL: 15 MINUTES

1 large ripe avocado, pitted, peeled, and coarsely chopped

½ cup packed fresh parsley

½ cup assorted fresh soft-leaf herbs, such as tarragon, basil, dill, and/or cilantro

2 tablespoons chopped fresh chives or green onions (green and white parts)

½ cup water, or more as needed

1 teaspoon grated lemon zest

¼ cup fresh lemon juice

2 tablespoons coconut aminos

2 tablespoons tahini

1 garlic clove, minced

¼ teaspoon salt (see Tip)

¼ teaspoon black pepper or red pepper flakes

This herby dressing makes an ideal dip for crudités or a dressing for hearty greens. It also stirs beautifully into chicken, tuna, or egg salad, since it is fairly thick.

In a food processor, combine all the ingredients. Cover and blend until smooth. If needed, stir in additional water 1 tablespoon at a time until dressing is desired consistency.

Store, covered, in the refrigerator for up to 3 days (it may darken slightly) or place in a freezer container or bag and freeze up to 1 month (thaw in the refrigerator overnight).

TIP: Traditional green goddess dressing usually calls for anchovies. You can add 1 or 2 salt-packed anchovies for that hit of salt and flavor. For a more pourable dressing, stir in more water.

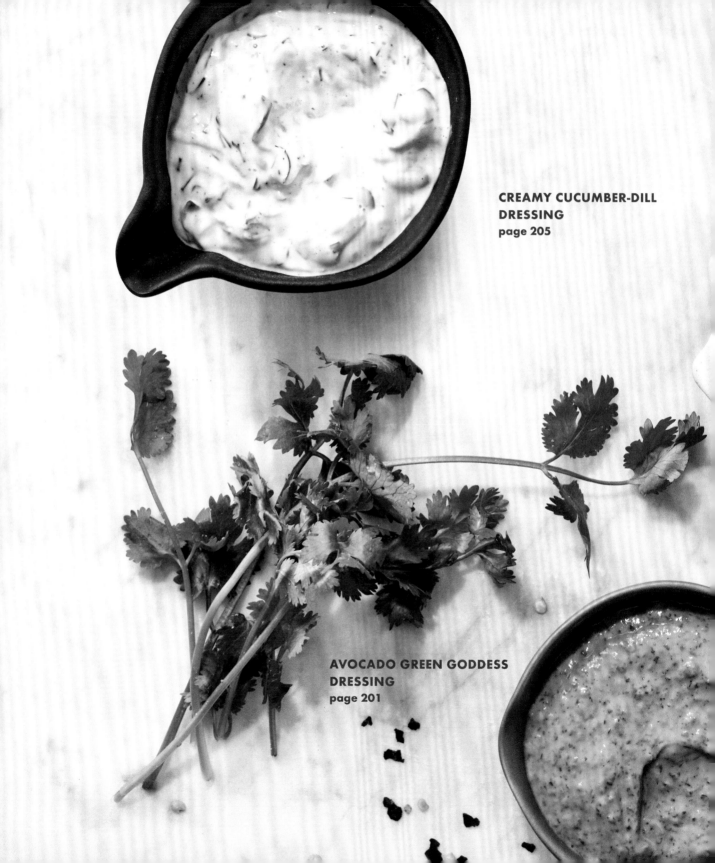

**CREAMY CUCUMBER-DILL
DRESSING**
page 205

**AVOCADO GREEN GODDESS
DRESSING**
page 201

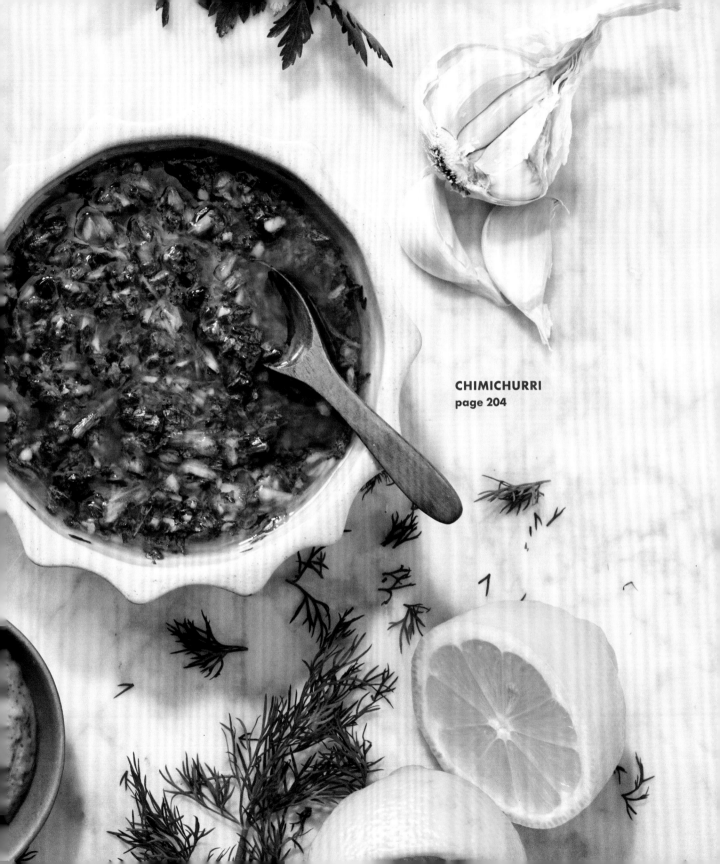

CHIMICHURRI
page 204

CHIMICHURRI

MAKES ABOUT 1 CUP • PREP: 15 MINUTES • TOTAL: 15 MINUTES

4 garlic cloves, coarsely chopped

1 shallot, sliced

½ cup lightly packed chopped fresh parsley

½ cup lightly packed chopped fresh cilantro

2 tablespoons chopped fresh oregano

½ teaspoon salt, plus more to taste

½ teaspoon red pepper flakes

⅓ cup extra-virgin olive oil

⅓ cup red wine vinegar

3 tablespoons water

This herby, zippy sauce originated in Argentina and appears often in Latin American cuisine. It's terrific spooned over grilled or roasted meats, poultry, fish and shellfish, eggs, or vegetables.

In a food processor, combine the garlic, shallot, parsley, cilantro, oregano, ½ teaspoon salt, and the red pepper flakes. Pulse until roughly chopped. Add the oil, vinegar, and water. Pulse to make a sauce that has some texture to it but is well blended. Taste and add more salt, if desired.

Transfer to a serving bowl.

TIP: Chimichurri can be made up to 3 days ahead of time. If made fresh, store in an airtight container in the refrigerator for 3 to 4 days. You can also freeze individual portions of chimichurri in ice cube trays or small freezer-safe containers. It can stay in your freezer for up to 3 months.

CREAMY CUCUMBER-DILL DRESSING

MAKES 1½ CUPS • PREP: 20 MINUTES • TOTAL: 20 MINUTES

½ English cucumber, coarsely grated

Salt

1 cup Whole30 Mayo (page 230) or Whole30-compatible mayonnaise

3 tablespoons minced green onions (green and white parts)

1 tablespoon chopped fresh dill

2 teaspoons Whole30-compatible Dijon mustard

1 teaspoon fresh lemon juice

Grated zest of ½ lemon

Cayenne or Whole30-compatible hot sauce of choice

This delicately flavored dressing is perfect mixed into the Potato and Green Bean Salad (page 197) or used as a sauce dolloped on grilled, baked, or poached fish.

Place the grated cucumber in a strainer and sprinkle with a little salt. Toss to coat and let stand for 15 minutes to draw out excess moisture.

Meanwhile, in a large bowl, whisk together the mayonnaise, green onions, dill, mustard, lemon juice and zest, and cayenne to taste.

Squeeze out the moisture from the cucumber and pat it as dry as possible with paper towels. Stir the cucumber into the mayonnaise mixture and let stand for 5 minutes before serving.

COFFEE BARBECUE SAUCE

MAKES 2⅓ CUPS • PREP: 15 MINUTES • COOK: 15 MINUTES + 10 MINUTES COOLING •
TOTAL: 40 MINUTES

1 medium onion, chopped

1 cup Whole30-compatible spicy ketchup (see Tip)

½ cup brewed espresso or strong coffee (see Tip)

½ cup apple cider vinegar

½ cup chopped pitted dates (preferably Medjool)

⅓ cup coconut aminos

3 garlic cloves, minced

2 teaspoons smoked paprika

2 teaspoons dry mustard

2 teaspoons chili powder

⅓ cup water, or more as needed

The coffee in this barbecue sauce isn't particularly pronounced, but it adds an amazing complexity of flavor. The sauce is spicy and smoky, with some tang from the vinegar and mild sweetness from the dates.

In a medium saucepan, combine the onion, ketchup, espresso, vinegar, dates, coconut aminos, garlic, paprika, mustard, and chili powder. Stir to combine.

Bring to a boil over medium-high heat, stirring occasionally. Reduce the heat and simmer, uncovered, for 15 minutes. Remove from the heat and let cool for 10 minutes.

Transfer the contents to a blender. Add the ⅓ cup water and blend until smooth. If desired, add additional water, 1 teaspoon at a time, until desired thickness.

TIP: While this recipe creates a brush-on thick sauce, you can thin it with a little bit of water, if desired.

If you can't find spicy ketchup, use any Whole30-compatible ketchup, and add cayenne until you achieve the desired level of spice.

If you don't have brewed espresso or coffee, mix 1 teaspoon instant coffee into ½ cup hot water and stir until dissolved.

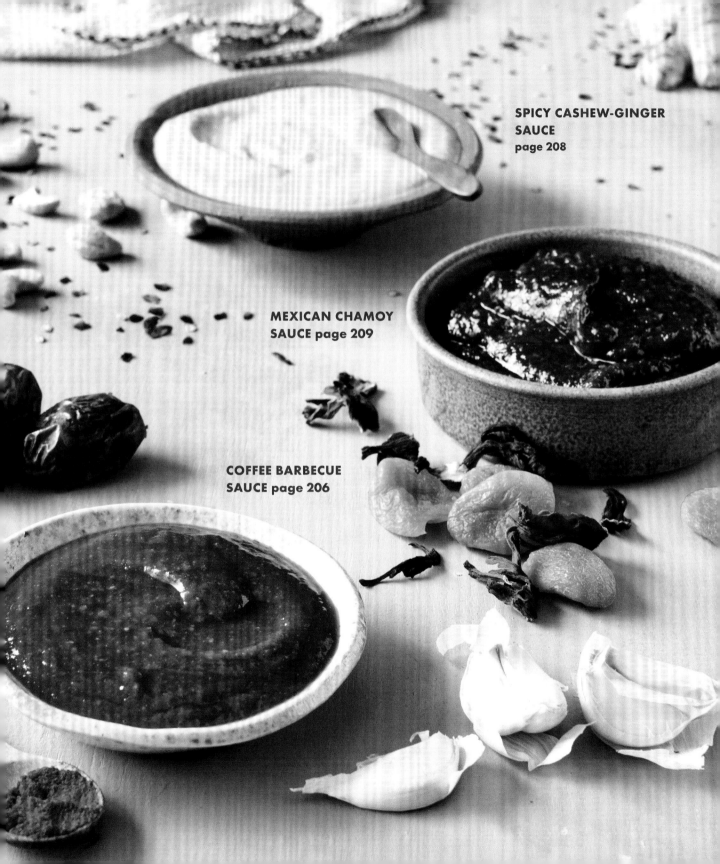

SPICY CASHEW-GINGER SAUCE page 208

MEXICAN CHAMOY SAUCE page 209

COFFEE BARBECUE SAUCE page 206

SPICY CASHEW-GINGER SAUCE

MAKES 1 CUP • PREP: 10 MINUTES • TOTAL: 10 MINUTES

½ cup unsweetened cashew butter (see Tip)

½ cup full-fat canned coconut milk

3 tablespoons fresh lime juice

1 tablespoon coconut aminos

1 garlic clove, minced

2 teaspoons peeled and grated fresh ginger (see Tip, page 130)

½ teaspoon red pepper flakes

½ teaspoon unseasoned rice vinegar or apple cider vinegar

¼ teaspoon salt

Enjoy this nutty, pleasantly spicy, sweet sauce as a dip for raw vegetables, drizzled over roasted vegetables, or as a sauce or dip for grilled chicken.

In a small bowl, whisk together all the ingredients.

Use immediately or store in an airtight container in the refrigerator for up to 1 week. To use, microwave for 15 to 20 seconds, or until it's easy to stir.

TIP: If you don't have cashew butter, you can use Whole30-compatible almond butter or sunflower seed butter.

MEXICAN CHAMOY SAUCE

MAKES 1 CUP • PREP: 5 MINUTES • COOK: 30 MINUTES • TOTAL: 35 MINUTES

⅓ cup dried apricots

⅓ cup pitted prunes

3 tablespoons dried hibiscus flowers (see Tip)

2 cups water, or more as needed

1 tablespoon chili powder

1 cinnamon stick

¼ teaspoon anise seeds

2 to 3 tablespoons fresh lime juice

Chamoy sauce is a bold, stone fruit–based Mexican sauce. It's thick, sweet, and spicy, and is delicious on grilled meats or roasted vegetables, like the Roasted Carrots and Parsnips with Chamoy and Pistachios (page 198).

In a medium saucepan, combine the apricots, prunes, hibiscus flowers, 2 cups water, the chili powder, cinnamon stick, and anise seeds. Bring to a boil over medium-high heat, then reduce the heat to medium-low and simmer for 30 minutes, or until fruit is very soft, stirring occasionally. (If the mixture starts to look dry during cooking, add more water ¼ cup at a time.) Let cool slightly and remove the cinnamon stick.

In a blender, puree the mixture with the lime juice until smooth; if the sauce is too thick, thin it with additional water.

Store in a tightly covered container in the refrigerator for up to 1 week.

TIP: Dried hibiscus flowers provide the chamoy with its characteristic tartness and dark red color. They can be found in the spice section of Mexican markets or from online sources. If you don't have the hibiscus flowers, substitute 3 tablespoons of Whole30-compatible dried cranberries instead.

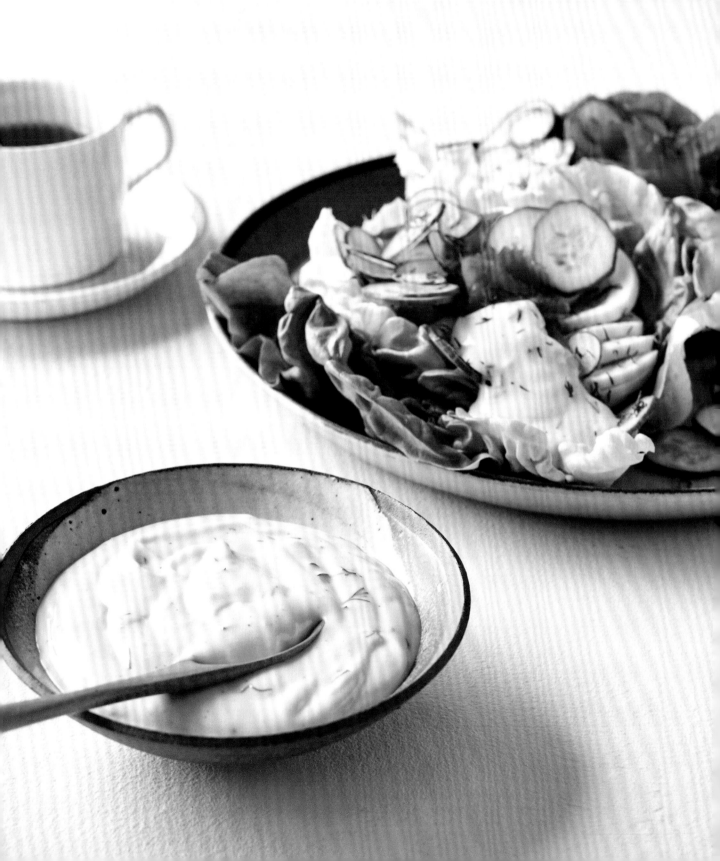

MOCK HOLLANDAISE

MAKES ABOUT 1 CUP • PREP: 5 MINUTES • COOK: 5 MINUTES • TOTAL: 10 MINUTES

2 tablespoons ghee or Clarified Butter (page 229)

1 cup Whole30 Mayo (page 230) or Whole30-compatible mayonnaise

2 tablespoons fresh lemon juice

½ teaspoon grated lemon zest

½ teaspoon dried dill

Pinches of salt and cayenne

Traditional hollandaise uses egg yolks and vigorous whisking to bring the thick, creamy mixture together. Our shortcut version allows you to enjoy Whole30 Eggs Benedict (see Tip) in a hurry by substituting mayo for the egg yolk.

In a small saucepan, melt the ghee over low heat. Whisk in the mayonnaise, lemon juice and zest, dill, salt, and cayenne. Gently heat through (do not boil). If desired, thin with a little hot water.

Serve warm with fish, vegetables, or use as a sauce for poached eggs.

TIP: To create a Whole30 version of eggs Benedict, dress 2 cups of baby spinach with Lemony Shallot-Mustard Vinaigrette (page 216) or your favorite Whole30-compatible vinaigrette. Plate the spinach and top with 2 crisp strips of Whole30-compatible bacon, 2 poached eggs (see page 124), and a generous dollop of this hollandaise. Add salt and pepper to taste.

REVAMPED RANCH DRESSING

MAKES 1½ CUPS • PREP: 15 MINUTES • TOTAL: 15 MINUTES

1 cup Whole30 Mayo (page 230) or Whole30-compatible mayonnaise

½ cup full-fat canned coconut milk

1 small garlic clove, minced

½ teaspoon onion powder

½ teaspoon salt

½ teaspoon black pepper

2 tablespoons finely chopped fresh dill

2 tablespoons finely chopped fresh chives

2 tablespoons finely chopped fresh curly-leaf parsley

1 tablespoon apple cider vinegar

Juice of ½ lemon

The Whole30 love for ranch dressing is real! Ranch is the most popular dressing in the country *and* in Whole30-land, and our version nails its tangy, herby flavor. We give you four versions here, each of which would be perfect as a dip for raw veggies, over roasted chicken or potatoes, or drizzled on a fresh green salad.

In a medium bowl, whisk together all the ingredients.

Use immediately, or store in an airtight container in the refrigerator for up to 1 week.

BUFFALO RANCH DRESSING: Whisk 1 to 2 tablespoons Whole30-compatible Buffalo-style hot sauce into the finished dressing.

BACON-DILL RANCH DRESSING: Double the dill and omit the parsley. Stir in ⅓ cup finely chopped cooked Whole30-compatible bacon.

CILANTRO-LIME RANCH DRESSING: Replace the dill, chives, and parsley with ½ cup fresh cilantro. Swap out the lemon juice for lime juice.

CREAMY TOMATILLO RANCH DRESSING: Add 2 diced husked tomatillos. Replace the dill, chives, and parsley with ½ cup fresh cilantro. Swap out the lemon juice for lime juice. Add ½ jalapeño (seeds removed and finely chopped), if you like a bit of spice.

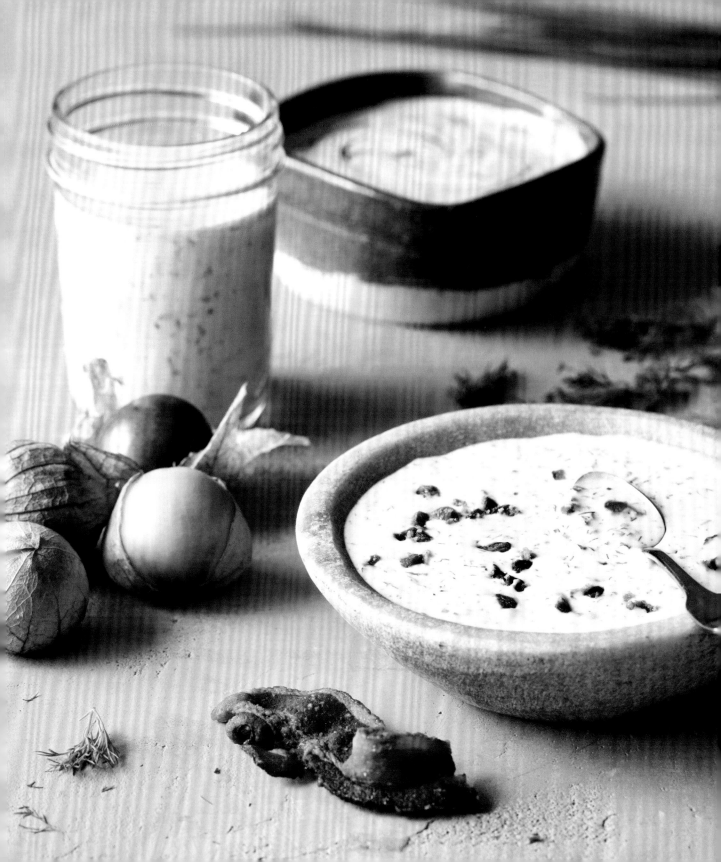

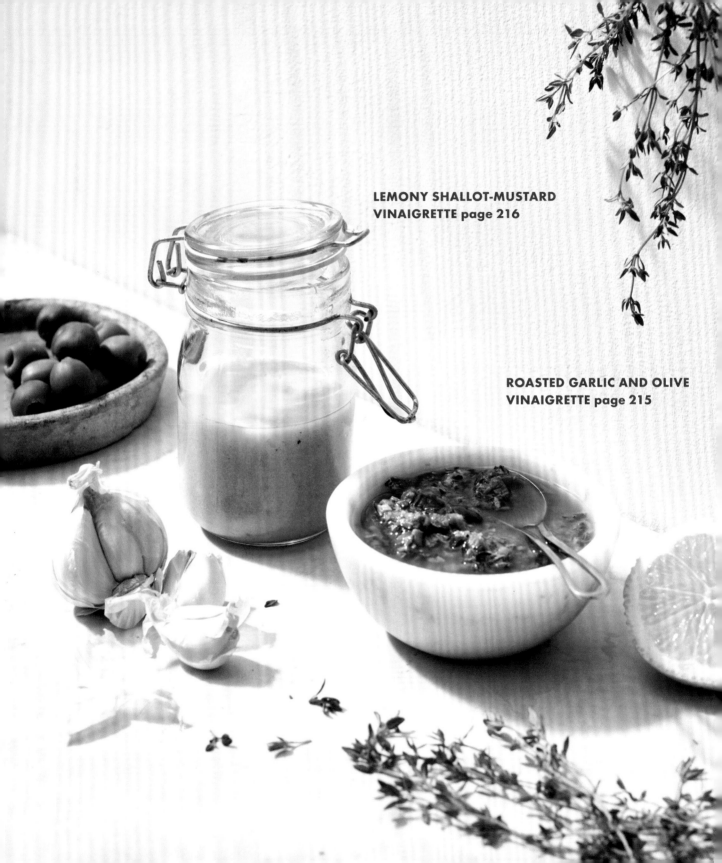

LEMONY SHALLOT-MUSTARD VINAIGRETTE page 216

ROASTED GARLIC AND OLIVE VINAIGRETTE page 215

ROASTED GARLIC AND OLIVE VINAIGRETTE

MAKES 1½ CUPS • PREP: 5 MINUTES + 5 TO 10 MINUTES RESTING •
ROAST: 20 MINUTES • TOTAL: 35 MINUTES

FOR THE ROASTED GARLIC

1 head of garlic (see Tip)

½ teaspoon extra-virgin
    olive oil

Pinch of salt

FOR THE VINAIGRETTE

½ cup sherry vinegar or
    balsamic vinegar (see Tip)

1 teaspoon Whole30-
    compatible Dijon mustard

1 tablespoon fresh thyme,
    or 1 teaspoon dried thyme

¼ teaspoon black pepper

1 cup extra-virgin olive oil

3 tablespoons finely chopped
    pitted green or Kalamata
    olives

This hearty, flavorful vinaigrette is robust enough to spoon over cooked vegetables, chicken, or fish. Of course, it's also a delicious salad dressing, particularly on heartier greens like spinach, arugula, or baby kale.

MAKE THE ROASTED GARLIC: Preheat the oven to 425°F. Cut a thick slice off the top of the head of garlic to reveal the individual cloves; leave the outer skin around the garlic head. Place the garlic head on a small square of foil, cut side up. Drizzle with the olive oil and sprinkle with the salt. Enclose the garlic in the foil and place in a shallow pan. Roast for 20 to 25 minutes, or until the garlic cloves are tender when pierced with a sharp knife. Let stand 5 to 10 minutes or until cool enough to handle.

Use your fingers to squeeze the garlic cloves from the heads. Use a fork to smash the garlic into a paste.

MAKE THE VINAIGRETTE: In a small jar with a lid, combine the roasted garlic, vinegar, mustard, thyme, pepper, and olive oil. Shake vigorously until emulsified. Add the olives and shake gently to incorporate. Store, covered, in the refrigerator for up to 2 weeks.

TIP: You can roast the garlic ahead to make the prep faster. Roast and smash as directed, then transfer to a small container and chill for up to 3 days (or freeze for up to 2 months). Bring the garlic to room temperature before using. Or, if you don't have time to roast the garlic, substitute 1 minced large garlic clove.
   If you prefer a savory, acidic vinaigrette, use the sherry vinegar; for a milder, slightly sweet vinaigrette, opt for the balsamic.

LEMONY SHALLOT-MUSTARD VINAIGRETTE

MAKES ½ CUP • PREP: 10 MINUTES + 10 MINUTES RESTING • TOTAL: 20 MINUTES

2 tablespoons finely chopped shallots

2 tablespoons fresh lemon juice

⅛ teaspoon sea salt, plus more to taste

2 teaspoons Whole30-compatible Dijon mustard

5 tablespoons extra-virgin olive oil

¼ teaspoon black pepper, plus more to taste

This fresh vinaigrette can brighten any salad and is delicious on delicate greens such as baby lettuces, spring mix, and buttery Bibb. This dressing pairs perfectly with the Roasted Beet Salad with Horseradish Cream on page 193.

In a small glass jar with a lid, stir together the shallots, lemon juice, and ⅛ teaspoon salt. Let stand 10 minutes.

Add the mustard, olive oil, and ¼ teaspoon pepper to the jar. Cover and shake vigorously until emulsified. Season to taste with additional salt and pepper, if desired.

TIP: The vinaigrette will stay fresh for up to 1 week in an airtight container in the refrigerator.

ORIGINAL WHOLE30 SNACKS

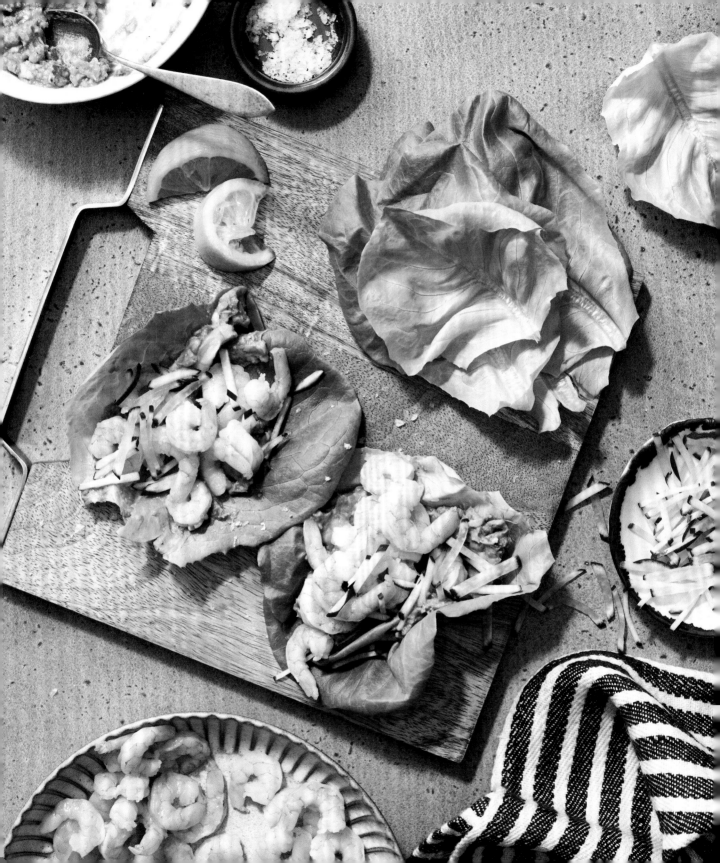

CREAMY AVOCADO, SHRIMP, AND RADISH WRAPS

SERVES 2 (4 ROLLS) • PREP: 15 MINUTES • TOTAL: 15 MINUTES

1 small ripe avocado, peeled and pitted

1 tablespoon fresh lemon juice

¼ teaspoon salt

⅛ teaspoon black pepper

8 Bibb lettuce leaves

1 cup frozen cooked extra-small (salad) shrimp, thawed (see Tip)

2 radishes, cut into matchsticks

1 tablespoon extra-virgin olive oil

Flaky sea salt

Whole30 pro tip: Keep cooked extra-small shrimp (often sold as "salad shrimp") in your freezer; they're fast to defrost, and when added to a salad or vegetable side, they make for an easy and protein-rich lunch, dinner, or snack.

In a small bowl, mash the avocado with the lemon juice, salt, and pepper to desired texture (leave some chunks or make it creamy).

On each of 2 plates, make 2 stacks of 2 Bibb lettuce leaves. Top each stack with some of the avocado mixture, then add the shrimp and matchstick radishes. Drizzle with the olive oil and sprinkle with the flaky salt.

Roll up and serve immediately.

TIP: To quickly thaw frozen shrimp, place them in a bowl and add cool water to cover. Let stand for 5 minutes, change the water, then let stand for another 5 minutes. Drain, then use.

GOLDEN MILK GREEN TEA SMOOTHIE

MAKES 1 • PREP: 10 MINUTES • TOTAL: 10 MINUTES

¼ (13.5-ounce) can full-fat coconut milk

1 ripe banana

1 to 2 scoops Whole30-compatible protein powder

1 tablespoon unsweetened almond butter

½ tablespoon peeled and grated fresh ginger, or ½ teaspoon ground ginger (see Tip, page 130)

½ teaspoon Whole30-compatible matcha powder (see Tip)

¼ teaspoon ground turmeric

¼ teaspoon ground cinnamon

¼ teaspoon ground cardamom

⅛ teaspoon black pepper

1½ cups ice cubes

This delicious smoothie is rich in protein and packed with healthy fats. Bright green matcha powder adds a pop of color, while the turmeric, cinnamon, and cardamom add warmth and comfort.

In a blender, combine the coconut milk, banana, protein powder, almond butter, ginger, matcha powder, turmeric, cinnamon, cardamom, and pepper. Add the ice. Cover and blend until smooth, then serve immediately.

TIP: Matcha is a traditional Japanese green tea made from finely powdered dried tea leaves. It has an earthy, grassy undertone with a slightly sweet finish. If you don't have matcha powder or don't like the taste, you can substitute spirulina powder, barley grass powder, or moringa powder. Or take the smoothie in a different flavor direction by using 100% cacao powder in place of the matcha—it pairs nicely with the turmeric and cinnamon.

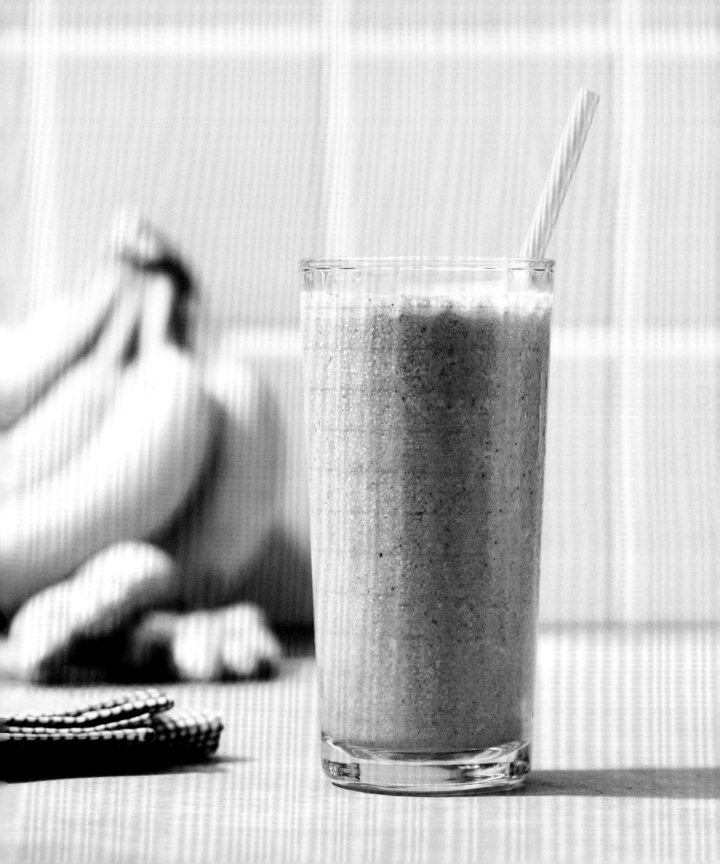

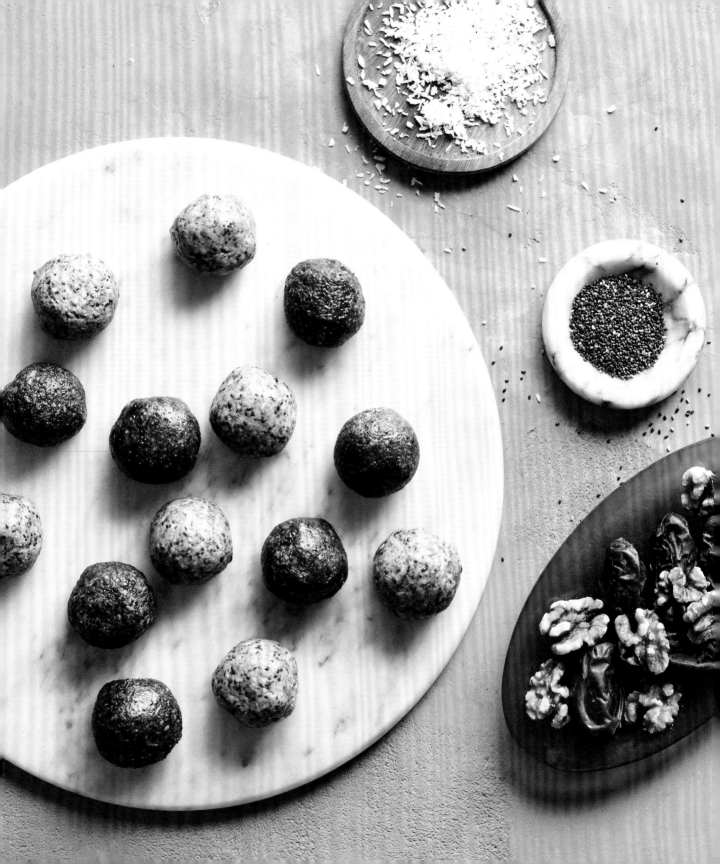

DATE-NUT ENERGY BALLS
WITH COLLAGEN

MAKES 12 TO 15 BALLS • PREP: 15 MINUTES • TOTAL: 15 MINUTES

¾ cup Whole30-compatible cashew butter or almond butter

½ cup unsweetened shredded coconut

½ cup nuts (walnuts, almonds, cashews, pistachios, pecans)

¼ cup Whole30-compatible collagen peptide powder

5 Medjool dates, pitted and coarsely chopped

2 tablespoons 100% cacao powder (optional)

2 tablespoons flaxseed meal

2 tablespoons chia seeds

1 teaspoon vanilla extract

¼ teaspoon salt

¼ teaspoon ground cinnamon

For energy on the go, pack a portion of these chewy fruit, nut, and seed bites to take to school, the office, the gym, and beyond.

In a food processor, combine the cashew butter, coconut, nuts, collagen powder, dates, cacao powder (if using), flaxseed meal, chia seeds, vanilla, salt, and cinnamon. Pulse until the mixture is blended and crumbly sticky.

Use a cookie scoop to shape the mixture into 12 to 15 balls, then roll each ball between your palms to smooth out. Store in an airtight container for up to 5 days in the refrigerator or up to 1 month in the freezer.

TUNA-STUFFED DEVILED EGGS

MAKES 12 (SERVES 2 TO 3) • PREP: 20 MINUTES • TOTAL: 20 MINUTES

6 hard-cooked eggs, peeled and halved lengthwise

6 tablespoons tuna packed in olive oil, drained and flaked (see Tip)

2 tablespoons Whole30 Mayo (page 230) or Whole30-compatible mayonnaise

2 tablespoons drained and rinsed capers

1 tablespoon fresh lemon juice

Salt and black pepper

Jarred roasted red peppers (optional)

Minced fresh parsley

Smoked paprika

This protein-packed twist on deviled eggs makes the perfect "emergency food" to have in your fridge. Snack on these between video calls, or eat a few extra halves as a quick lunch.

Separate the yolks from the whites of the eggs and place the yolks in a small bowl. Mash well with a fork, then gently fold in the tuna, mayonnaise, capers, and lemon juice. Season to taste with salt and pepper.

Spoon the yolk mixture into the white halves, dividing evenly. Thinly slice a roasted red pepper (if using) and drape a sliver on top of each stuffed egg. Sprinkle the eggs with parsley and paprika, then serve.

TIP: Tuna packed in olive oil (not water) makes a huge different in the flavor here. If you have only tuna pouches or cans of tuna packed in water, drizzle a little extra-virgin olive oil into the tuna and mayo mixture to add some richness.

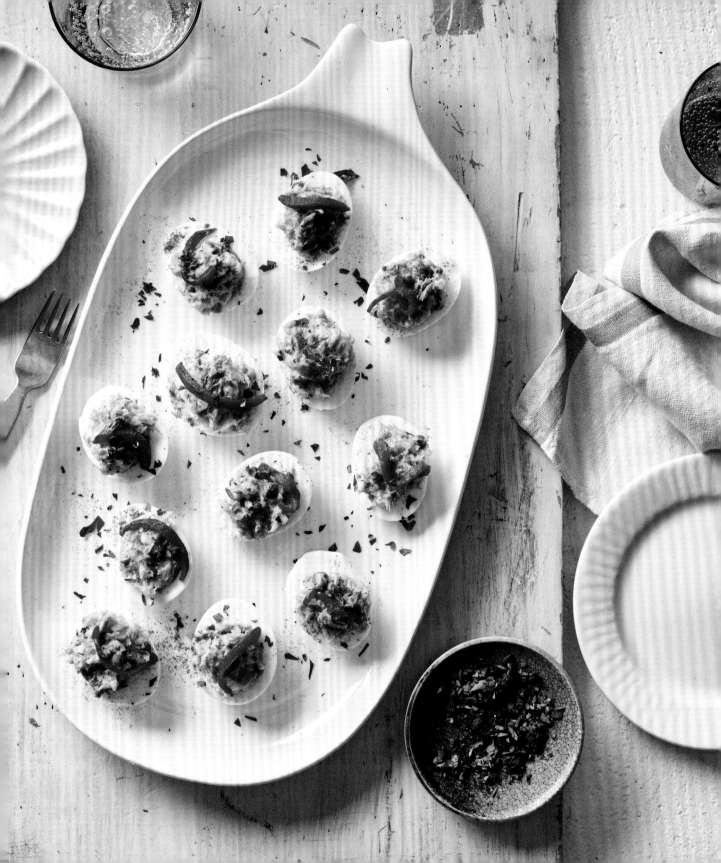

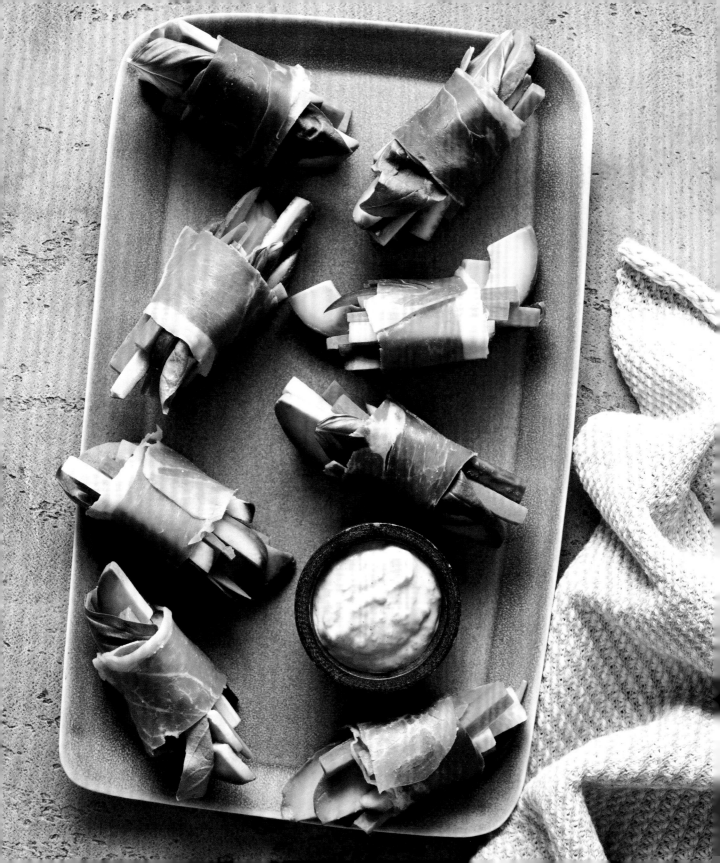

VEGGIE-STUFFED PROSCIUTTO SNACK ROLLS

MAKES 8 (SERVES 2) • PREP: 20 MINUTES • TOTAL: 20 MINUTES

We want our snacks to look like mini-meals, which is why these veggie-forward, portable rolls offer a healthy dose of protein and natural fats. The content of these rolls is flexible, so use whatever you have in the refrigerator.

FOR THE AIOLI DIPPING SAUCE

2 tablespoons Whole30 Mayo (page 230) or Whole30-compatible mayonnaise

1 teaspoon balsamic vinegar

1 teaspoon grated lemon zest or fresh juice

1 small garlic clove, crushed

Pinch of cayenne, Aleppo pepper flakes, or black pepper

FOR THE SNACK ROLLS

1 small avocado, halved and pitted

4 slices prosciutto

8 large basil leaves

1 medium carrot, peeled and cut into 2-inch sticks

¼ medium cucumber, cut into 2-inch sticks (see Tip)

MAKE THE SAUCE: In a small bowl, stir together the mayonnaise, vinegar, lemon zest, garlic, and cayenne.

MAKE THE SNACK ROLLS: With the skin on, cut each avocado half into 8 thin slices lengthwise. Use a spoon to carefully remove the slices from the skin.

With a kitchen scissors, halve each slice of prosciutto lengthwise into 2 strips. Divide the avocado slices and the carrot and cucumber sticks into 8 bundles.

Place 1 basil leaf near one end of a prosciutto strip. Place one bundle crosswise on top of the basil leaf. Roll the prosciutto strip up and around the bundle to form a tight roll. Repeat with the remaining prosciutto strips, basil leaves, and bundles. Serve with the dipping sauce (see Tip).

TIP: If making ahead, brush the avocado with lemon juice to keep it from turning brown. If desired, swap out the carrot or cucumber for bell pepper, celery, jicama, or cooked asparagus. Add some thin pickle slices for even more zesty flavor. Double the prosciutto for even more protein! You can also replace the dipping sauce with Revamped Ranch Dressing (page 212) or Avocado Green Goddess Dressing (page 201).

FOUNDATIONAL RECIPES

CLARIFIED BUTTER

MAKES 3 CUPS • PREP: 3 MINUTES • COOK: 20 MINUTES • TOTAL: 23 MINUTES

1 pound unsalted butter

Clarified butter is the technique of simmering butter slowly at a low temperature to separate the milk solids from the pure butter oil. It's perfect for flavoring dishes or cooking, even on high heat. Making your own clarified butter is a low-cost alternative to purchasing ghee (a variation of clarified butter popular in the culinary traditions of India and the Middle East).

Cut the butter into 1-inch cubes and add to a small pot or saucepan. Place the pot on medium-low heat and allow the butter to melt, then come to a simmer without stirring. As the butter simmers, foamy white dairy solids will rise to the surface. With a spoon or ladle, gently skim the dairy solids off the top and discard, leaving just the pure clarified butter in the pot.

Once you've removed the majority of the milk solids, strain the butter through cheesecloth into a glass storage jar, discarding the remaining milk solids and the cheesecloth. Allow the butter to cool before storing.

TIP: Clarified butter can be stored in the refrigerator or at room temperature for 1 month.

WHOLE30 MAYO

MAKES 1½ CUPS • PREP: 10 MINUTES • TOTAL: 30 MINUTES

1 ¼ cups light olive oil, avocado oil, or high-oleic safflower or sunflower oil

1 large egg

½ teaspoon dry mustard

½ teaspoon salt

Juice of ½ lemon

Homemade mayonnaise is a staple in the Whole30 kitchen. It is the base for an unlimited number of sauces and dressings. It also holds together chicken, tuna, salmon, or egg salads, and it coats meat and seafood before cooking or grilling. All ingredients should be at room temperature before you begin (see Tip).

Place ¼ cup of the oil, the egg, mustard, and salt in a blender, food processor, or large bowl. Blend thoroughly. While the food processor or blender is running (or while mixing in a bowl with an immersion blender), slowly drizzle in the remaining cup oil. When you've added all the oil and the mixture has emulsified, add the lemon juice, blending on low to incorporate.

Transfer the mayonnaise to a glass jar and refrigerate. The mayonnaise will last in the fridge for about 7 days after the expiration date for the eggs. (Check the date on your egg carton before you pull one out for your mayo, then add a week and write that date on your jar.)

> **TIP:** The key to this emulsion is making sure all ingredients are at room temperature. Leave the egg out on the counter for 1 hour, or let it sit in a bowl of hot water for 5 minutes before mixing. And if you keep your lemons in the fridge, pull one out the night before.
>
> The slower you add the oil, the thicker and creamier the emulsion will be. You can slowly pour the oil by hand from a spouted measuring cup, or use a plastic squeeze bottle to slowly drizzle it into the bowl, food processor, or blender. If using an immersion blender, pump the stick up and down a few times toward the end to whip some air into the mixture, making it even fluffier.

CHICKEN BONE BROTH

MAKES 4 QUARTS • PREP: 15 MINUTES • COOK: 12 TO 24 HOURS • TOTAL: 12 TO 24 HOURS

6 quarts cold water

1 carcass from 3- to 4-pound chicken

2 medium carrots, roughly chopped

3 celery stalks, roughly chopped

2 medium onions, roughly chopped

2 to 3 garlic cloves, roughly smashed

1 bunch fresh parsley

1 fresh thyme sprig

2 tablespoons apple cider vinegar

10 black peppercorns

1 teaspoon salt

Bone broth is a Whole30 staple, not just as a cooking ingredient! You'll find many people drinking a mug of broth in the morning or afternoon, just as they would coffee or tea. It's a rich source of vitamins, minerals, and collagen, and a mug of bone broth can add a boost of protein and comforting warmth to your day.

Fill a large stockpot with the cold water, and set on high heat. Add all the ingredients to the pot and bring the water to a boil. Cover and reduce the heat to low. Simmer the broth for 12 to 24 hours without stirring. (Note, you can also do this in a slow cooker. Set the temperature to high until the liquid boils, then turn down to low and simmer for 12 to 24 hours.)

Remove the pot from the heat and pour the broth through a fine-mesh strainer. Discard the vegetables, herbs, and bones. Transfer the stock to multiple containers to speed up the cooling—don't freeze or refrigerate while hot. Allow the broth to sit in the fridge (uncovered) for several hours, until the fat rises to the top and hardens. Scrape off the fat with a spoon and discard.

A properly prepared broth will look jiggly when cold; that's the gelatin from the collagen in the bones. Heating the broth gently will return it to a liquid.

Transfer to quart or pint glass containers (see Tip). Store refrigerated broth for 3 to 4 days, or freeze for up to 1 year (see Tip).

> **TIP:** For an easy way to add small amounts of broth to recipes, pour some of the broth in an ice cube tray and freeze, then transfer the cubes to a container and store in the freezer. One cube is about 1 fluid ounce (2 tablespoons) of broth.
>   You can store larger amounts of the broth in glass mason jars, but be sure to let the broth cool before transferring to the glass, and make sure you leave enough space for the broth to expand upon freezing.
>   Experiment with using different herbs, spices, and vegetables in your broth. Try adding green onions, leeks, shallots, mushrooms, chard, parsnips, garlic, red pepper flakes, bay leaves, rosemary, sage, or ginger. Avoid using broccoli, turnips, cabbage, Brussels sprouts, green peppers, kale, collard greens, or mustard greens, as they can make your broth bitter. Skip the potatoes, too, as they can leave broth cloudy.

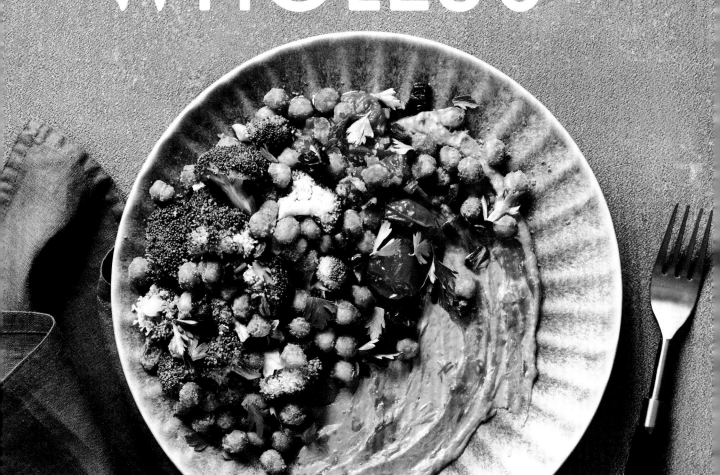

PART 5
THE PLANT-BASED WHOLE30

The Plant-Based Whole30 is our vegan elimination program. During the elimination phase, you eat beans, lentils, and peas; minimally processed forms of soy; plant-based protein powders; vegetables and fruit; natural plant-based fats; and herbs, spices, and seasonings. You don't count or restrict calories, track your intake, or limit your portions. You eat real, whole foods to satiety, inspired by the delicious, satisfying, and diverse recipes starting on page 244.

The following is a summary of the rules. For a detailed description of the Plant-Based Whole30 Program Rules, return to page 38.

PLANT-BASED WHOLE30 PROGRAM RULES (QUICK REFERENCE)

Plant-Based Whole30 elimination—30 days

By definition, the Plant-Based Whole30 elimination phase assumes you will also not be eating any animal protein, animal fats, or animal-based dairy.

- Added sugar (real or artificial)
- Alcohol (wine, beer, cider, liquor, etc.)
- Grains (wheat, oats, rice, corn, quinoa, etc.)
- Soy (highly processed forms)
- The Pancake Rule (baked goods, pasta, cereal, chips, and fries)
- The Scale Rule (weighing yourself or taking measurements)

The Fine Print (exceptions)

These foods *are* allowed during the Plant-Based Whole30 elimination phase:

- Rice found in fermented soy (listed as an ingredient in miso or tempeh)
- Cooking oils (regardless of the source)
- Coconut aminos
- Alcohol-based botanical extracts (such as vanilla, lemon, or lavender)

Harissa Chickpea Bowl, page 272

- Cane, Champagne, red wine, rice, sherry, and white wine vinegar
- Iodized salt (which contains dextrose as a stabilizer)

Plant-Based Whole30 reintroduction—6+ days

- Added sugar (optional)
- Return to the Plant-Based Whole30 elimination phase for 2 to 3 days
- Non-gluten grains
- Return to the Plant-Based Whole30 elimination phase for 2 to 3 days
- Animal protein (optional)
- Return to the Plant-Based Whole30 elimination phase for 2 to 3 days
- Animal-sourced dairy (optional)
- Return to the Plant-Based Whole30 elimination phase for 2 to 3 days
- Gluten-containing grains
- Return to the Plant-Based Whole30 elimination phase for 2 to 3 days
- Alcohol (optional)
- Return to the Plant-Based Whole30 elimination phase for 2 to 3 days

PLANT-BASED WHOLE30 MEAL TEMPLATE

One of the benefits of the Whole30 is that the program gets you back in touch with your body's natural "hungry" and "full" signals. Most participants find by the second week of their Whole30, they're able to tune into their body for cues, and use their energy, focus, hunger, and mood to help them build an individual meal plate that suits their needs, activity levels, and schedule.

Until then, here is a general meal template for the Plant-Based Whole30. Use this as a starting place if you're not sure how much to eat. Treat this template as a *minimum;* that is, you won't be eating less than the quantities recommended here.

Meal recommendations

Eat 4 meals a day. Base each meal on a plant-based protein source, ensuring each meal contains at least 15 grams of protein:

- Cooked beans or lentils: ½ to 1 cup
- Whole or less-processed soy (tofu, tempeh, edamame): 4 to 6 ounces
- Plant-based protein powder: 1 to 2 scoops*

Can be mixed into smoothies, soups, stews, curries, or puddings

Fill the rest of your plate with vegetables. Add a serving of fruit, if you choose. Add plant-based fats in these recommended minimum amounts per meal:

- Cooking oils (olive oil, avocado oil, etc.): 1 to 2 thumb-sized portions
- Butters (nut butter, coconut butter, etc.): 1 to 2 thumb-sized portions
- Coconut (shredded or flaked): 1 to 2 open (heaping) handfuls
- Olives: 1 to 2 open (heaping) handfuls
- Nuts and seeds: 1 small handful
- Avocado: ½ to 1 avocado
- Coconut milk: Between ¼ and ½ of one (13.5-ounce) full-fat can

Your schedule, hunger levels, or activity levels may require a snack between meals. For each snack, include at least two of the three macronutrients (protein, fat, and carbs) for satiety. Make your snack as big as you need to tide you over, but not so big that you're too full to eat your next scheduled meal. (See page 239 for snack ideas.)

If your activity levels necessitate a pre-workout or post-workout meal, follow the general guidelines on page 76, and work with your athletic trainer or sports nutritionist to ensure you are fueling your activities appropriately.

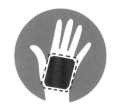

TOFU/TEMPEH

VEGETABLES

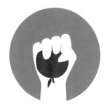

FRUIT

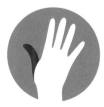

OILS & BUTTER

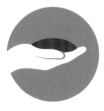

COCONUT & OLIVES

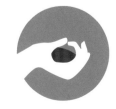

NUTS & SEEDS

PLANT-BASED WHOLE30 SHOPPING LIST

LEGUMES

Use dried, canned, or pre-sprouted beans and lentils.

BEANS AND PEAS

- [ ] Adzuki beans
- [ ] Black (turtle) beans
- [ ] Black chickpeas (kaala chana)
- [ ] Black-eyed peas (lobia)
- [ ] Chickpeas (garbanzo beans)
- [ ] Cranberry beans
- [ ] Fava (broad) beans
- [ ] Great northern beans
- [ ] Kidney beans (red, white)
- [ ] Lima (butter) beans
- [ ] Lupini beans
- [ ] Mung beans (moong dal)
- [ ] Navy (haricot) beans
- [ ] Peas (English, garden, green, snow, sugar snap, yellow)
- [ ] Pinto beans
- [ ] Red kidney beans (rajma)
- [ ] Split peas
- [ ] White chickpeas (kabuli chana)

LENTILS

- [ ] Bengal gram (chana dal)
- [ ] Black (Beluga)
- [ ] Black gram (urad dal)
- [ ] Brown
- [ ] Green
- [ ] Puy (French green)
- [ ] Red (masoor dal)
- [ ] Split pigeon peas (toor dal)
- [ ] Yellow

SOY

- [ ] Edamame
- [ ] Miso
- [ ] Natto
- [ ] Soy nuts
- [ ] Tempeh
- [ ] Tofu

PLANT-BASED PROTEINS

Read your labels and avoid protein sources with incompatible ingredients (like added sweeteners, quinoa, or rice bran).

- [ ] Hemp seed protein powder
- [ ] Pea protein powder
- [ ] Plant-based "meat" (ground)
- [ ] Plant-based "meat" (other)
- [ ] Plant-based protein "crumbles"
- [ ] Plant-based protein powders (mixed)
- [ ] Pumpkin seed protein powder
- [ ] Sunflower seed protein powder
- [ ] Watermelon seed protein powder

VEGETABLES

All vegetables but corn are compatible with the Plant-Based Whole30 elimination phase. Use fresh, frozen, or canned vegetables.

- [ ] Artichokes
- [ ] Arugula
- [ ] Asparagus
- [ ] Beets
- [ ] Bok choy
- [ ] Broccoli rabe
- [ ] Broccoli/broccolini
- [ ] Brussels sprouts
- [ ] Cabbage
- [ ] Calabaza
- [ ] Callaloo
- [ ] Carrots
- [ ] Cassava
- [ ] Cauliflower
- [ ] Celery
- [ ] Chard
- [ ] Chayote
- [ ] Chile peppers (jalapeño, poblano, serrano, etc.)
- [ ] Cucumber
- [ ] Eggplant
- [ ] Endive
- [ ] Fennel (anise)
- [ ] Frisee (curly endive)
- [ ] Garlic
- [ ] Green beans
- [ ] Green onion
- [ ] Greens (beet, collard, dandelion, mustard, Swiss chard, turnip, etc.)
- [ ] Hearts of palm
- [ ] Jicama
- [ ] Kale
- [ ] Leeks
- [ ] Lettuce (all types, including Bibb, butter, romaine)
- [ ] Microgreens
- [ ] Mushrooms (all types)
- [ ] Nopal (prickly pear)
- [ ] Nori
- [ ] Okra
- [ ] Onions
- [ ] Parsnips
- [ ] Peppers, bell
- [ ] Peppers, dried (all types)
- [ ] Potatoes (all types)
- [ ] Pumpkin
- [ ] Radishes
- [ ] Rhubarb
- [ ] Romanesco
- [ ] Rutabaga
- [ ] Shallots
- [ ] Spinach

- ☐ Sprouts
- ☐ Squash (acorn, butternut, delicata, kabocha, spaghetti, summer, etc.)
- ☐ Sweet potato/yams
- ☐ Tomatillos
- ☐ Tomatoes
- ☐ Turnips
- ☐ Zucchini

FRUITS

All fruit is compatible with the Whole30 elimination phase. Use fresh, frozen, or canned fruit (without added sugar).

- ☐ Apples (all types)
- ☐ Apricots
- ☐ Bananas
- ☐ Blackberries
- ☐ Blueberries
- ☐ Cherries
- ☐ Cranberries
- ☐ Currants (all types)
- ☐ Dates
- ☐ Dried fruit (all types)
- ☐ Elderberries
- ☐ Figs
- ☐ Gooseberries (Cape gooseberries)
- ☐ Grapefruit
- ☐ Grapes (all types)
- ☐ Kiwifruit
- ☐ Kumquats
- ☐ Lemons
- ☐ Limes
- ☐ Mango
- ☐ Melon (all types)
- ☐ Nectarines
- ☐ Oranges (all types)
- ☐ Papaya
- ☐ Pawpaw
- ☐ Peaches
- ☐ Pears (all types)
- ☐ Persimmons
- ☐ Pineapple
- ☐ Plantains
- ☐ Plums
- ☐ Pomegranates
- ☐ Raisins
- ☐ Raspberries
- ☐ Salmonberries
- ☐ Strawberries
- ☐ Tangerines
- ☐ Xoconostle
- ☐ Yuzu (citrus)

PLANT-BASED FATS

All cooking oils (regardless of their source) are compatible with the Whole30 elimination phase.

COOKING
- ☐ Avocado oil
- ☐ Canola oil
- ☐ Coconut oil
- ☐ Corn oil
- ☐ Cultured oil
- ☐ Soybean oil
- ☐ Sunflower oil

EATING
- ☐ Avocado
- ☐ Coconut butter
- ☐ Coconut (flakes, shredded)
- ☐ Coconut milk (canned)
- ☐ Olives (all types)
- ☐ Ghee (plant-based)

- ☐ Grapeseed oil
- ☐ Olive oil (light, extra-virgin)
- ☐ Palm oil
- ☐ Safflower oil
- ☐ Sesame oil (toasted/untoasted)

NUTS AND SEEDS
- ☐ Almonds/almond butter
- ☐ Brazil nuts
- ☐ Cashews/cashew butter
- ☐ Chia seeds
- ☐ Flax seeds
- ☐ Hazelnuts/hazelnut butter
- ☐ Hemp seeds (hearts)
- ☐ Macadamia/macadamia butter
- ☐ Pecans/pecan butter
- ☐ Pine nuts
- ☐ Pistachios
- ☐ Pumpkin seeds/pepitas
- ☐ Sesame seeds/tahini
- ☐ Sunflower seeds/sunflower butter
- ☐ Walnuts

HERBS, SPICES, SEASONINGS

Make sure your spices and spice blends are free from cornstarch, rice bran, added sugar, or other incompatible ingredients.

- ☐ Aleppo pepper flakes
- ☐ Allspice (whole/ground)
- ☐ Ancho chile powder
- ☐ Anise seeds
- ☐ Baharat (spice blend)
- ☐ Basil (fresh/dried)
- ☐ Bay leaves (fresh/dried)
- ☐ Black pepper (ground)
- ☐ Cacao powder (100%)
- ☐ Caraway seeds
- ☐ Cardamom seeds
- ☐ Cayenne
- ☐ Celery seeds
- ☐ Chervil (French parsley)
- ☐ Chili powder
- ☐ Chinese five-spice powder
- ☐ Chipotle powder
- ☐ Chives (fresh/dried)
- ☐ Cilantro (fresh/dried)
- ☐ Cinnamon (stick/ground)
- ☐ Cloves (whole/ground)
- ☐ Coriander (seeds/ground)
- ☐ Creole seasoning (blend)
- ☐ Cumin (seeds/ground)
- ☐ Curry powder (blend)
- ☐ Dill (fresh/dried)
- ☐ Everything bagel seasoning
- ☐ Galangal
- ☐ Garam masala
- ☐ Garlic powder
- ☐ Ginger (fresh/ground)
- ☐ Harissa (paste/sauce)
- ☐ Hibiscus flowers (dried)
- ☐ Hing (asafetida)
- ☐ Horseradish (fresh/prepared)

- [ ] Italian seasoning
- [ ] Lemongrass (fresh/ dried)
- [ ] Liquid smoke
- [ ] Matcha powder
- [ ] Mint (fresh/dried)
- [ ] Mustard (powder)
- [ ] Nutmeg
- [ ] Onion powder
- [ ] Oregano (fresh/dried)
- [ ] Paprika (sweet/ smoked)
- [ ] Parsley (fresh/dried)
- [ ] Peppercorns (black, pink)
- [ ] Red pepper flakes
- [ ] Rosemary (fresh/ dried)
- [ ] Sage (fresh/dried)
- [ ] Salt
- [ ] Sumac (ground)
- [ ] Tajin (chile blend)
- [ ] Tarragon (fresh/ dried)
- [ ] Thai basil
- [ ] Thyme (fresh/dried)
- [ ] Truffle salt
- [ ] Turmeric (whole/ ground)
- [ ] Urfa biber (chile flakes)
- [ ] Vanilla (bean/ extract)
- [ ] Wasabi powder
- [ ] Za'atar (blend)

PANTRY AND FRIDGE ITEMS

This is one category in which reading labels is paramount. Better yet, just look for Whole30 Approved® products, and skip the label-reading!

- [ ] Almond flour
- [ ] Arrowroot powder
- [ ] Beet kvass
- [ ] Broth (vegetable)
- [ ] Capers
- [ ] Coconut aminos
- [ ] Coconut flour
- [ ] Cream cheese (dairy-free)
- [ ] Hot sauce
- [ ] Hummus
- [ ] Ketchup (no-sugar)
- [ ] Kimchi
- [ ] Mayonnaise (vegan)
- [ ] Mustard (all types)
- [ ] Nutritional yeast
- [ ] Olives (canned)
- [ ] Peppers, roasted (jarred)
- [ ] Pickled vegetables (jalapeño, red onion, etc.)
- [ ] Pickles
- [ ] Preserved lemons
- [ ] Pumpkin (canned)
- [ ] Queso (dairy-free)
- [ ] Ricotta (dairy-free)
- [ ] Salad dressing (vegan)
- [ ] Sauerkraut
- [ ] Sun-dried tomatoes
- [ ] Sweet potato (canned)
- [ ] Tapioca, instant
- [ ] Tapioca starch
- [ ] Squash, butternut (canned)
- [ ] Tomato paste
- [ ] Tomato sauce
- [ ] Tomatoes (canned, crushed, diced, stewed)
- [ ] Vinegar (apple cider, balsamic, cane, Champagne, red wine, rice, sherry, white, white wine)
- [ ] Yogurt (dairy-free)

BEVERAGES

Look for hidden sources of added sugar, especially in flavored waters or teas, and avoid oat-based non-dairy products.

- [ ] Apple cider/juice
- [ ] Club soda
- [ ] Coconut water
- [ ] Coffee
- [ ] Coffee creamer (non-dairy)
- [ ] Fruit juice (other than orange or apple)
- [ ] Kombucha
- [ ] Milk (non-dairy)
- [ ] Mineral water
- [ ] Orange juice
- [ ] Seltzer water
- [ ] Sparkling tea
- [ ] Sparkling water
- [ ] Tea (brewed)
- [ ] Tomato juice
- [ ] Vegetable juice (such as celery or vegetable blends)

PLANT-BASED WHOLE30 FAQ

Why does the Plant-Based Whole30 eliminate _____?

The first question many people have after reading the rules is, "Wait, I thought whole grains were *healthy*?" To which I respond, "Healthy for whom, and in what context?" There are no universally healthy foods. Not even broccoli! (Just ask my dad, who gets terrible gas and bloating every time he tries to eat it raw.) Our bodies are unique, and we all respond to foods and ingredients differently. If you're sensitive to the gluten in bread, the artificial sweetener in your non-dairy creamer, or the fermentable carbohydrates in beans, it won't feel health-promoting when *you* consume them.

Please visit our website (whole30.com) for detailed articles and references supporting these elimination groups.

On the flip side, there are no universally *unhealthy* foods. Remember, Whole30 doesn't eliminate foods because they're "bad," and we certainly don't believe everyone needs to avoid them. These food groups have been shown in both the scientific literature and our fifteen-plus years of clinical experience to be commonly problematic—to varying degrees. I don't know if or how they're problematic for you—and neither do you, until you eliminate them, reintroduce them, and compare your experience. What you choose to do with those learnings is completely up to you.

In summary:

- **Added sugar, real and artificial:** In the right context, added sugar can have health-promoting properties, making foods taste delicious and fueling your activities, mood, and energy levels. However, research overwhelmingly demonstrates that excess sugar consumption has a negative impact on cravings, blood sugar regulation and metabolism, digestion and gut health, systemic inflammation, and risk for chronic disease. While artificial sweeteners aren't believed to promote blood sugar dysregulation in the same way as natural forms of sugar, they can contribute to headaches, migraines, irritability, increased sugar cravings, gas, and bloating. Avoiding all forms of added sugar during your Whole30 elimination will help you become more aware of added sugar in your diet and help you identify which forms of sugar, in what amounts, and in what context work best for your body.

- **Alcohol:** Recent studies show that even small amounts of alcohol can have a negative effect on health—everything from cravings to blood sugar regulation and hormonal balance (particularly sex hormones), gut health, and systemic inflammation, particularly impacting the nervous system and brain. In addition, alcohol inhibits your judgment concerning all kinds of decisions, including food choices. Reintroduction will help you identify when, how often, in what amounts, and in what form alcohol may be "worth it" for you going forward.

- **Grains:** Whole grains provide fiber, vitamins, minerals, and other nutrients. Whole-grain foods can also help maintain healthy cholesterol levels and blood pressure, and assist in lowering the risk of diabetes, heart disease and other conditions. (In many studies, replacing refined grains with whole grains has been found to reduce inflammation, perhaps owing to their high fiber content.) However, there are different protein structures in grains that are particularly resistant to digestion and can improperly cross the gut barrier. This can trigger not only digestive issues but also an immune response that promotes systemic inflammation. You may be familiar with *gluten,* a protein component of wheat, rye, or barley that can be especially problematic. However, non-gluten grains like corn or pseudo-cereals like quinoa contain other proteins to which people can be similarly sensitive. Inflammation can also be the result of impaired metabolic health or blood sugar control. When grains (especially refined versions) are consumed in excess, it can be difficult to keep blood sugar within a healthy range. We replace all grains with fiber-rich, nutrient-dense vegetables and fruit during the Whole30 elimination to help you identify if or how grains may be impacting your health and how you feel.

- **Highly processed forms of soy:** Although limited research is available on highly processed forms of soy (like textured soy protein, textured vegetable protein, soy protein isolate, and soy protein concentrate), studies suggest that most do not offer the same health benefits as whole, unprocessed forms. Some research also suggests that highly processed soy products may have less favorable effects on the immune system compared to natural soy products. In addition, our registered dietitians agree that patients experience more issues (like joint pain, swelling, or gastrointestinal distress) from highly processed forms of soy, versus soy in its whole form. For these reasons, we include only minimally processed soy in the program and eliminate highly processed forms.

What are some snack ideas for the Plant-Based Whole30?

Here are some ideas for snacks or mini-meals for your Plant-Based Whole30. Some require a bit of planning and preparation (like roasting a tray of chickpeas). Others are more grab-and-go, like veggie sticks and guacamole. All contain at least two macronutrients to keep you satiated and energized.

- Edamame + fruit
- Banana + unsweetened nut butter
- Crispy roasted chickpeas + pistachios
- Lupini beans + veggies + tahini
- Apple slices + hummus
- Smoothie (see page 242)

You can also serve a small leftover portion of last night's dinner as a snack! Snacks don't have to be grab-and-go options; a small bowl of black bean chili, a slice of tofu frittata, or a bowl of Muhammara (page 341) with some roasted veggies would also work just as well.

What are some on-the-go ideas for the Plant-Based Whole30?

Here are some easy on-the-go ideas for your Plant-Based Whole30. Not every option will be a good fit for your situation—you can't exactly blend a smoothie on an airplane—but you can certainly leave one in the freezer at the office as a quick mini-meal between Zoom calls. Make sure your on-the-go items also fit the rules of the Plant-Based Whole30 elimination phase.

- Protein: Edamame, crispy chickpeas, lupini beans, smoothie, hummus
- Carbs: Fruit, sliced veggies, baby food pouches, applesauce, dried fruit, fruit-and-nut bars
- Fat: Avocado or guacamole, coconut flakes, olives, nuts and seeds, nut butter, coconut butter, salad dressing, nut "cheese" or dips

Smoothies (see page 242) generally contain plant-based protein powder, carbs from fruit and veggies, and healthy fats from coconut milk or nut butters, making them well-balanced on-the-go meals or snacks. In fact, many of these ideas (like dried fruit-and-nut bars or hummus) are good sources of at least two macronutrients.

Will I get enough protein on the Plant-Based Whole30?

During the Plant-Based Whole30 elimination phase, you use legumes (beans, lentils, soy, and peanuts) as your primary protein sources. Nuts and seeds, plant-based protein powders, and plant-based meat alternatives provide additional essential amino acids and protein.

The recommended dietary allowance (RDA) of protein is 0.8 grams per kilogram (about 0.36 grams per pound of body weight per day. That works out to (on average) 54 grams of protein a day for a 150-pound adult. Keep in mind, however, that the RDA is the amount of a nutrient you need to meet your basic nutritional requirements. In other words, it's the minimum amount you need *to keep from getting sick,* not the amount you should be eating to optimize your health.

Your body, activity levels, and health context all play a role in your ideal protein needs. It's highly likely that 54 grams a day won't be adequate if you're an athlete, live an active lifestyle, or

OPTIMIZE YOUR PROTEIN

While the lower end of this range *may* meet the nutrient needs for sedentary individuals, our registered dietitians recommend aiming for a minimum of 1 gram per kilogram (0.45 grams per pound) of body weight to better support satiety, strength, and general health. On average, that translates to a protein intake of around 70 grams a day—and *that* is the minimum amount we're recommending per day on the Plant-Based Whole30.

simply have a larger body or more muscle mass. Active individuals typically require protein in amounts closer to 1.2 to 1.8 grams per kilogram, or 0.54 to 0.82 grams per pound of body weight per day to support muscle protein synthesis, tissue maintenance, and repair.

If this is your context, you'll likely need to include a compatible protein powder at least once a day to supplement your protein needs, and you'll shoot for the higher range of plant-based protein sources at each meal. This looks like 1 cup of cooked beans or lentils or 6 to 7 ounces of tofu or tempeh at each meal, along with higher-protein nuts and seeds. (Visit whole30.com for our Plant-Based Protein Table.)

You'll notice the majority of our Plant-Based recipes serve 3, which is an odd number for most cookbooks. This was intentional! For those who need more protein, we've deliberately included an extra portion to help boost your protein intake. (And if you're cooking for one, you've got built-in leftovers—bonus!)

In general, aim for a minimum of 15 grams of protein from your main protein source at each of your four meals. Use nuts and seeds, dressings and sauces (like tahini or hummus), and compatible plant-based protein powders to provide additional protein.

I thought I wasn't supposed to weigh, measure, or track my food?

It's *really* important to consume enough protein to support your health and performance, whether you're active or not. Plant-based protein sources aren't generally as dense as animal proteins, and most don't contain adequate amounts of all nine essential amino acids. If you're already eating a vegan diet, you likely know how to ensure your meals include adequate protein intake and a variety of amino acids.

If you're an omnivore, however, and plant-based eating is new, you'll have to pay more attention to your protein sources to ensure you're eating enough—at least at first. This doesn't mean you need to run all your ingredients through a calorie tracker, though. As you begin your Whole30 elimination phase, make sure your meals are centered on protein, and include enough of that protein source to meet your needs. After a week or two, you'll be familiar with the serving sizes you need and the extra touches you can add to dishes to boost their protein content.

In summary, all the recipes in this book meet or exceed our protein recommendations per serving. However, if your protein needs are higher, you may need to adjust your serving size, add a supplementary protein smoothie to your day, or include more of the protein called for in the recipe.

Do I have to eat complete proteins with every meal?

The quick answer is "Nope, just eat a variety of foods in the elimination phase." Here's the longer answer:

"Complete protein" means the protein source contains an adequate amount of all nine essential amino acids. These amino acids cannot be made by the body and must be provided by the foods we eat. On the Plant-Based Whole30, soy (like tofu or tempeh) is a source of complete protein. (Some resources also list pea protein, hemp, and chia as complete, although they are all low in at least one of the essential amino acids.) Other plant proteins, like those found in beans, lentils, nuts, and seeds, are "incomplete," meaning they lack one or more of the essential amino acids.

Eating a variety of amino acids (and ensuring adequate amounts of all the essential amino acids) is important, but that doesn't mean you need to include a complete protein in every meal. Over the course of your day, your body can combine the amino acids from the various foods you eat to perform all the tasks they are needed to do, from breaking down food to growing and repairing body tissue.

To ensure adequate protein and intake of essential amino acids, make sure your Plant-Based Whole30 includes a variety of protein sources (including soy products, beans, lentils, peas, nuts, and seeds) over the course of your daily and weekly meals. You may also choose to supplement with a compatible plant-based protein powder made from pea protein, hemp, or chia.

How do I use a plant-based protein powder during the elimination phase?

Plant-based protein powders can provide a protein boost to meals, and they are an easy way to increase your overall protein intake. Read the labels carefully, as many plant-based protein "blends" include incompatible ingredients for the Whole30, like sweeteners, rice bran, or other grain-derived ingredients.

Here are several ways you can use plant-based protein powders:

- Blended into a smoothie (keep reading for our smoothie formula and see page 340 for a sample recipe)
- Blended into chia puddings (see page 342)
- 1 scoop of powder mixed into a soup or stew (before cooking)
- 1 scoop of powder mixed into guacamole or hummus

Visit whole30.com/whole30-approved to see a complete list of Whole30 Approved® plant-based protein powders.

How do I make a Plant-Based Whole30 smoothie?

Smoothies are a great way to add more protein to your day, and they can be an easy, portable source of energy when you're on the go. You can use fresh or frozen ingredients here. Be sure all the ingredients in your smoothie are compatible with the Plant-Based Whole30 elimination phase! Here is a general template:

Liquids: 8 to 12 fluid ounces (1 to 1½ cups)

- Full-fat canned coconut milk (also counts as added fat)
- Unsweetened soy or nut milk
- Brewed unsweetened tea
- Vegetable broth
- Water/ice

Protein: 15 grams, minimum

- Plant-based protein powder
- Tofu*

Silken tofu provides the best texture, but extra-firm or super-firm provides the most protein

Fat: 1 serving, minimum

- Avocado
- Seeds (chia, hemp, pumpkin, ground flaxseed, etc.)
- Nut butter, seed butter, or coconut butter
- Coconut flakes

Fruit: ½ to 1 cup

- Berries (up to 1 cup)
- Apple, pear, or peach (up to 1 cup)
- Pineapple or mango (up to ½ cup)
- Unsweetened acai puree (up to ½ cup)
- Banana (up to 1 small)

Veggies: 1 cup, minimum

- Leafy greens
- Mashed pumpkin
- Mashed butternut squash
- Mashed sweet potato
- Cauliflower rice
- Zucchini

Boosts: optional or to taste

- Cinnamon
- Chai seasoning
- Turmeric

- 100% cacao powder
- Sea salt
- Fresh herbs (mint, basil)

I'm not used to eating this much soy, beans, and lentils. Do you have any tips for digestion?

Digestive distress is more common on the Plant-Based Whole30 compared to the Original. The amount of legumes you need to meet your protein needs may provide more fiber or fermentable carbohydrates than your digestive tract is accustomed to. This is especially true if you have a soy allergy, you need to limit your soy consumption, or you weren't consuming many soy products, beans, or lentils prior to beginning your Plant-Based Whole30. (In which case, your body may not be producing many of the digestive enzymes needed to break down legumes.)

These tips can help you better prepare your body for Day 1 of the Plant-Based Whole30, increase enzymatic production, and reduce gas, bloating, and other digestive symptoms during the elimination phase.

- Gradually increase your consumption of beans and lentils before you begin the Whole30. Start off small, adding just ¼ cup to your meals, and increase your consumption slowly. This will help to encourage enzymatic production in your gut.
- During the elimination phase, include more fermented soy products and plant-based meats in your meals, and fewer legumes, lentils, and other forms of soy.
- Choose smaller varieties of beans and lentils, like split peas, adzuki beans, or green lentils. These may prove easier to digest than larger beans, like kidney, garbanzo, or black beans.

- Choose fermented versions of soy, like tempeh or miso, as the fermentation process may aid digestion.
- Soak dried beans and lentils before cooking. Soaking can break down some of the complex carbohydrates that cause gas and bloating, help the beans cook more quickly, and lead to a more tender texture. Dried beans should soak for 12 to 24 hours; then drain and rinse them before cooking. You can also quick-soak beans by adding them to a pot, covering with 1 to 2 inches of water, bringing to a boil, then cooking for 5 minutes. Let the beans sit in the pot for 1 hour, then drain and rinse before completing the cooking.
- Rinse and drain canned beans at least once before consuming. The draining can also help remove excess starches that can contribute to digestive issues.
- Sprout legumes and lentils before cooking them. (Or purchase sprouted beans from your local grocer or online market.) Sprouting can help to improve digestion and nutrient absorption. You'll find tips for sprouting beans, lentils, and chickpeas on pages 268, 283, and 349, respectively.
- Cook dried beans thoroughly. Well-cooked beans will be easier to digest.
- Add tempering agents to your meals. Garlic, ginger, turmeric, kombu (a type of seaweed), and asafoetida (an Indian spice also known as hing) have anti-flatulent properties.
- Use other plant-based proteins, such as whole forms of soy and unsweetened protein powder, to help you meet your protein needs with fewer legumes and lentils.
- Ask your healthcare provider if using a digestive enzyme supplement is appropriate for you. When used with meals, this supplement can help your body adjust to the increased fiber content in your diet and the specific carbohydrates in legumes.

PLANT-BASED WHOLE30 RECIPES

BREAKFASTS

opposite: Good-Day Tofu Eggs, Greens, and Hash Browns, page 252

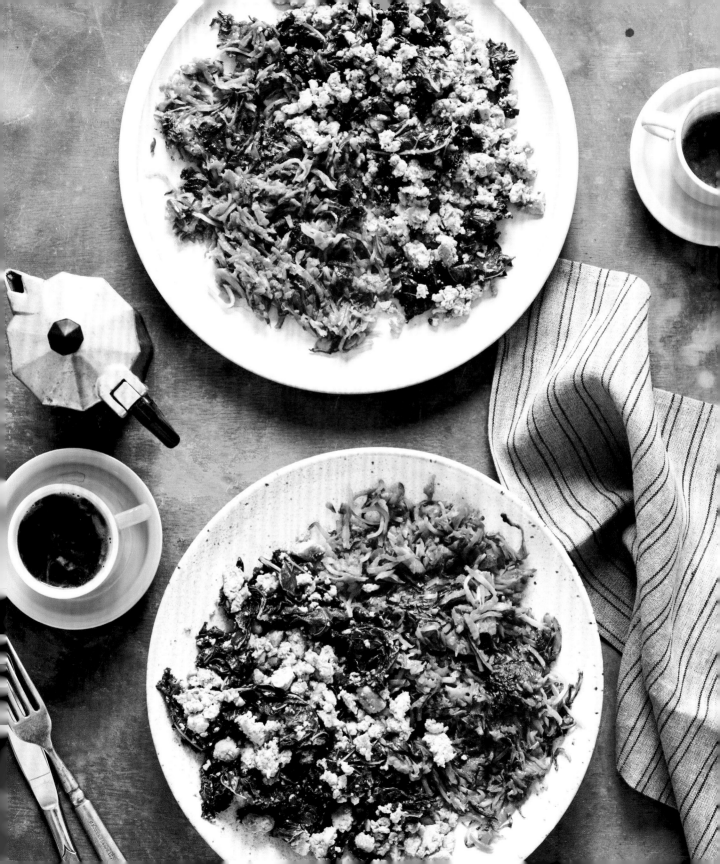

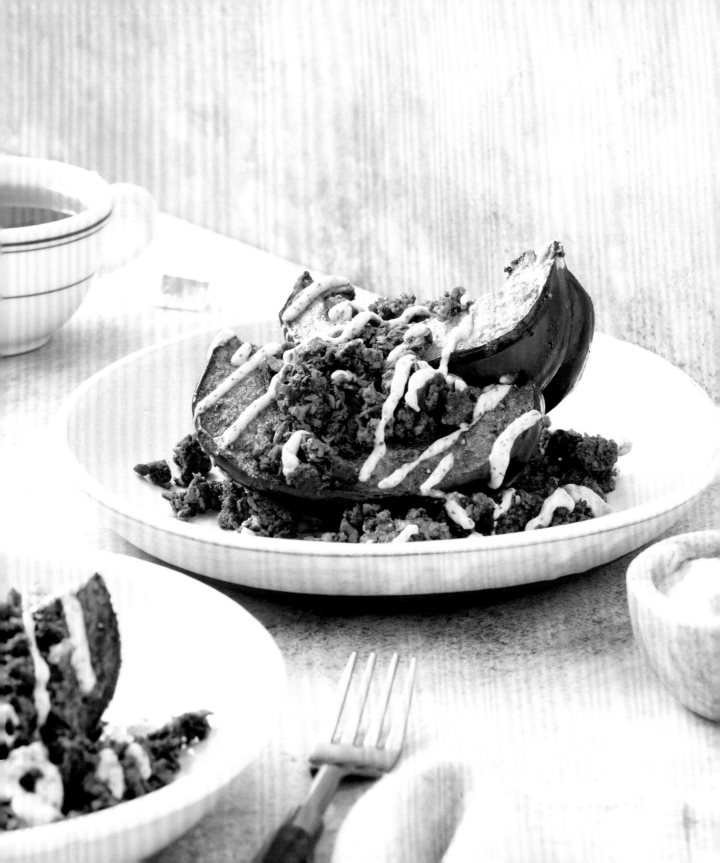

ACORN SQUASH AND CHORIZO WITH AVOCADO SAUCE

SERVES 2 TO 3 • PREP: 15 MINUTES • BAKE: 20 MINUTES • COOK: 5 MINUTES •
TOTAL: 40 MINUTES

FOR THE ACORN SQUASH

3 tablespoons extra-virgin olive oil

¾ teaspoon ground cinnamon

½ teaspoon ground cumin

½ teaspoon paprika

½ teaspoon salt

¼ teaspoon black pepper

1 medium acorn squash, cut into quarters and seeds removed

⅛ teaspoon cayenne

FOR THE AVOCADO SAUCE

1 large ripe avocado, halved, pitted, peeled, and chopped

¼ cup lightly packed fresh cilantro

3 tablespoons Plant-Based Whole30 Mayo (page 230) or Plant-Based Whole30–compatible mayonnaise

3 tablespoons water, or more as needed

2 tablespoons fresh lime juice (see Tip)

½ teaspoon salt

FOR THE CHORIZO AND SERVING

1 (10-ounce) package Plant-Based Whole30–compatible chorizo

1 teaspoon extra-virgin olive oil

The flavors of this hearty breakfast dish complement each other beautifully. The mild spiciness of the plant-based chorizo is balanced with the sweetness of the squash and the cool creaminess of the buttery avocado sauce.

MAKE THE SQUASH: Preheat the oven to 425°F. Line a large rimmed baking sheet with parchment.

In a small bowl, stir together the olive oil, cinnamon, cumin, paprika, salt, and pepper, and brush the mixture on the flesh of the squash. Place the squash, cut side down, on the baking sheet. Bake until the squash is tender, about 20 minutes. Let cool while preparing the avocado sauce and chorizo.

MAKE THE AVOCADO SAUCE: In a food processor, combine the avocado, cilantro, mayonnaise, 3 tablespoons water, lime juice, and salt. Process until smooth. If the sauce is too thick, add additional water, 1 teaspoon at a time.

Cook the chorizo and serve: In a large nonstick skillet, cook the chorizo in the olive oil until heated through and slightly browned, 8 to 10 minutes.

Spread the squash on a serving platter and spoon the chorizo over it. Drizzle with the avocado sauce.

> **TIP:** The avocado sauce will keep in the fridge for 4 to 5 days, if you want to make a double batch.
>
> The lime juice helps prevent oxidation and keeps it from browning, but you can also press a piece of plastic wrap onto the top of the sauce, then cover it tightly. (A mason jar works well here.)

CREAMY GARAM MASALA SPLIT PEAS

SERVES 3 • PREP: 10 MINUTES • COOK: 35 MINUTES • TOTAL: 45 MINUTES

1½ cups yellow or red split peas

1 tablespoon coconut oil or extra-virgin olive oil

2 large shallots, finely chopped

1 red bell pepper, cored, seeded, and chopped

2 teaspoons garam masala

1 teaspoon nutritional yeast

1 teaspoon salt

2½ cups Vegetable Broth (page 351) or Plant-Based Whole30–compatible vegetable broth

½ cup canned full-fat coconut cream (see Tip)

Chopped fresh cilantro and/ or mint

Garam masala is an Indian spice blend made with a number of spices, including cloves, cinnamon, cardamom, cumin seeds, coriander seeds, nutmeg, bay leaf, mace, and black peppercorns. The spices are first toasted to bring out their aroma, then ground to a powder. Coconut cream nicely balances the warming flavors of garam masala, while a garnish of fresh herbs brightens the plate.

Using a strainer, rinse the split peas under cool running water until the water runs clear, then drain. (See Tip.)

In a large saucepan, heat the coconut oil over medium heat. Add the shallots and bell pepper and cook until tender, 3 to 5 minutes. Stir in the split peas, garam masala, nutritional yeast, and salt. Stir in the broth. Bring to a boil, then reduce the heat, cover, and simmer until the split peas are tender, 30 to 40 minutes.

Stir in the coconut cream, then spoon into bowls or onto plates. Top the servings with the fresh herbs.

TIP: Rinsing the split peas helps remove any dust and dirt. You don't need to soak split peas, as they cook relatively quickly.

If you can't find canned coconut cream, it's easy to make your own. Place a can of full-fat coconut milk in the fridge for 1 hour, until the cream solidifies on top and separates from the water. Scoop out the solid cream and reserve the water for use in a smoothie.

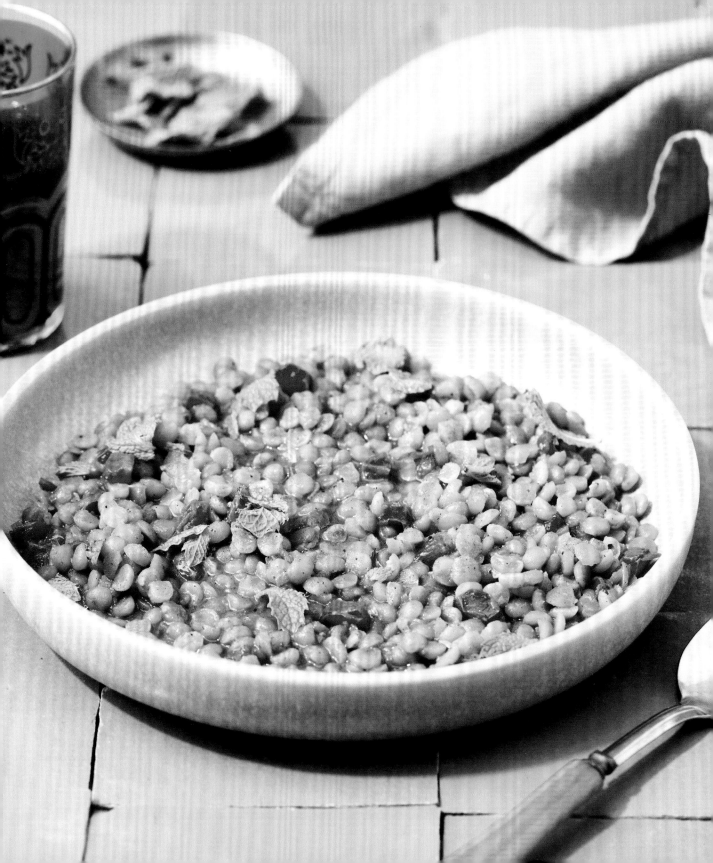

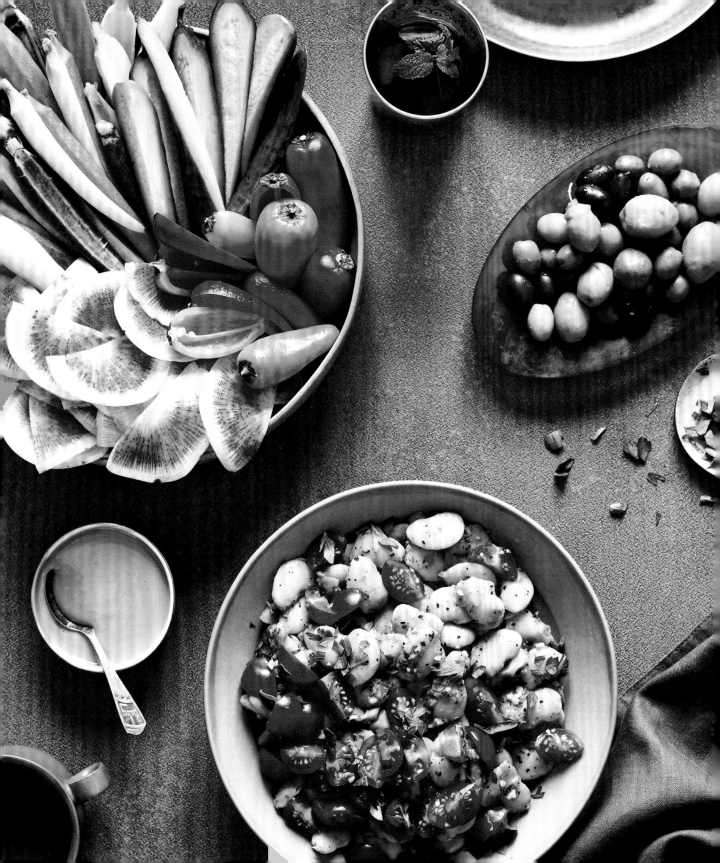

EGYPTIAN-INSPIRED BUTTER BEANS WITH VEGGIES

SERVES 3 • PREP: 10 MINUTES • COOK: 5 MINUTES • TOTAL: 15 MINUTES

2 (13- to 15-ounce) cans butter beans, rinsed and drained

¼ cup extra-virgin olive oil

1 tablespoon fresh lemon juice

2 garlic cloves, minced

1 teaspoon Urfa chile flakes or ½ teaspoon Aleppo pepper flakes or red pepper flakes (see Tip)

1 teaspoon cumin seeds, crushed

½ teaspoon salt

9 cherry tomatoes, quartered

¼ cup chopped fresh parsley

¾ cup tahini

Assorted vegetables, such as halved baby bell peppers, radishes, and sliced cucumber

Assorted olives

This recipe was inspired by ful medames, a classic breakfast dish of stewed seasoned fava beans. The dish originated in ancient Egypt, but is now popular throughout Africa and Asia. Canned or frozen fava beans are hard to find, and fresh favas are available only in the spring. We've adapted the flavors of ful medames to canned butter beans to make this dish more accessible year-round.

In a medium saucepan, warm the butter beans over medium heat, about 5 minutes. Remove from the heat and stir in the olive oil, lemon juice, garlic, Urfa chile flakes, cumin, and salt. If desired, lightly mash the beans.

Spoon the butter beans onto a serving platter and top with the tomatoes and parsley. Serve with the tahini, assorted vegetables, and olives.

TIP: Urfa (sometimes called urfa biber) is a Turkish chile that has a dark burgundy color and a smoky/sweet/sour/fruity flavor with a modest amount of heat. Aleppo pepper flakes add more of a fruity flavor, and a mild level of spice. If you have neither, red pepper flakes will work in a pinch, but will add more heat to the dish.

GOOD-DAY TOFU EGGS, GREENS, AND HASH BROWNS

SERVES 3 • PREP: 15 MINUTES • COOK: 10 MINUTES • TOTAL: 25 MINUTES

FOR THE TOFU EGGS AND GREENS

1 (16-ounce) block super-firm tofu, drained (see Tip)

3 tablespoons nutritional yeast

¾ teaspoon coarse black salt (see Tip)

½ teaspoon ground turmeric

¼ teaspoon smoked paprika

2 tablespoons extra-virgin olive oil

4 cups lightly packed torn curly kale

1 teaspoon apple cider vinegar

1 teaspoon Plant-Based Whole30–compatible Dijon mustard

¼ teaspoon salt

⅛ teaspoon black pepper

FOR THE HASH BROWNS AND SERVING

2 tablespoons extra-virgin olive oil

1 (12-ounce) bag frozen root-vegetable hash browns or potato hash browns

½ teaspoon salt

½ teaspoon black pepper

Plant-Based Whole30–compatible hot sauce (optional)

Seasonings of nutritional yeast, black salt, turmeric, and smoked paprika make these tofu eggs far more interesting than your usual morning scramble. Serve with a side of kale seasoned with vinegar and mustard, along with colorful root-vegetable hash browns.

MAKE THE TOFU EGGS AND GREENS: Finely crumble the tofu into a medium bowl. In a small bowl, stir together the nutritional yeast, black salt, turmeric, and paprika. Sprinkle the seasoning over the tofu and stir to combine.

In an extra-large skillet, heat 1 tablespoon of the olive oil over medium heat. Add the seasoned tofu and cook, stirring, until the tofu is heated through, 3 to 4 minutes.

Push the tofu to the edge of the skillet, creating an empty center. Add the remaining tablespoon oil to the center, then add the kale and use tongs to toss until wilted, about 2 minutes. Sprinkle the kale with the vinegar, mustard, salt, and pepper and toss to coat.

MAKE THE HASH BROWNS: In another large skillet, heat the olive oil over medium heat. Once the oil is hot, add the hash browns to the skillet and spread evenly in the pan. Cook without stirring until the bottom is golden brown, 5 to 6 minutes. Using a large spatula, turn the hash browns over and cook until golden brown on the other side, about 3 minutes more. Sprinkle with the salt and pepper.

Serve: Spoon the hash browns and tofu eggs onto serving plates. Add the kale and serve with the hot sauce (if using).

> **TIP:** You don't have to press the tofu before you scramble it, as any water left after draining will evaporate in the cooking process.
>
> Using black salt (also called lava salt) in the tofu egg mixture approximates the sulfury flavor of natural eggs. Of course, you can always substitute table salt or sea salt.

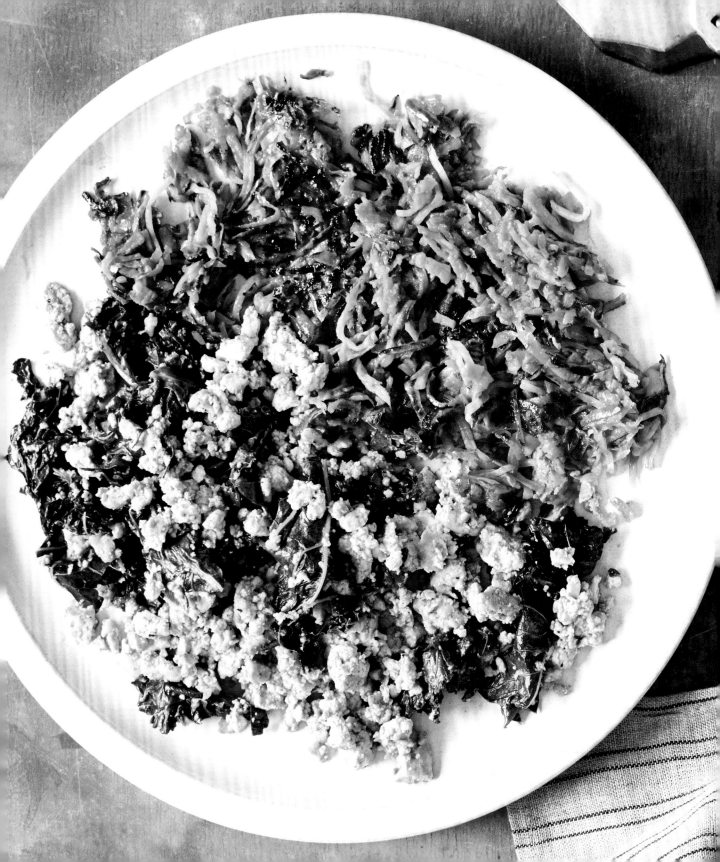

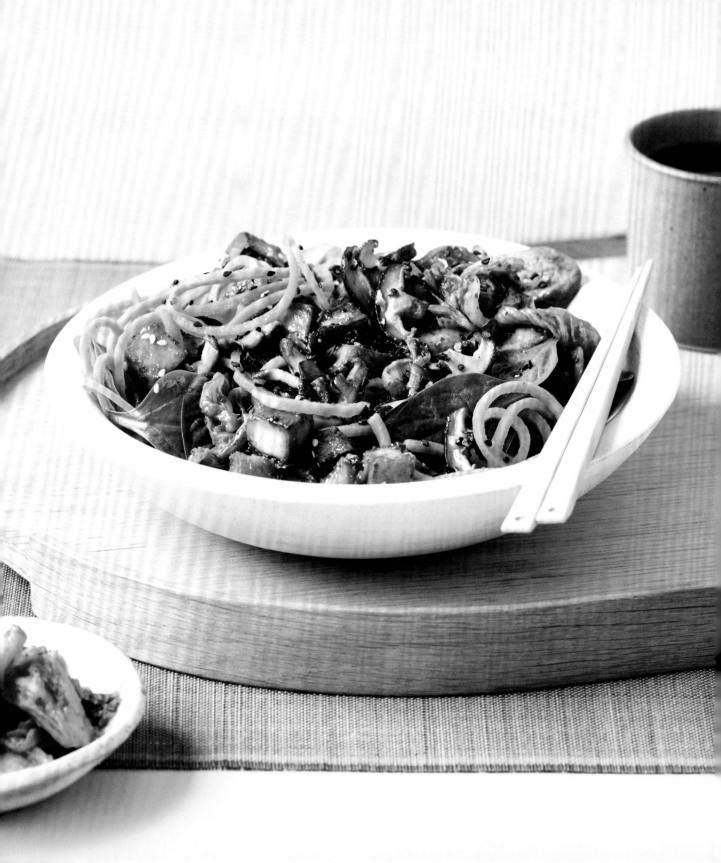

KOREAN-INSPIRED BREAKFAST BOWL

SERVES 3 • PREP: 20 MINUTES • BAKE/COOK: 25 MINUTES • TOTAL: 45 MINUTES

FOR THE SAUCE

¼ cup coconut aminos

¼ cup water

3 tablespoons unseasoned rice vinegar

3 tablespoons toasted sesame oil

1 tablespoon fresh orange juice

2 teaspoons red pepper flakes

FOR THE TOFU

1 (14-ounce) block super-firm tofu, drained, pressed, and diced (see Tip)

1 tablespoon extra-virgin olive oil

1 tablespoon coconut aminos

1 tablespoon arrowroot powder

1 teaspoon sesame seeds

FOR THE SALAD AND SERVING

3 tablespoons extra-virgin olive oil

2 garlic cloves, minced

1 (5-ounce) container fresh shiitake mushrooms, stems trimmed and caps thinly sliced

¼ teaspoon salt

¼ teaspoon black pepper

1 (10-ounce) package of butternut squash noodles or sweet potato noodles

1 (5-ounce) package baby spinach

1 cup Plant-Based Whole30–compatible kimchi

1 teaspoon black sesame seeds

This beautiful bowl may look a bit daunting, but it comes together quite easily. The tofu roasts in the oven while you make the salad, and the toasty sweet sauce whips up in just 2 minutes.

MAKE THE SAUCE: In a small bowl, stir together the coconut aminos, water, vinegar, sesame oil, orange juice, and red pepper flakes. Set aside.

MAKE THE TOFU: Prehcat the oven to 400°F. Line a large rimmed baking sheet with parchment.

In a medium bowl, combine the tofu, olive oil, and coconut aminos, and toss to combine. Sprinkle the arrowroot over the tofu and toss to coat. Arrange the tofu in an even layer on the baking sheet and sprinkle with the sesame seeds. Bake until golden, 15 to 20 minutes.

MAKE THE SALAD: Meanwhile, in a large skillet, heat 2 tablespoons of the olive oil over medium heat. Add the garlic and cook until sizzling, about 2 minutes (do not let the garlic brown). Add the mushrooms and cook until lightly browned, 3 to 4 minutes. Lightly sprinkle with the salt and pepper. Transfer the mushrooms to a bowl and cover to keep warm.

In the same skillet, add the remaining tablespoon olive oil and warm over medium heat. Add the noodles and cook, tossing occasionally, until just tender, 5 to 8 minutes.

Serve: In 3 shallow serving bowls, arrange the spinach and then add the tofu, mushrooms, and noodles. Top with the kimchi, drizzle with the sauce, and sprinkle with the sesame seeds.

TIP: Pressing the tofu before you bake, pan-fry, air-fry, or grill it allows you to remove most of the excess moisture. This helps the tofu better absorb the flavors of marinades and seasonings and is the key to getting lightly crisped edges. The longer your tofu is pressed, the more firm it becomes. Ideally, press the tofu for 30 to 60 minutes before cooking, but even a quick press will help. To press a block of tofu, wrap it in a tea towel and place on a cooling rack over a baking sheet to help contain the moisture. Put a heavy object (like a cast-iron pan or gallon water jug) on top of the tofu block and allow it to sit for the desired length of time.

LION'S MANE MUSHROOMS AND ASPARAGUS WITH HERBED RICOTTA

SERVES 3 • **PREP: 15 MINUTES** • **COOK: 5 MINUTES** • **TOTAL: 20 MINUTES**

3 tablespoons extra-virgin olive oil

1 (10-ounce) package Plant-Based Whole30–compatible lion's mane mushroom crumbles or pork, or Good-Day Tofu Eggs (page 252)

6 asparagus spears, trimmed and cut into 2-inch pieces

1 (8-ounce) container Plant-Based Whole30–compatible ricotta

1 teaspoon grated lemon zest

1 tablespoon fresh lemon juice

1 small garlic clove, minced

1 tablespoon finely chopped fresh tarragon

¼ teaspoon salt

1 tablespoon finely chopped fresh chives

Chopped or sliced cantaloupe or honeydew melon

Lion's mane mushrooms have long been used in traditional Chinese medicine and Asian cultures to support the digestive tract. Those attributes may be a side benefit to their role here as a hearty companion to sautéed asparagus, served on a bed of lemony herbed plant-based ricotta.

In a large nonstick skillet, heat 1 tablespoon of the olive oil over medium heat. Add the mushroom crumbles and the asparagus and cook until the crumbles are heated through and the asparagus is crisp-tender, 4 to 5 minutes. Set aside.

In a food processor, combine the ricotta, remaining 2 tablespoons olive oil, lemon zest and juice, and garlic and process until smooth. Transfer to a small bowl and stir in the tarragon and salt.

Divide the ricotta mixture among 3 shallow serving bowls. Top with the crumble-asparagus mixture, then sprinkle with the chives and serve with the sliced melon.

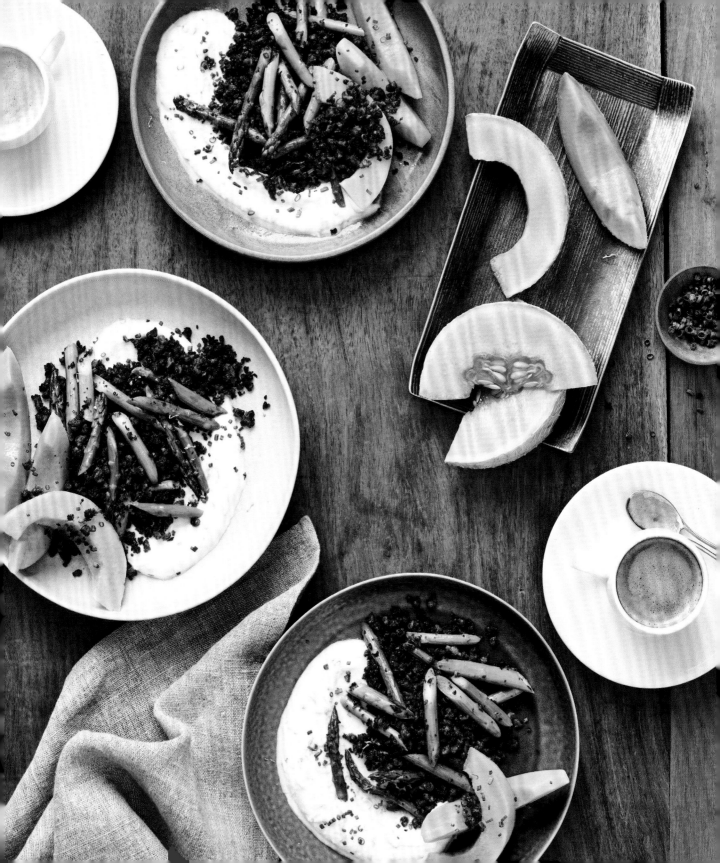

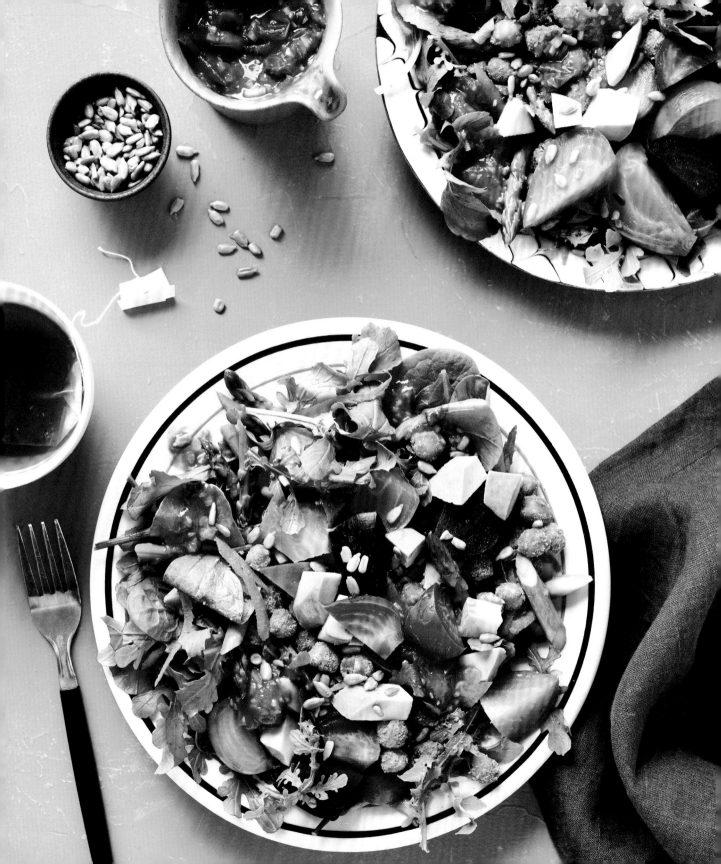

POWERHOUSE SALAD

SERVES 3 • PREP: 10 MINUTES • COOK: 5 MINUTES • TOTAL: 15 MINUTES

9 asparagus spears, trimmed and cut into 2-inch pieces

1 (5-ounce) package power greens or spinach and arugula

1 cup coarsely shredded carrots

3 cups Roasted Chickpea Meat (page 349)

1 cup sliced or matchstick-cut cooked beet (see Tip)

1 large avocado, halved, seeded, and chopped

Charred Tomato Dressing (page 327) or Plant-Based Whole30–compatible balsamic vinaigrette

3 tablespoons roasted and salted sunflower seeds

There's a lot going on this salad, and it's all good! If you have a batch of Roasted Chickpea Meat on hand, the asparagus needs just a few minutes of prep. The shredded carrots, beets, and dressing can all be bought prepared. Or roast your own beets and mix your own dressing to make this a more budget-friendly meal.

Place a steamer basket in a medium saucepan or skillet filled with water just below the basket. Bring to a boil and add the asparagus. Reduce the heat, cover, and steam until asparagus is crisp-tender, 2 to 3 minutes. Immediately transfer the asparagus to a small bowl filled with ice water to stop the cooking.

In a large bowl, toss together the greens and carrots. Add the asparagus.

Divide the mixture among 3 shallow serving bowls or plates. Add the chickpea meat, beet, and avocado. Drizzle the salads with the dressing and sprinkle with the sunflower seeds.

TIP: If you can't find cooked beets in the produce section of your local grocery store, it's easy to roast your own. Preheat the oven to 375°F. Scrub the outside of the beets under cool running water—no need to peel. Trim the tops and bottoms, then set the beets upright on their flat bottoms and slice vertically into 1-inch pieces. (Slice small beets in half, larger beets into 4 to 6 pieces.) Toss in a bowl with 1 tablespoon extra-virgin olive oil, then place on a parchment-lined baking sheet in a single layer; do not crowd. Sprinkle with salt. Roast for 35 to 45 minutes, turning once or twice with a spatula, until beets are easily pierced with a fork.

ROASTED VEGGIES AND WHITE BEANS WITH ZHUG

SERVES 3 • PREP: 15 MINUTES • BAKE: 15 MINUTES • TOTAL: 30 MINUTES

6 fingerling potatoes, quartered lengthwise

9 asparagus spears, trimmed and cut into 1- to 2-inch pieces (see Tip)

1 large shallot, cut into wedges

9 radishes, halved

1 Bartlett pear, cored and sliced (see Tip)

⅓ cup Plant-Based Whole30–compatible balsamic vinaigrette

2 (15-ounce) cans white beans, rinsed and drained

2 tablespoons chopped fresh tarragon

Zhug (page 336)

This sheet-pan breakfast features an array of spring vegetables, like fingerling potatoes, asparagus, and radishes. The pear gets deliciously caramelized while baking, adding a pop of sweetness. But the star of this meal is the zhug—a bright and spicy herb sauce that originated in Yemen. It gives the dish amazing flavor and aroma.

Preheat the oven to 400°F. Line 2 large rimmed sheet pans with parchment.

Arrange the potatoes, asparagus, shallot, radishes, and pear on one sheet pan in a single layer and brush with some of the vinaigrette.

In a large bowl, toss together the beans and remaining dressing until well coated. Arrange the beans in a single layer on the second baking sheet.

Bake until the vegetables are tender and the beans are heated through, about 15 minutes.

Serve the vegetables on individual plates, add the beans, and sprinkle with the tarragon. Drizzle generously with zhug.

TIP: You can replace the pear with apple in this dish, if desired. Choose an apple that is firm, crisp, and mildly sweet; Honeycrisp, Jazz, Fuji, or Pink Lady would all work well.

You can substitute green beans or sugar snap peas for the asparagus.

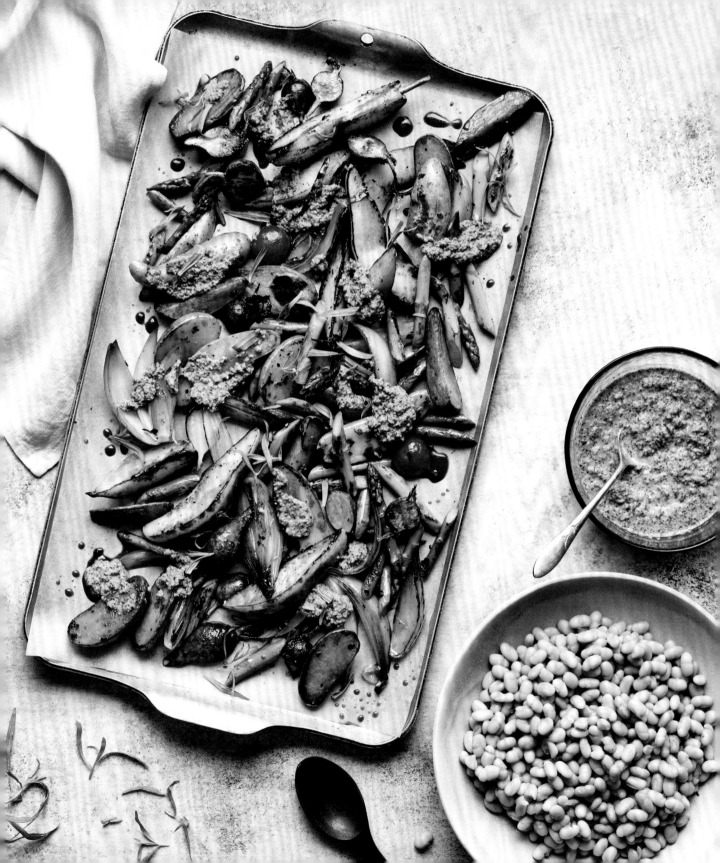

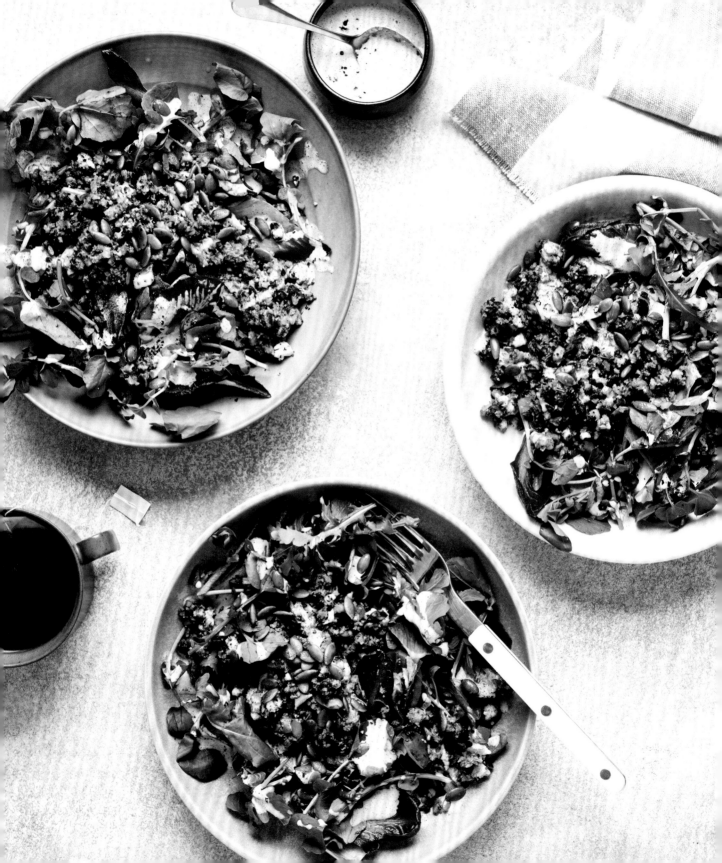

SMOKY CAULIFLOWER, WALNUT, AND BLACK BEAN CRUMBLE WITH GREENS

SERVES 3 • PREP: 10 MINUTES • BAKE: 5 MINUTES • COOK: 5 MINUTES • TOTAL: 20 MINUTES

1½ cups chopped walnuts

2 (15-ounce) cans black beans, drained and rinsed

2 cups cauliflower florets

¼ cup nutritional yeast

3 tablespoons avocado oil, coconut oil, or extra-virgin olive oil

¼ cup chili powder

¼ cup ground cumin

2 tablespoons dried oregano

1 teaspoon salt

1 tablespoon extra-virgin olive oil

1 (5-ounce) package salad greens

Creamy Ancho Chile Dressing (page 329)

Roasted and salted pepitas (pumpkin seeds)

The base of this dish is a taco "meat" made with toasted walnuts, black beans, and cauliflower. Combined with greens and the ancho dressing, this hearty, flavorful meal is the kind of breakfast that keeps you well satisfied and your taste buds happy.

Preheat the oven to 350°F. Arrange the walnuts in a single layer on a large rimmed baking sheet. Bake, stirring once, until fragrant and golden, 5 to 8 minutes. Let cool.

In a food processor, combine the toasted walnuts, the black beans, cauliflower, nutritional yeast, avocado oil, chili powder, cumin, oregano, and salt. Pulse until nuts are finely chopped and mixture is combined (be careful to not overprocess).

In a large skillet, heat the olive oil over medium heat. Add the cauliflower mixture and cook until heated through, 3 to 5 minutes.

Divide the salad greens among 3 serving plates and top with the crumble. Drizzle with the dressing and sprinkle with the pepitas.

TIP: The crumble can be made up to 5 days ahead. Store in an airtight container in the refrigerator until use, or freeze up to 1 month.

TEMPEH AVOCADO TOAST

SERVES 2 TO 3 • PREP: 10 MINUTES + 20 MINUTES MARINATING • COOK: 5 MINUTES •
TOTAL: 35 MINUTES

1 (8-ounce) package tempeh, drained

3 tablespoons extra-virgin olive oil

2 teaspoons smoked paprika

1 teaspoon ground cumin

1 garlic clove, minced

½ teaspoon salt

¼ teaspoon black pepper

1 (8-ounce) container Plant-Based Whole30–compatible cream cheese

1 avocado, halved, pitted, and sliced

Everything bagel seasoning

Fresh berries

This Whole30 take on the popular brunch dish swaps the bread for protein-packed tempeh. Soaking it in a smoked paprika–spiced marinade and pan-frying it in olive oil gives the tempeh a crisp and "toasted" flavor. Topped with plant-based cream cheese and avocado, this is a rich, creamy, and deeply satisfying dish.

Place a vegetable steamer in a large skillet; add water to just below the steamer basket. Bring the water to a boil, then add the tempeh to the steamer. Reduce the heat to maintain a simmer, cover, and steam the tempeh for 10 minutes. Transfer the tempeh to a cutting board and cut into 6 even slices (this will be the "toast").

In a resealable plastic bag, combine 2 tablespoons of the olive oil, the smoked paprika, cumin, garlic, salt, and pepper. Seal the bag and massage to combine the marinade. Add the tempeh and seal the bag again. Marinate for 20 to 30 minutes, then drain the tempeh and discard marinade.

In a large skillet, heat the remaining tablespoon olive oil over medium heat. Add the tempeh slices and cook until browned, turning once halfway, about 5 minutes.

Spread the cream cheese on one side of the 6 tempeh slices and top with the avocado slices. Sprinkle with the bagel seasoning. Serve with the berries on the side.

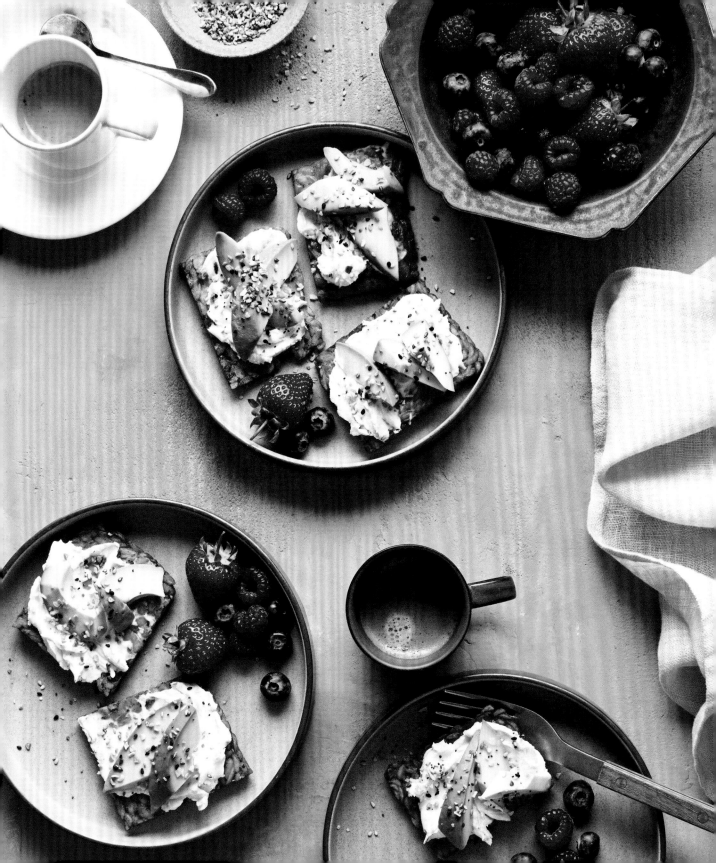

PLANT-BASED WHOLE30 LUNCHES

CRISPY TOFU AND BROCCOLI BITES WITH SPICY PEANUT SAUCE

SERVES 3 • PREP: 10 MINUTES • COOK: 15 MINUTES • TOTAL: 25 MINUTES

2 tablespoons coconut oil or extra-virgin olive oil

1 (16-ounce) block super-firm tofu, drained, pressed, and diced (see Tip, page 255)

3 cups broccoli florets

¾ cup Spicy Peanut Dressing (page 332; see Tip)

9 butter lettuce leaves

⅓ cup chopped roasted and salted cashews or peanuts

2 tablespoons chopped fresh chives

Lime wedges

Plant-Based Whole30–compatible hot sauce

This recipe looks simple, but it packs in a ton of flavor and texture, and it is easy to customize to your desired heat level.

In a large skillet, heat the coconut oil over medium heat. Add the tofu and broccoli and cook until the tofu is browned and the broccoli is tender, about 15 minutes. Stir in the peanut dressing.

Fill the lettuce leaves with the saucy tofu and broccoli, then sprinkle with the cashews and chives. Serve with the lime wedges and the hot sauce.

TIP: You could add any hearty veggie to this dish to use up the last of what's in your produce drawer. The peanut dressing pairs especially well with carrots, cauliflower, Brussels sprouts, sweet potato, cabbage, or bell peppers.

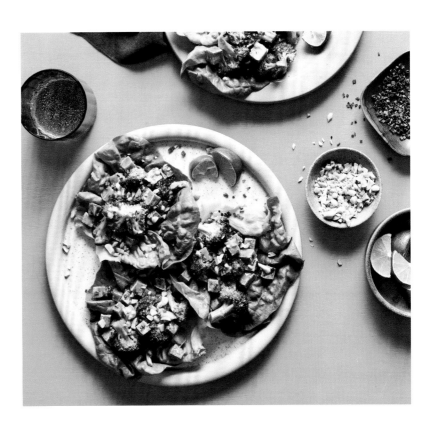

COCONUT-GINGER BLACK BEANS

SERVES 3 • PREP: 10 MINUTES • COOK: 15 MINUTES • TOTAL: 25 MINUTES

1 teaspoon coconut oil or extra-virgin olive oil

1½ teaspoons coriander seeds

½ teaspoon cumin seeds

1 (2-inch) piece fresh ginger, peeled and grated (see Tip)

1 (13.5-ounce) can full-fat coconut milk

1 cup Plant-Based Whole30–compatible almond milk

2 (15-ounce) cans black beans, rinsed and drained, or 3 cups cooked sprouted beans (see Tip)

1 (10-ounce) package frozen diced sweet potato

1½ teaspoons salt

½ teaspoon black pepper

6 ounces fresh green beans, trimmed and sliced

1 red bell pepper, cored, seeded, and chopped

1 teaspoon grated lime zest

Coconut flakes, toasted

This warming bowl is like a cross between a curry and a stew, and it is packed with colorful veggies. A topping of toasted coconut flakes adds crunch and flavor.

In a large pot, heat the coconut oil over medium heat. Add the coriander seeds and cumin seeds and cook, stirring occasionally, until toasted and fragrant, 1 to 2 minutes. Add the ginger and cook, stirring, for 30 seconds.

Stir in the coconut milk, almond milk, black beans, sweet potato, salt, and pepper and bring to a boil over medium-high heat. Reduce the heat to low and simmer, uncovered, for 10 minutes. Stir in the green beans, bell pepper, and lime zest. Cook until vegetables are tender, about 4 minutes.

Spoon the mixture into shallow serving bowls and top with the coconut flakes.

TIP: To sprout beans, place 1 cup of dried beans in a 1-quart canning jar. Add water to cover, then cover the opening with a piece of cheesecloth and secure the cheesecloth with the jar ring or with a tightly fitted rubber band. Place the jar out of sunlight to sit for 12 hours. During that time, rinse and drain the beans through the cheesecloth twice, adding cool water to cover each time. At the end of the 12 hours, drain off the water, then rinse and drain 2 to 3 times daily until you see short sprouts emerging, usually in 3 to 4 days. Store the sprouted beans, covered, in the refrigerator to impede further sprouting.

When cooking sprouted beans, begin to check for tenderness at the halfway point in the cooking time called for in a recipe; 1 cup of dried beans makes about 3 cups cooked sprouted beans.

Here are two tips for grating ginger: First, use a microplane (not a cheese grater), as it's less likely the ginger will get stuck in the holes. Second, keep a piece of fresh ginger in your freezer! Frozen ginger is much easier to grate, and it thaws in seconds in the pan. You can also buy minced ginger in a jar, which makes it easy to add to any recipe. A 1-inch piece of fresh ginger equates to 1 tablespoon of minced ginger.

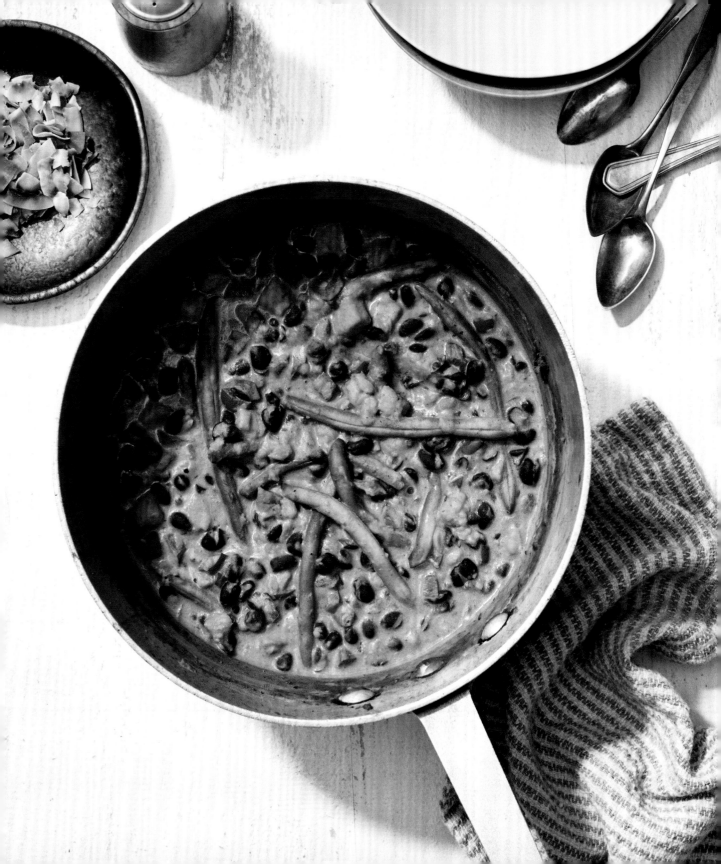

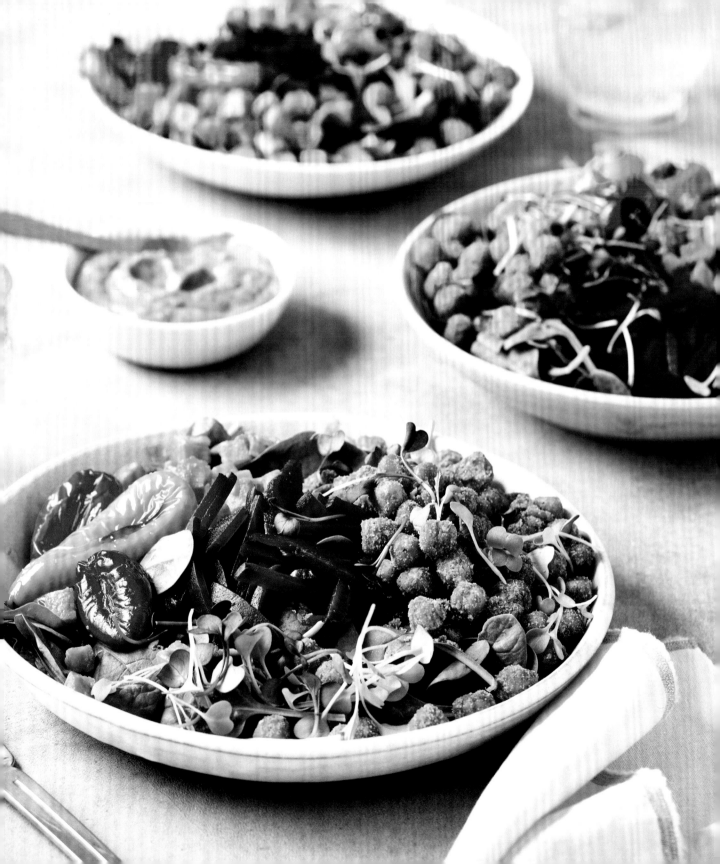

FEELIN' GOOD BOWL

SERVES 3 • PREP: 30 MINUTES • BAKE: 10 MINUTES • TOTAL: 40 MINUTES

FOR THE GREEN SAUCE

1 ripe avocado, halved, pitted and chopped

½ cup water

½ cup lightly packed chopped fresh cilantro

1 small jalapeño, halved, seeded, and sliced

2 tablespoons fresh lime juice

1 garlic clove, minced

½ teaspoon salt

½ teaspoon ground coriander

½ teaspoon ground cumin

FOR THE SALAD AND SERVING

9 mini bell peppers

1 large (8- to 10-ounce) sweet potato, peeled and diced

1 tablespoon extra-virgin olive oil

½ teaspoon salt

¼ teaspoon black pepper

1 (5-ounce) package baby spinach

3 cooked beets, sliced into matchsticks (see Tip, page 304)

3 cups Roasted Chickpea Meat (page 349) or Plant-Based Whole30– compatible mushroom crumbles

Microgreens (such as broccoli sprouts)

This gorgeous arrangement of vegetables, greens, and crispy Roasted Chickpea Meat offers a rainbow of color and nutrition. Pile on the flavor with a generous dollop of the garlicky avocado sauce.

MAKE THE GREEN SAUCE: In a food processor, combine the avocado, water, cilantro, jalapeño, lime juice, garlic, salt, coriander, and cumin. Process until blended and almost smooth. Refrigerate in an airtight container for up to 2 days.

MAKE THE SALAD AND SERVE: Preheat the oven to 400°F. Line a large rimmed baking sheet with parchment.

Arrange the peppers on one side of the baking sheet and the sweet potato on the other. Drizzle the peppers and sweet potato with the olive oil and sprinkle with the salt and pepper. Bake until the peppers are shriveling and browned and the potato cubes are tender, about 20 minutes.

Divide the spinach among 3 plates or shallow bowls. Arrange the roasted peppers and sweet potato, beets, and chickpea meat on the spinach. Top with the microgreens, then drizzle with the sauce.

HARISSA CHICKPEA BOWL

SERVES 3 • PREP: 10 MINUTES • COOK: 10 MINUTES • TOTAL: 20 MINUTES

1 tablespoon extra-virgin olive oil

1 (1-pint) container cherry tomatoes

1 shallot, finely chopped

3 cups broccoli florets

½ teaspoon salt

½ teaspoon black pepper

¾ cup tahini

2 tablespoons Plant-Based Whole30–compatible harissa sauce

3 cups Roasted Chickpea Meat (page 349)

2 Medjool dates, pitted and chopped

¼ cup chopped fresh parsley

1 lemon, cut into wedges

Assorted olives

This hearty bowl turns the sauce-on-top paradigm on its head. Harissa-spiced tahini is smeared on the bottom of the bowl, so you can scoop it up with every bite of the veggie and chickpea mixture. A sprinkle of chopped dates adds a touch of sweetness to the heat.

In a large skillet, heat the olive oil over medium heat. Add the tomatoes and shallot and cook, covered and undisturbed, until slightly browned on the bottom, 2 to 3 minutes. Stir, cover, and cook until the tomatoes collapse and release their juices, 3 to 5 minutes.

Meanwhile, place a vegetable steamer in a large skillet; add water to just below the steamer basket. Bring the water to a boil and add the broccoli. Reduce the heat to low, cover, and steam the broccoli until tender, 5 to 6 minutes. Drain the broccoli and season with salt and pepper.

In a small bowl, stir together the tahini and harissa. Smear the spiced tahini on the bottom of 3 shallow serving bowls, then add the tomatoes and then the broccoli. Heat a portion of the chickpea meat, and crumble it over the vegetables. Top with the dates and parsley. Serve with the lemon wedges and olives.

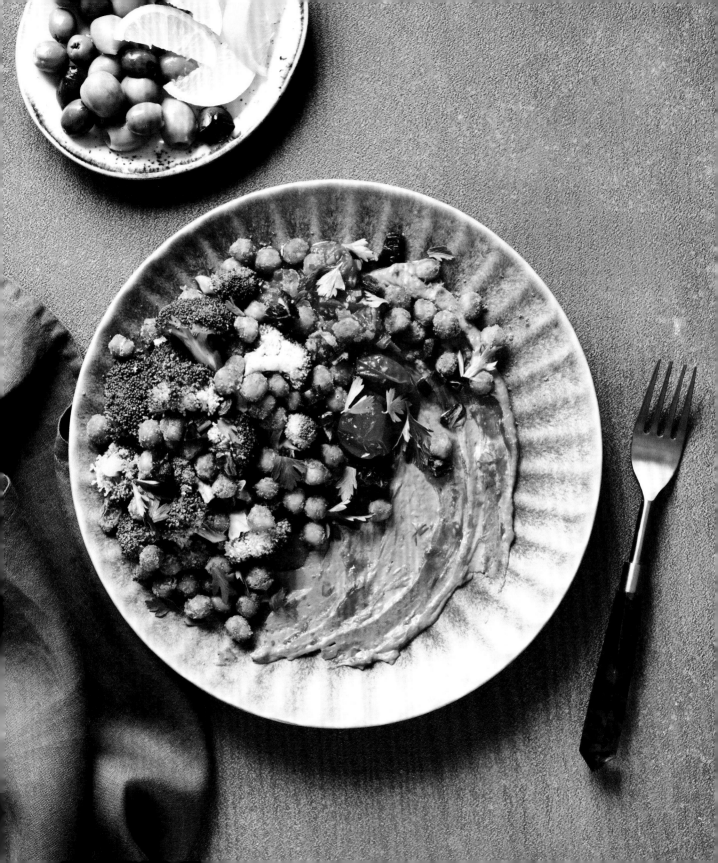

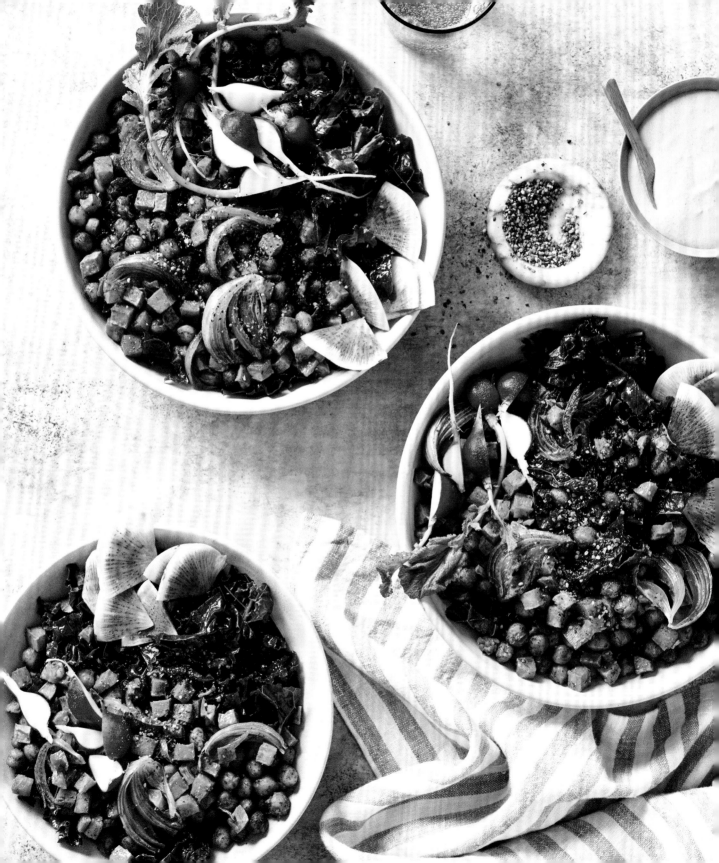

MACROBIOTIC BOWL

SERVES 3 • PREP: 15 MINUTES • BAKE: 30 MINUTES • TOTAL: 45 MINUTES

2 (15.5-ounce) cans chickpeas, rinsed, drained, and blotted dry

1 large (8- to 10-ounce) sweet potato, peeled and diced

1 small red onion, cut into wedges

4 tablespoons extra-virgin olive oil

1½ teaspoons salt

1 teaspoon paprika

½ teaspoon ground cinnamon

½ teaspoon ground cumin

¼ teaspoon ground black pepper

¼ teaspoon ground turmeric

1 (10-ounce) package curly kale

3 radishes, trimmed and quartered

Turmeric-Ginger Dressing (page 333)

1 tablespoon hemp hearts, toasted (see Tip)

The macrobiotic diet was brought to the United States in the 1950s, but it originated in the practice of Zen Buddhism in Japan. This eye-catching bowl doesn't include grains, but it is loaded with vegetables and dressed with a vibrant ginger dressing. Enjoy every bite mindfully!

Preheat the oven to 400°F. Line 2 large rimmed baking sheets with parchment.

Spread the chickpeas on one baking sheet and the sweet potato and onion on the other. Drizzle the chickpeas with 1 tablespoon of the olive oil and the vegetables with 2 tablespoons of the oil; toss to coat.

In a small bowl, stir together the salt, paprika, cinnamon, cumin, pepper, and turmeric. Sprinkle the seasoning over the chickpeas and vegetables, and toss to coat. Bake both sheets 20 to 30 minutes, until the sweet potato cubes are tender and browned and the chickpeas are golden or slightly darker.

Meanwhile, place the kale in a large bowl and drizzle with the remaining tablespoon olive oil. Massage for 1 minute to soften.

Arrange the chickpeas, roasted vegetables, kale, and radishes in 3 shallow serving bowls. Drizzle with the dressing and sprinkle with the hemp hearts.

TIP: Toasting hemp hearts adds a nice crunch and lightly toasted flavor to your dish. To toast, place the hemp hearts in a dry skillet or pan over low heat. Shake the pan until they just start to color, then remove when they're a light golden brown.

MUSHROOM SAUCE OVER BUTTERNUT SQUASH NOODLES

SERVES 3 • PREP: 10 MINUTES • COOK: 15 MINUTES • TOTAL: 25 MINUTES

2 tablespoons extra-virgin olive oil

1 (10-ounce) package Plant-Based Whole30–compatible mushroom crumble or pork

1 small onion, finely chopped

1 garlic clove, minced

1 (15-ounce) can Great Northern beans, rinsed and drained

½ (28-ounce) can crushed tomatoes

1 (14.5-ounce) can fire-roasted diced tomatoes

2 teaspoons balsamic vinegar

1 teaspoon Italian seasoning

½ teaspoon salt

¼ teaspoon black pepper

1 (10-ounce) package butternut squash noodles (see Tip)

Plant-Based Whole30–compatible ricotta

Chopped fresh basil

This dish features a hearty sauce you can enjoy over veggie noodles. If you can't find butternut squash noodles, substitute sweet potato noodles or spaghetti squash (see Tip).

In a large, preferably nonstick, skillet, heat 1 tablespoon of the olive oil over medium heat. Add the mushroom crumble, onion, and garlic and cook until onion is tender and the mushroom crumble is heated through, about 5 minutes. Add the beans and mash slightly. Stir in the tomatoes, vinegar, Italian seasoning, salt, and pepper and bring to a boil. Reduce the heat and simmer, covered, for 15 minutes.

Meanwhile, in another large skillet, heat the remaining tablespoon olive oil over medium heat. Add the noodles and cook, using tongs to occasionally toss to coat in the oil, until tender, 5 to 7 minutes.

Divide the noodles among 3 serving plates. Spoon the sauce over the noodles, and top with dollops of the ricotta. Sprinkle with the basil and serve.

TIP: If you're substituting spaghetti squash, cut the squash into 1½-inch *rings*, not in half. (This gives you longer noodles that are far more spaghetti-like.) Preheat the oven to 400°F. Scrape the inside of the rings with a spoon to remove the seeds. Brush the squash with olive oil, then place the rings on a parchment-lined baking sheet. Bake for 30 to 35 minutes. Let cool, then use a fork to separate the spaghetti strands from the skin.

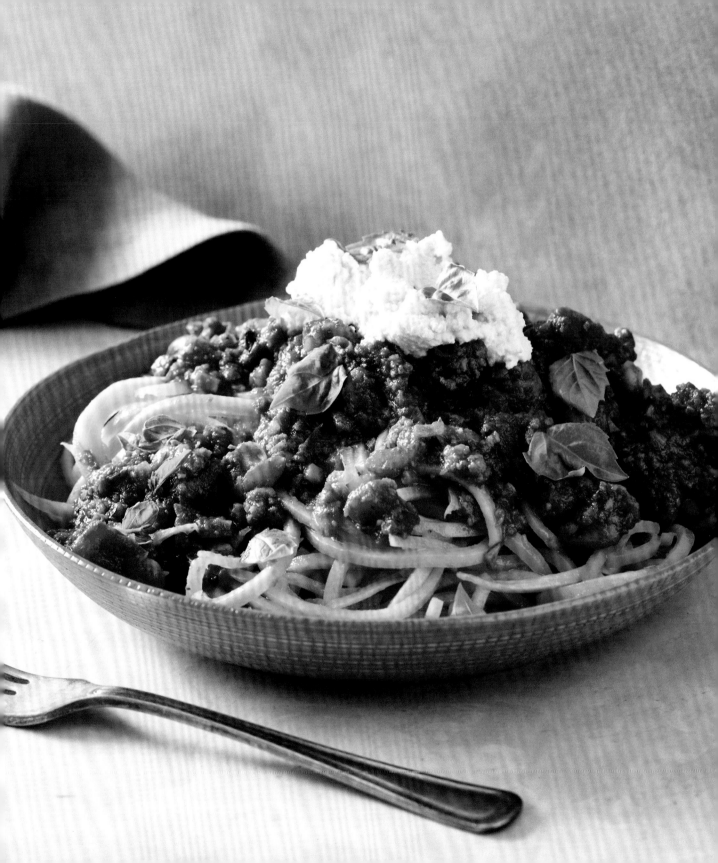

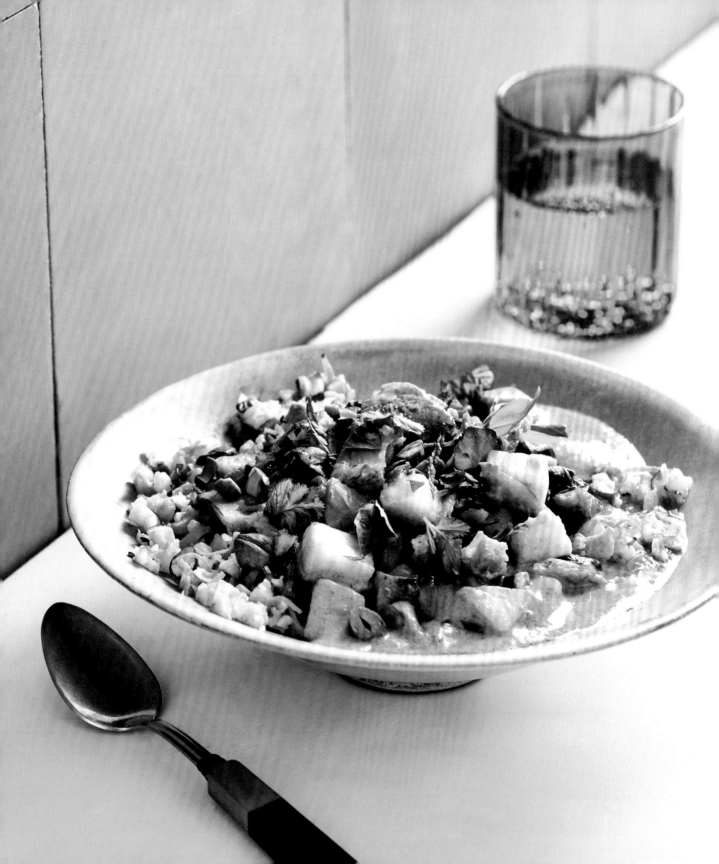

PANANG CURRY BOWL

SERVES 3 • PREP: 15 MINUTES • COOK: 10 MINUTES • TOTAL: 25 MINUTES

1 tablespoon coconut oil

1 (10-ounce) package Plant-Based Whole30–compatible chicken or pork or 1 (16-ounce) block super-firm tofu, drained, pressed, and diced (see Tip, page 255)

1 shallot, finely chopped

1 (1-inch) piece fresh ginger, peeled and minced (see Tip, page 268)

1 (13.5-ounce) can full-fat coconut milk

½ cup Vegetable Broth (page 351) or Plant-Based Whole30–compatible vegetable broth

2 teaspoons grated lime zest

1 tablespoon fresh lime juice

1 to 2 tablespoons Plant-Based Whole30–compatible Panang curry paste (see Tip)

1 teaspoon salt

1 baby bok choy, sliced in half lengthwise

½ cup chopped fresh pineapple

Vegan Cauliflower Rice (recipe follows)

Chopped fresh basil, cilantro, and/or mint

¼ cup chopped roasted cashews

TIP: Substitute a red curry paste if Panang is not available.

Panang curry is a type of red curry that originated in northern Thailand. It has a mild, sweet, and nutty flavor. Panang curry is traditionally cooked with meat or poultry, but this dish is adaptable to your choice of plant-based protein.

In a large skillet, heat the coconut oil over medium heat. Add the chicken, shallot, and ginger and cook until browned, 5 to 7 minutes.

Stir in the coconut milk, broth, lime zest and juice, curry paste, and salt. Add the bok choy and pineapple; cook until heated through, about 5 minutes.

Divide the cauliflower rice among 3 serving bowls. Ladle the curry over the cauliflower, then top with the herbs and cashews.

VEGAN CAULIFLOWER RICE

SERVES 2 TO 3 • PREP: 5 MINUTES • COOK: 10 MINUTES • TOTAL: 15 MINUTES

2 tablespoons coconut oil

2 green onions, thinly sliced, green and white parts separated

1 garlic clove, minced

1 small carrot, finely shredded

1 (10- to 12-ounce) bag frozen cauliflower rice

½ teaspoon salt

¼ teaspoon black pepper

In a medium nonstick skillet, heat the coconut oil over medium heat. Add the white parts of the green onions, the garlic, and the carrot. Cook, stirring frequently, until the garlic is fragrant and the carrot and green onion are slightly softened, 2 to 3 minutes.

Break up any lumps of frozen cauliflower rice by gently whacking the sealed bag on the countertop. Add the cauliflower to the skillet and cook, stirring, occasionally, until it is tender (but not mushy) and lightly browned, 6 to 8 minutes.

Stir in the green parts of the green onions, the salt, and the pepper.

SALSA MACHA TACOS

SERVES 3 • PREP: 10 MINUTES • COOK: 5 MINUTES • TOTAL: 15 MINUTES

1 teaspoon extra-virgin olive oil

1 (10-ounce) package Plant-Based Whole30–compatible chicken or pork

9 Bibb lettuce leaves

Salsa Macha (page 330)

3 radishes, trimmed and thinly sliced

1 avocado, halved, pitted, and sliced

¼ cup chopped fresh cilantro

1 lime, cut into wedges

Cucumber slices

Plant-Based Whole30 Sour Cream (recipe follows) or Plant-Based Whole30–compatible plain yogurt

The sauce—a spicy, nutty, garlicky salsa—is the secret ingredient in these simple plant-based tacos. Plant-based sour cream provides a dash of coolness and a lovely creamy texture.

In a medium skillet over medium heat, heat the olive oil, then add the plant-based meat and cook until heated through and browned, 8 to 10 minutes.

Spoon about ¼ cup of the meat on each lettuce leaf. Top with some of the salsa, then add the radish, avocado, and cilantro. Fold the leaves and place 3 on each of 3 serving plates. Serve with the lime wedges and additional salsa. Offer cucumber slices and sour cream on the side.

PLANT-BASED WHOLE30 SOUR CREAM

In a small bowl, combine 1 cup raw cashews and water to cover. Soak overnight. Drain the cashews. In a food processor, combine the cashews, ⅓ cup water, 1 teaspoon apple cider vinegar, ½ teaspoon fresh lemon juice, and ⅛ teaspoon salt. Cover and blend until smooth, adding more water as necessary, 1 teaspoon at a time, to reach desired consistency. Makes about 1 cup.

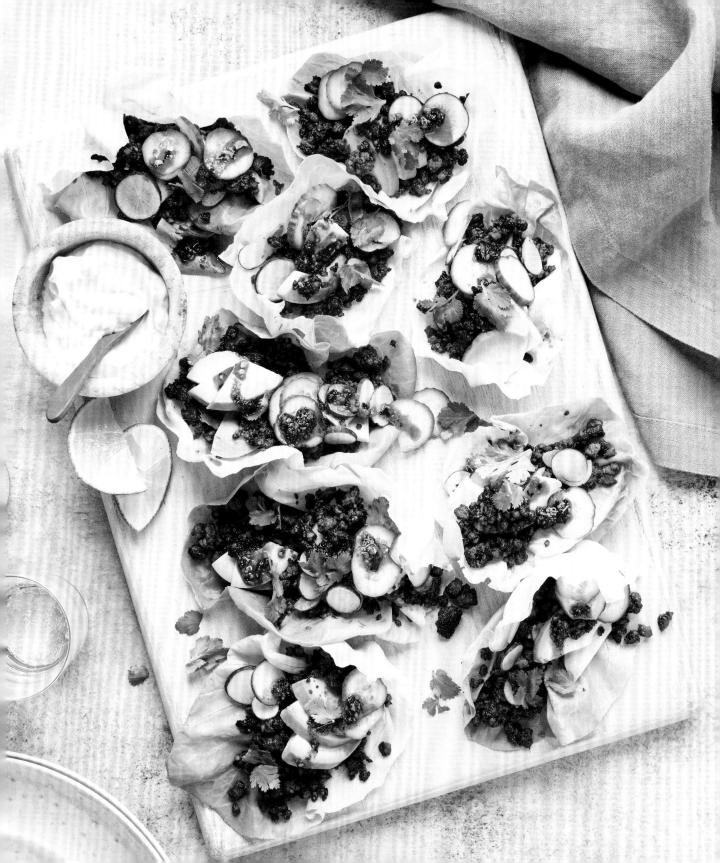

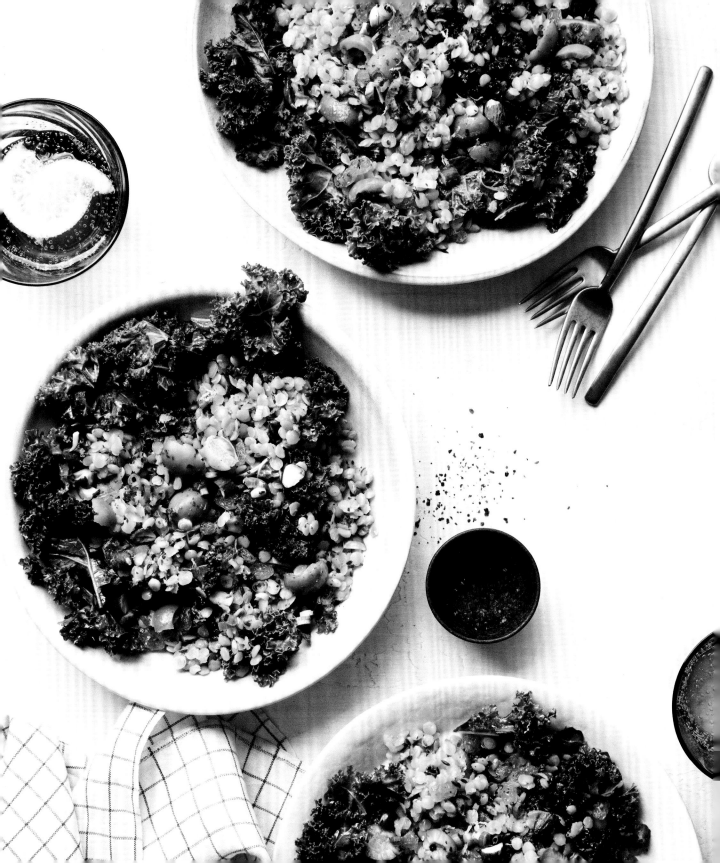

SPROUTED LENTIL AND KALE SALAD

SERVES 3 • PREP: 10 MINUTES • COOK: 10 MINUTES • TOTAL: 20 MINUTES

1½ cups lentils, any type (see Tip)

3 cups water

1 teaspoon salt

1 (10-ounce) package curly kale

3 teaspoons extra-virgin olive oil

2 green onions, sliced (green and white parts)

½ cup coarsely chopped almonds

1 teaspoon cumin seeds

3 teaspoons grated lemon zest

½ teaspoon Aleppo pepper flakes or ¼ teaspoon red pepper flakes

10 pitted Castelvetrano or other buttery olives, quartered

2 tablespoons golden raisins or chopped Medjool dates

This high-fiber salad is a fabulous blend of flavors and textures. Aleppo pepper flakes bring the heat, golden raisins deliver the sweet, olives provide buttery bites of briny goodness, and toasted almonds add nuttiness and crunch.

In a large saucepan, combine the lentils, water, and ½ teaspoon of the salt. Bring to a boil over medium heat. Reduce the heat to low, cover, and simmer until lentils are tender, 10 to 15 minutes for sprouted lentils and about 30 minutes for dried lentils. Drain.

Meanwhile, place the kale in a large bowl and drizzle with 2 teaspoons of the olive oil. Using your fingers, gently massage the kale until it just begins to wilt, 1 to 2 minutes. Sprinkle with the remaining ½ teaspoon salt.

In a large skillet, heat the remaining teaspoon olive oil over medium heat. Add the green onions, almonds, and cumin seeds and cook until the almonds are lightly toasted, about 2 minutes. Remove from the heat and add the lemon zest, Aleppo pepper flakes, olives, and raisins. Add the warm lentils and stir to combine.

Divide the kale among 3 serving plates or shallow bowls, and top with the lentil mixture.

TIP: For increased nutritional density and digestibility, and a shorter cook time, use purchased sprouted lentils or sprout your own. Sprouting lentils is generally a 3-day process. On Day 1, place ¾ cup red, green, and/or black lentils in a 1-quart glass canning jar. Add water to cover and cover with cheesecloth and the jar ring or a tight-fitting rubber band. Let stand 12 hours out of sunlight, rinsing and draining the lentils twice, then adding 2 cups cool water. On the morning of Day 2, drain and rinse the lentils again with cool water but then let stand without adding water. Rinse and drain the lentils every 6 hours. Let stand without water overnight. On the morning of Day 3, you should see some sprouts; the lentils are now ready to eat. If not, continue rinsing and draining until sprouts are visible. Store, covered, in the refrigerator to slow further sprouting. Yields 1½ to 2 cups sprouted lentils. When using sprouted lentils, reduce the cook time to 10 to 15 minutes.

SUSHI BOWL

SERVES 3 • PREP: 15 MINUTES + 30 MINUTES MARINATING • STEAM: 10 MINUTES •
COOK: 5 MINUTES • TOTAL: 1 HOUR

FOR THE PICKLE

½ cup water

½ cup unseasoned rice vinegar

1 cup thinly sliced carrots

1 (1-inch) piece fresh ginger, peeled and thinly sliced into matchsticks

FOR THE TEMPEH

1 (8-ounce) package tempeh (see Tip)

¼ cup coconut aminos

¼ cup unseasoned rice vinegar

1 (2-inch) piece fresh ginger, peeled and grated (see Tip, page 268)

2 tablespoons fresh orange juice

2 teaspoons toasted sesame oil

FOR SERVING

1 tablespoon coconut oil or extra-virgin olive oil

Vegan Cauliflower Rice (page 279), warm

1 avocado, pitted, peeled, and thinly sliced

1 medium cucumber, peeled and sliced

3 tablespoons crumbled wakame or nori

1 tablespoon sesame seeds, toasted

Think of this as a deconstructed vegan sushi roll you can eat with a fork. The seaweed serves as a crumbled topping instead of a wrap, and the "rice" is cauliflower. Make the quick-pickled carrots first, so they have time to tenderize and take on as much flavor as possible.

MAKE THE QUICK PICKLE: In a small saucepan, bring the water and vinegar to a boil over medium-high heat. Place the carrot and ginger in a small bowl; pour the water-vinegar liquid over the carrot and ginger. Cover and refrigerate for 30 minutes or up to 3 days (see Tip). Just before serving, drain the carrot and ginger, discarding the liquid.

MAKE THE TEMPEH: Place a vegetable steamer in a large skillet; add water to just below the steamer basket. Bring the water to a boil, then add the tempeh to the steamer. Reduce the heat to low, cover, and steam the tempeh for 10 minutes. Transfer the tempeh to a cutting board and cut into bite-sized pieces.

In a medium bowl, mix the coconut aminos, vinegar, ginger, orange juice, and sesame oil. Reserve 3 tablespoons for serving, and add the tempeh to the marinade; mix to coat well and let marinate for 30 minutes. Drain the tempeh and discard marinade.

Serve: In a large skillet, heat the coconut oil. Add the tempeh and cook, stirring occasionally, until heated through, 5 to 8 minutes.

Divide the cauliflower rice among 3 shallow serving bowls. Arrange the tempeh, avocado, and cucumber on the cauliflower, then also add the pickled carrot and ginger. Drizzle with the reserved marinade and sprinkle with the wakame and sesame seeds.

TIP: Not a big fan of tempeh? You can also use drained and pressed extra-firm tofu. Follow the directions for marinating, but skip the steaming.

Pickled carrots and ginger can be stored in an airtight container or mason jar in the fridge for up to 2 weeks.

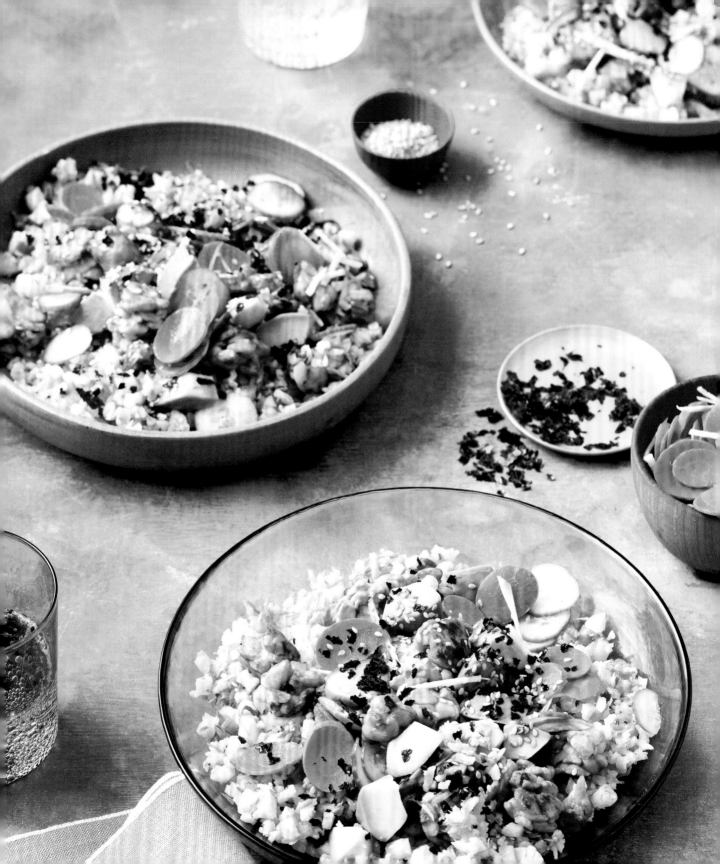

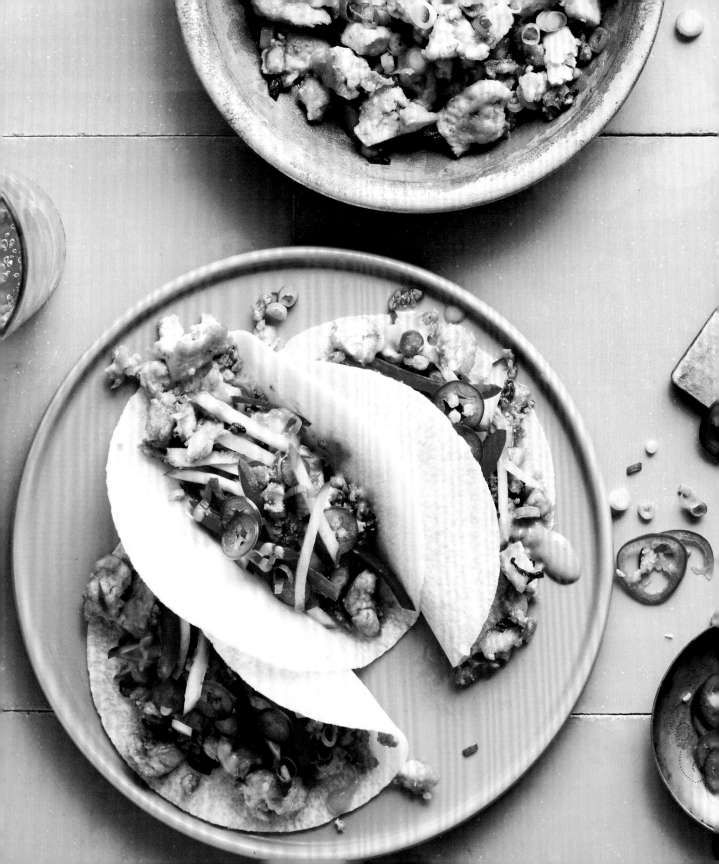

THAI-INSPIRED JICAMA WRAPS

SERVES 3 • PREP: 10 MINUTES • COOK: 5 MINUTES • TOTAL: 15 MINUTES

1 (16-ounce) block super-firm tofu, drained and pressed (see Tip, page 255)

2 green onions, finely chopped (green and white parts)

2 tablespoons nutritional yeast

¾ teaspoon salt

¾ teaspoon black pepper

1 tablespoon coconut oil, avocado oil, or extra-virgin olive oil

1 medium cucumber, cut into matchsticks

1 red bell pepper, cored, seeded, and cut into matchsticks

12 jicama tortillas (see Tip)

Spicy Peanut Dressing (page 332)

1 serrano chile, seeded and thinly sliced (optional)

You can buy fresh jicama tortillas at many supermarkets. These make for a quick lunch, especially if you have the dressing already made. In fact, the rich dressing contrasts perfectly with the fresh, crunchy jicama.

Finely crumble the tofu into a medium bowl. Add the green onions. In a small bowl, stir together the nutritional yeast, salt, and pepper. Sprinkle the seasoning over the tofu and stir to combine.

In a large skillet, heat the oil over medium heat. Add the tofu and cook, stirring occasionally, until heated through, about 3 minutes.

Divide the tofu, cucumber, and bell pepper among the tortillas and drizzle each with the dressing. Top with the chile slices (if using) and serve.

> **TIP:** Create your own tortillas by slicing a whole jicama (get the largest one you can find) with a mandoline. You could also use savoy cabbage leaves or any firm lettuce leaves in place of the jicama tortillas.

PLANT-BASED WHOLE30 DINNERS

WHITE BEAN CHILI

SERVES 6 • PREP: 10 MINUTES • COOK: 15 MINUTES • TOTAL: 25 MINUTES

2 tablespoons extra-virgin olive oil

1 (10-ounce) package Plant-Based Whole30–compatible chorizo or chicken

1 small yellow onion, chopped

1 medium carrot, peeled and chopped

2 garlic cloves, minced

2 (15-ounce) cans Great Northern beans, rinsed and drained

2 cups Vegetable Broth (page 351; see Tip) or Plant-Based Whole30–compatible vegetable broth

2 (4-ounce) cans diced mild green chiles

1 teaspoon ground cumin

1 teaspoon dried oregano

Salt and black pepper

1 small zucchini, chopped

1 green onion, finely chopped (green and white parts)

Plant-Based Whole30 Sour Cream (page 280) or Plant-Based Whole30–compatible sour cream or plain yogurt

Chopped fresh cilantro

Chopped avocado

Lime wedges

If you like your chili spicy, use the plant-based chorizo. If you prefer flavors on the milder side, opt for a plant-based chicken.

In a large saucepan or pot, heat the olive oil over medium heat. Stir in the chorizo, onion, carrot, and garlic and cook, stirring occasionally, until the vegetables are softened, about 3 minutes. Stir in the beans, broth, chiles, cumin, oregano, and salt and pepper to taste. Bring to a boil, reduce the heat to low, cover, and simmer 10 minutes. Add the zucchini and cook, uncovered, until tender, about 2 minutes more.

Ladle the chili into bowls, then top with the green onion, sour cream, cilantro, and avocado. Serve with lime wedges.

TIP: To make this dish creamier, substitute 1 cup full-fat coconut milk for 1 cup of the broth.

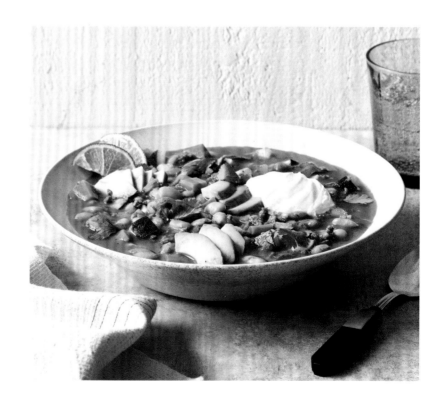

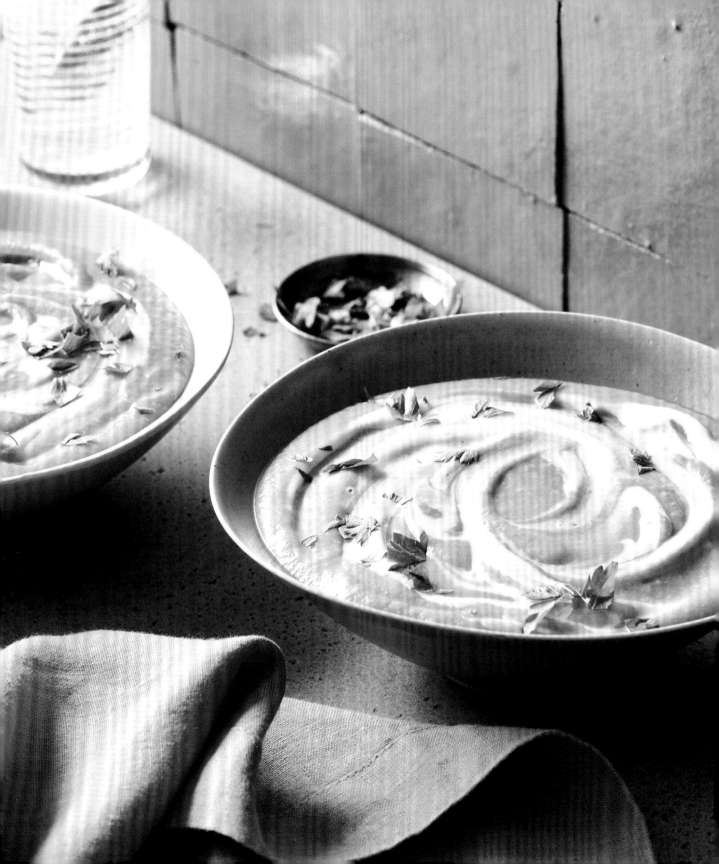

CREAMY SWEET POTATO–GINGER RED LENTIL SOUP

SERVES 4 • PREP: 10 MINUTES • COOK: 20 MINUTES • TOTAL: 30 MINUTES

1 tablespoon coconut oil or extra-virgin olive oil

2 large shallots, chopped

1 (2-inch) piece fresh ginger, peeled and finely chopped

4½ cups Vegetable Broth (page 351) or Plant-Based Whole30–compatible vegetable broth

1 pound sweet potatoes, peeled and chopped

1½ cups red lentils (see Tip)

2 teaspoons ground turmeric

2 teaspoons ground coriander

2 teaspoons ground cumin

1 teaspoon paprika

1 teaspoon salt

1 cup full-fat canned coconut milk

2 tablespoons fresh lemon juice

Plant-Based Whole30–compatible plain yogurt

Chopped fresh parsley

The flavor of ginger in this pretty soup has a presence but isn't overwhelming. This makes a nice big batch, so freeze the extra for a busy day in the future.

Melt the coconut oil in a large saucepan or pot over medium heat. Stir in the shallots and cook, stirring occasionally, until tender, 3 to 4 minutes. Add the ginger and cook until fragrant, about 30 seconds. Stir in the broth, sweet potatoes, lentils, turmeric, coriander, cumin, paprika, and salt and bring to a boil. Reduce the heat to low, cover, and simmer until the sweet potatoes and lentils are tender, 20 to 30 minutes.

Stir in the coconut milk and lemon juice. Carefully transfer the soup to a blender and let cool briefly, then blend until smooth.

Ladle the soup into 4 serving bowls and top with dollops of yogurt and a sprinkling of parsley.

TIP: For a shorter cook time, use purchased sprouted lentils or sprout your own. Sprouting lentils is generally a 3-day process; see Tip, page 283, for instructions. When using sprouted lentils, reduce the cook time to 10 to 15 minutes.

CREOLE-STYLE RED BEANS OVER CAULIFLOWER RICE

SERVES 4 • PREP: 10 MINUTES • COOK: 25 MINUTES • TOTAL: 35 MINUTES

2 tablespoons extra-virgin olive oil

1 medium onion, chopped

1 green bell pepper, cored, seeded, and chopped

2 celery stalks, trimmed and chopped

3 garlic cloves, minced

1 (10-ounce) package Plant-Based Whole30–compatible chorizo

1 (15-ounce) can red kidney beans, rinsed and drained

1 cup Vegetable Broth (page 351) or Plant-Based Whole30–compatible vegetable broth

2 teaspoons Creole seasoning (see Tip)

2 bay leaves

Vegan Cauliflower Rice (page 279), warm

3 tablespoons chopped fresh parsley

Plant-Based Whole30–compatible hot sauce

The plant-based chorizo gives a serious kick to this vegan version of the Creole classic. Red beans may be in the name, but you can swap in any type of bean you prefer.

In a large skillet, heat the olive oil over medium heat. Add the onion, bell pepper, celery, and garlic, and cook, stirring occasionally, until vegetables are softened, 2 to 3 minutes. Push the vegetables to the edge, creating an empty center. Add the chorizo and cook, stirring frequently, until the plant-based meat is heated through, 3 to 4 minutes.

Stir in the beans, broth, seasoning, and bay leaves and bring to a boil. Reduce the heat to low, cover, and simmer for 15 minutes. Remove and discard the bay leaves.

Place the cauliflower rice on 4 serving plates. Spoon the bean mixture over the cauliflower, then sprinkle with parsley and serve with the hot sauce.

> **TIP:** You can find Creole seasoning at most grocery stores, but you can also make your own using common spices. Mix 5 tablespoons paprika, 2 tablespoons salt, 2 tablespoons onion powder, 2 tablespoons garlic powder, 2 tablespoons dried oregano, 2 tablespoons dried basil, 1 tablespoon dried thyme, 1 tablespoon black pepper, 1 tablespoon white pepper, and ½ to 1 tablespoon cayenne. Store in an airtight container for up to 6 months.

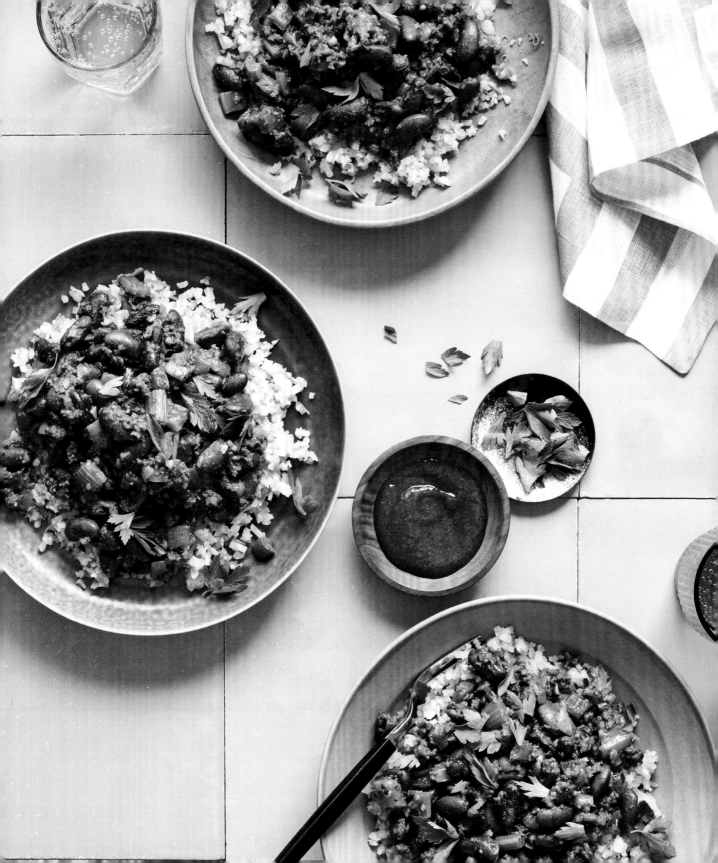

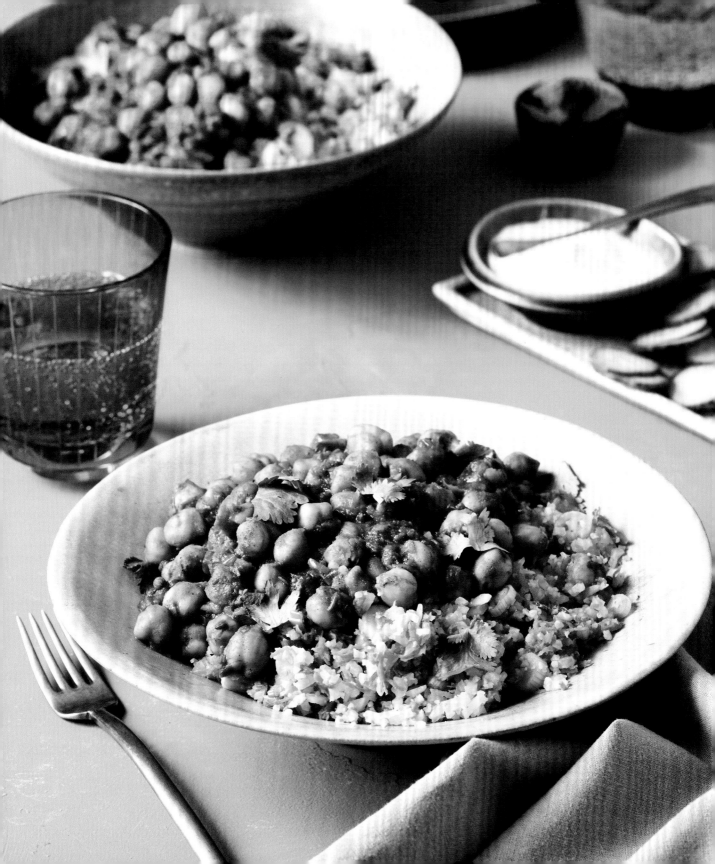

GARAM MASALA–SPICED VEGETABLES AND CHICKPEAS

SERVES 3 • PREP: 10 MINUTES • COOK: 15 MINUTES • TOTAL: 25 MINUTES

1 tablespoon coconut oil or extra-virgin olive oil

1 teaspoon cumin seeds

1 teaspoon coriander seeds

1 (1-inch) piece fresh ginger, peeled and grated (see Tip, page 268)

2 garlic cloves, minced

1 large onion, finely chopped

2 Roma (plum) tomatoes, finely chopped

2 tablespoons tomato paste

2 teaspoons garam masala

1 teaspoon ground turmeric

1 teaspoon salt

2 (15-ounce) cans chickpeas, rinsed and drained (see Tip)

1 cup Vegetable Broth (page 351) or Plant-Based Whole30–compatible vegetable broth

Vegan Cauliflower Rice (page 279), warm

Chopped fresh cilantro

Sliced cucumber

Plant-Based Whole30–compatible plain yogurt

One of the most popular dishes in northern India is a curry called chana masala, or chickpeas simmered in a spicy onion and tomato gravy. This recipe is inspired by that dish, but we've simplified it a bit and are using canned chickpeas to make it a 25-minute meal.

In a large saucepan or skillet, heat the coconut oil over medium heat. Stir in the cumin, coriander seeds, ginger, and garlic and cook, stirring often, until fragrant and lightly toasted, 4 to 5 minutes. Stir in the onion and cook until softened, 2 to 3 minutes. Stir in the tomatoes, tomato paste, garam masala, turmeric, and salt. Cook until the tomatoes are tender, 4 to 5 minutes. Stir in the chickpeas and broth, cover, and cook until the chickpeas are heated through, about 4 minutes.

Divide the cauliflower rice among 3 serving bowls and top each with some of the chickpea and vegetable mixture. Sprinkle with the cilantro. Serve the cucumber and yogurt on the side.

TIP: Alternatively, you can use dried chickpeas in this dish. Place 1½ cups of dried chickpeas in a large bowl and cover generously with water. (The chickpeas will soak up much of the water, eventually doubling in size.) Cover the bowl with a dish towel and let soak overnight. Using a colander, drain the water from the chickpeas and rinse thoroughly before cooking.

INDIAN-STYLE SHEET-PAN VEGGIES AND CHICKPEAS

SERVES 3 • PREP: 10 MINUTES • BAKE: 20 MINUTES • TOTAL: 30 MINUTES

2 cups cauliflower florets

2 cups broccoli florets

1 medium sweet potato, peeled and chopped

1 medium yellow onion, chopped

2 (15-ounce) cans chickpeas, rinsed and drained

½ cup olive oil

1 tablespoon ground cumin

1 tablespoon ground turmeric

2 teaspoons ground coriander

2 teaspoons yellow mustard seeds

1 teaspoon salt

1 teaspoon red pepper flakes

1½ cups Plant-Based Whole30–compatible plain yogurt

1 teaspoon fresh lemon juice

1 small garlic clove

⅛ teaspoon salt

Chopped fresh cilantro, mint, and basil

Roasted and lightly salted pistachios

Cauliflower, broccoli, sweet potato, onion, and chickpeas are tossed with a generous amount of well-spiced oil, then roasted and served topped with fresh herbs, pistachios, and a lemony-garlicky yogurt sauce. Mustard seeds in the mix provide both flavor and crunch.

Preheat the oven to 400°F. Line 2 large rimmed baking sheets with parchment.

Spread out the cauliflower, broccoli, sweet potato, and onion on one baking sheet and the chickpeas on the other. In a small bowl, stir together the olive oil, cumin, turmeric, coriander, mustard seeds, salt, and red pepper flakes. Drizzle the seasoned oil over the vegetables and the chickpeas and toss to coat.

Bake for about 20 minutes, until the vegetables are tender and the chickpeas are slightly browned. Carefully pour the chickpeas onto the vegetables and stir to combine.

In a small bowl, stir together the yogurt, lemon juice, garlic, and salt.

Divide the vegetable mixture among 3 shallow serving bowls and top with the herbs and pistachios. Serve with the yogurt sauce.

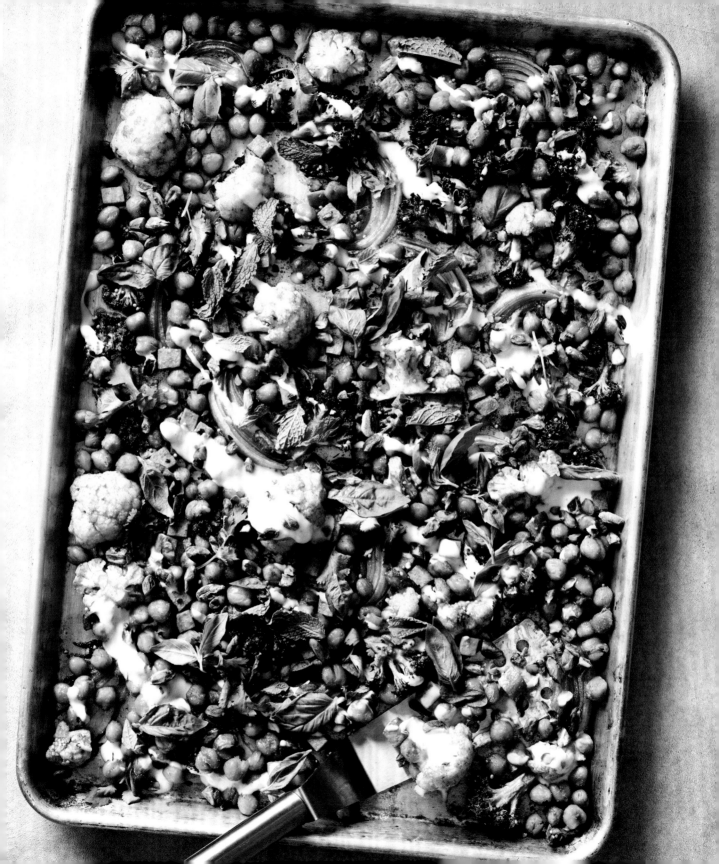

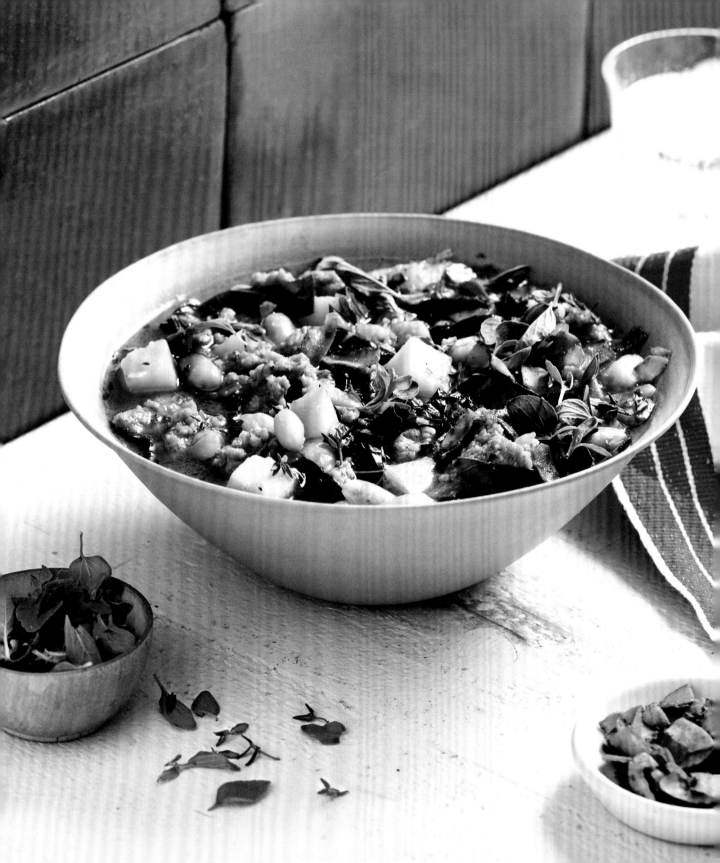

ITALIAN WHITE BEAN AND GREENS SOUP

SERVES 3 TO 4 • PREP: 10 MINUTES • COOK: 15 MINUTES • TOTAL: 25 MINUTES

1 tablespoon extra-virgin olive oil

1 small onion, chopped

2 garlic cloves, minced

4 cups Vegetable Broth (page 351) or Plant-Based Whole30–compatible vegetable broth

1 (15-ounce) can white beans, rinsed and drained

1 (10-ounce) package plant-based pork or mushroom crumbles

1 pound Yukon Gold potatoes, scrubbed and chopped

2 tablespoons nutritional yeast

2 teaspoons dried Italian herbs

1 teaspoon salt

½ teaspoon black pepper

½ teaspoon red pepper flakes (optional)

6 collard greens or kale leaves, stems trimmed, leafy portions cut into ribbons

Coconut-Almond Bacon (page 313)

Chopped fresh herbs, such as oregano, basil, and thyme

There are lots of variations on an Italian-style soup of white beans, sausage, and sturdy winter greens. This one is every bit as hearty and satisfying, but it's 100 percent plant based. Italian-style plant-based pork provides heft and protein, nutritional yeast contributes the umami, and a topping of Coconut-Almond Bacon adds smokiness and crunch.

In a large saucepan, heat the olive oil over medium heat. Add the onion and garlic and cook until tender, 4 to 5 minutes. Stir in the broth, beans, plant-based meat, potatoes, nutritional yeast, Italian herbs, salt, pepper, and red pepper flakes (if using). Bring to a boil. Reduce the heat to low, cover, and simmer until the potatoes are almost tender, 8 to 10 minutes. Stir in the collard greens and simmer, again covered, until tender, 3 minutes.

Divide the mix among 4 serving bowls. Top the servings with the bacon and fresh herbs.

TIP: This hearty soup makes a *great* breakfast. It's warm, filling, and easy to reheat in the morning. You can also store leftovers in a mason jar and take it to work for a quick lunch. Or make a double batch and freeze the leftovers in single-serving portions in a quart-sized freezer bag or glass storage container. Just leave room for the soup to expand as it freezes.

LENTIL BOLOGNESE

SERVES 3 • PREP: 15 MINUTES • COOK: 30 MINUTES • TOTAL: 45 MINUTES

4 tablespoons extra-virgin
   olive oil

1 small onion, finely chopped

1 medium carrot, peeled and
   finely chopped

1 celery stalk, finely chopped

2 garlic cloves, minced

1 (8-ounce) package fresh
   cremini mushrooms, finely
   chopped

1 (28-ounce) can crushed
   tomatoes

2 cups Vegetable Broth
   (page 351) or Plant-Based
   Whole30–compatible
   vegetable broth

1 cup brown lentils

2 tablespoons balsamic
   vinegar

2 teaspoons Italian seasoning

1 teaspoon salt

½ teaspoon black pepper

2 (10.7-ounce) packages
   zucchini noodles or
   3 medium zucchini,
   spiralized

Plant-Based Whole30–
   compatible ricotta

Chopped fresh basil

This lentil-based bolognese served over zoodles will become an instant family favorite. A dollop of plant-based ricotta adds a touch of creaminess.

In a large pot, heat 2 tablespoons of the olive oil over medium heat. Stir in the onion, carrot, celery, and garlic. Cook, stirring occasionally, until softened, 4 to 5 minutes. Stir in the mushrooms and cook until lightly browned, 3 to 4 minutes. Add the tomatoes, broth, lentils, vinegar, Italian seasoning, salt, and pepper and bring to a boil. Reduce the heat to low, cover, and simmer, stirring twice, until the lentils are tender and the sauce has thickened, 20 to 25 minutes.

In a large skillet, heat the remaining 2 tablespoons oil over medium heat. Add the zucchini noodles and cook, tossing, until tender, 2 to 3 minutes.

Spoon the bolognese over the zucchini noodles and top with the ricotta and fresh basil.

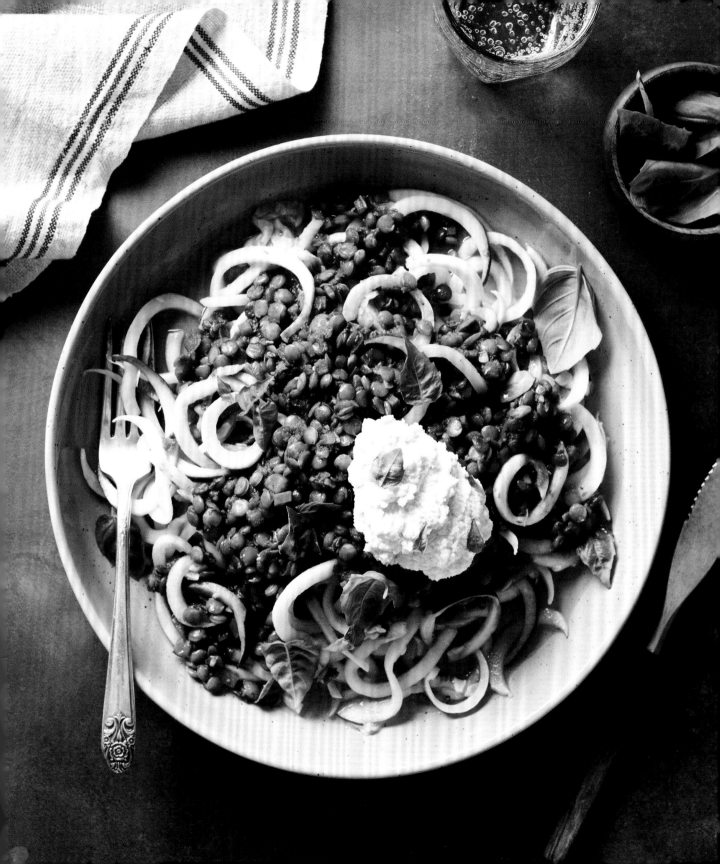

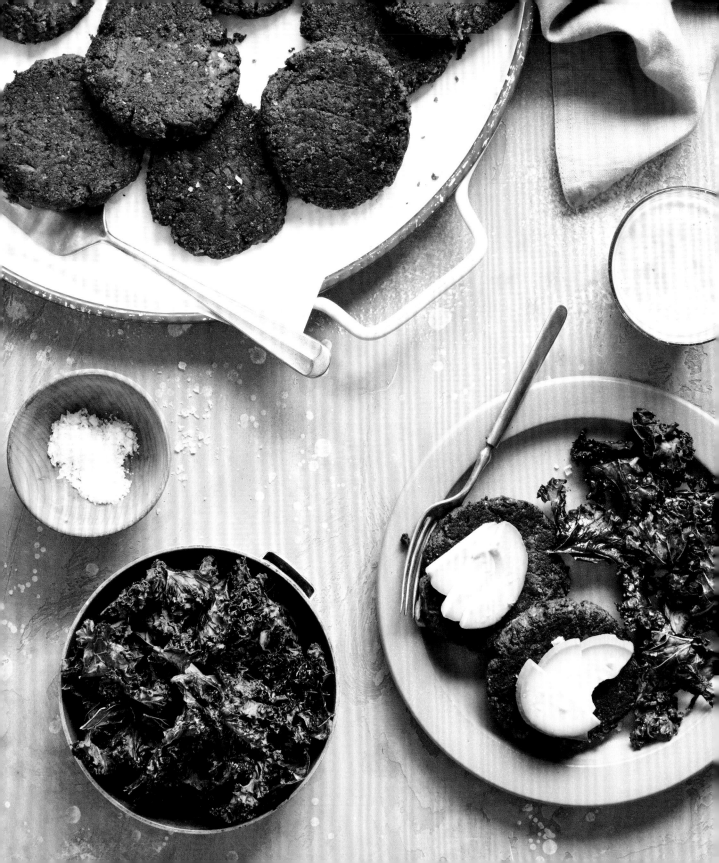

MUSHROOM–BLACK BEAN PATTIES

SERVES 4 • PREP: 10 MINUTES + 1 HOUR CHILLING • COOK: 10 MINUTES •
TOTAL: 1 HOUR 20 MINUTES

¼ cup plus 1 tablespoon ground flaxmeal

3 tablespoons extra-virgin olive oil, plus more if needed

1 (12- to 15-ounce) jar roasted red bell peppers, thoroughly drained and chopped

1 (8-ounce) package fresh cremini mushrooms, chopped

2 garlic cloves, minced

1 small onion, chopped

1 teaspoon salt

½ teaspoon black pepper

1 (15-ounce) can black beans, rinsed and drained

½ cup walnut halves

¼ cup coconut flour

1 tablespoon balsamic vinegar

1 tablespoon coconut aminos

1 teaspoon smoked paprika

1 teaspoon Plant-Based Whole30–compatible hot sauce

¼ to ½ avocado, sliced

TIP: Uncooked patties can be stored in an airtight container in the refrigerator up to 3 days.

A flax "egg" helps to hold these knife-and-fork veggie patties together, while pan-frying gives them a crisp crust. Serve these with a cold Power-Up Smoothie (page 340) and crisp Truffled Kale Chips (page 345).

First, make the flax egg. In a small bowl, combine 1 tablespoon of the ground flaxmeal and 2½ tablespoons of water. Let stand, stirring occasionally, while you chop and cook the vegetables.

In a large skillet, heat 1 tablespoon of the olive oil over medium-high heat. Add the peppers, mushrooms, garlic, onion, salt, and black pepper. Cook, stirring frequently, until vegetables are tender, mushrooms have browned, and most of the liquid has evaporated, 5 to 8 minutes. Transfer the vegetables to a fine-mesh sieve, hold it over the sink, and press gently with the back of a large spoon to extract any excess liquid. Let the vegetables cool for 10 minutes.

In a food processor, combine the flax egg, beans, walnuts, coconut flour, balsamic vinegar, coconut aminos, paprika, and hot sauce. Add the cooked vegetables and pulse in 5-second intervals until mixture is well combined but retains some texture (8 to 10 pulses).

Spray a large rimmed baking sheet lightly with extra-virgin olive oil spray.

Pour the remaining ¼ cup flaxmeal onto a plate. Using a ⅓ cup measure, scoop the bean mixture (overfilling the measuring cup slightly). Use your hands to gently shape each portion into a ball, then roll the ball in flaxmeal. Flatten to a ½-inch-thick patty on the prepared baking sheet. Repeat until the mixture is gone and you have about 10 evenly sized patties. Refrigerate, uncovered, for 1 hour.

In a large nonstick skillet, heat the remaining 2 tablespoons olive oil over medium-high heat. Transfer 2 to 3 cold patties to the skillet and cook until browned on the bottom, 3 to 4 minutes. Carefully flip the patties and cook until they are heated through, an additional 3 to 4 minutes, adding more oil to the pan if necessary.

Serve the patties with the avocado slices.

ROASTED VEGGIES AND BLACK BEANS WITH MUHAMMARA

SERVES 3 • PREP: 15 MINUTES • BAKE: 15 MINUTES • TOTAL: 30 MINUTES

½ cup extra-virgin olive oil

6 tablespoons fresh lemon juice

1 large garlic clove, minced

½ teaspoon salt

¼ teaspoon black pepper

6 fingerling potatoes, quartered lengthwise

10 ounces Brussels sprouts, trimmed and halved

1 (5-ounce) package fresh cremini mushrooms, quartered

1 medium onion, cut into wedges

4 medium beets, steamed and quartered (see Tip)

4 carrots, peeled and cut into 2-inch pieces

2 (15-ounce) cans black beans, rinsed and drained

2 tablespoons chopped fresh chives

Muhammara (page 341)

Muhammara is a roasted red pepper and walnut spread with origins in Syria—and it's the real star of this simple sheet-pan supper. This dish is quite versatile, so feel free to use a different type of potato, swap broccoli or cauliflower for the Brussels sprouts, or add a different type of beans.

Preheat the oven to 400°F. Line 2 large rimmed baking sheets with parchment.

In a large bowl, whisk together the olive oil, lemon juice, garlic, salt, and pepper. Measure out and reserve 3 tablespoons of the dressing. Add the potatoes, Brussels sprouts, mushrooms, onion, beets, and carrots to the bowl and toss to combine. Arrange the seasoned vegetables on one baking sheet in a single layer.

Pour the reserved dressing into the bowl and stir in the beans. Arrange beans on the second baking sheet in a single layer. Bake until the vegetables are tender and the beans are heated through, about 15 minutes.

Spoon the vegetables and beans onto 3 serving plates. Sprinkle with the chives and serve with the Muhammara.

TIP: You may be able to find cooked beets in the produce section, but steaming your own beets is easy. Scrub the beets, then trim the greens and any roots. Place the beets in a steamer basket above 2 inches of water. Bring the water to a boil, then reduce the heat to low, cover, and simmer for 30 minutes, or until beets are easily pierced with a fork. Once cool, rub off the skins and cut the beets into quarters. Note: Beet juice stains anything it touches, so peel them in the sink or over parchment, and wear gloves to protect your hands.

You can also use golden beets in this recipe, which would impart a slightly sweeter flavor to the dish.

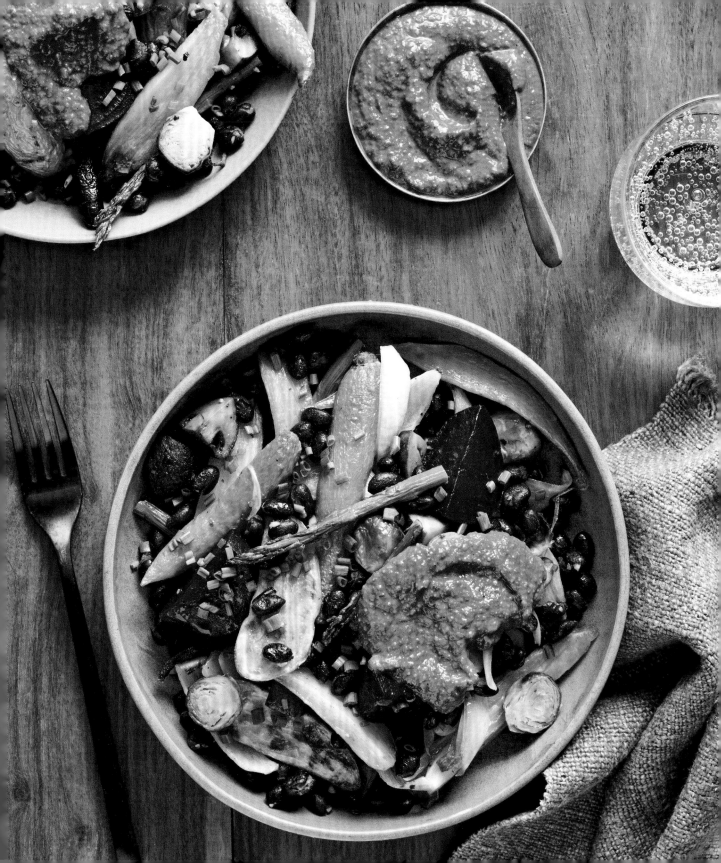

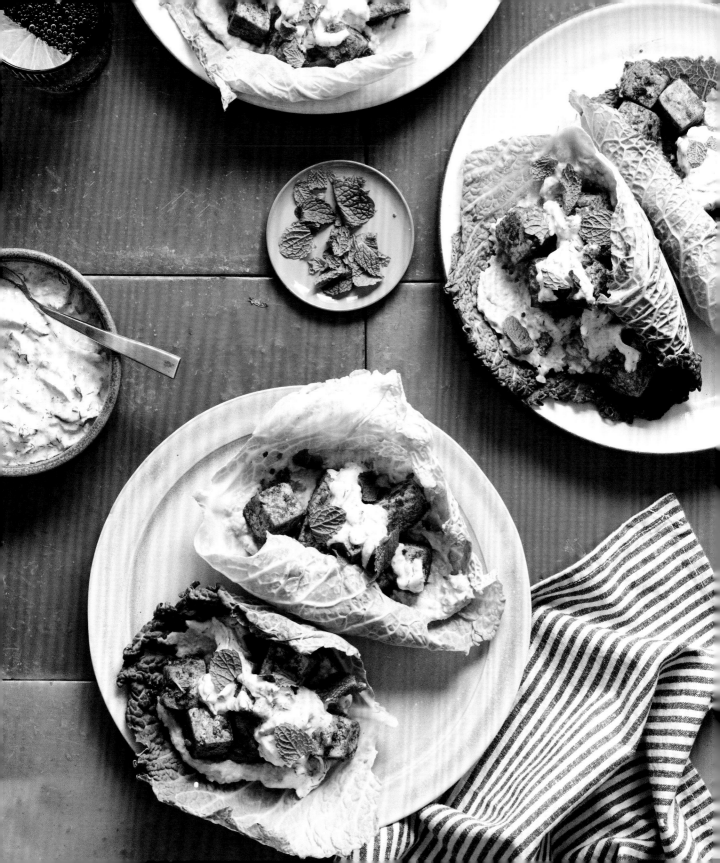

SHAWARMA-INSPIRED TOFU WRAPS

SERVES 3 • PREP: 10 MINUTES + 30 MINUTES MARINATING • COOK: 5 MINUTES •
TOTAL: 45 MINUTES

FOR THE TZATZIKI

½ cup Plant-Based Whole30 Sour Cream (page 280) or Plant-Based Whole30–compatible plain yogurt

¼ cup shredded radishes

¼ cup shredded cucumber

1 tablespoon chopped fresh dill

1 teaspoon fresh lemon juice

⅛ teaspoon salt

1 small garlic clove, minced

FOR THE TOFU

1 (16-ounce) block super-firm tofu, drained, pressed, and diced (see Tip, page 255)

⅓ cup extra-virgin olive oil

2 tablespoons fresh lemon juice

1 tablespoon apple cider vinegar

3 garlic cloves, minced

1 teaspoon paprika

1 teaspoon ground cumin

1 teaspoon salt

½ teaspoon ground cinnamon

½ teaspoon red pepper flakes

1 tablespoon coconut oil

FOR SERVING

⅔ cup Plant-Based Whole30–compatible hummus

9 Bibb lettuce or savoy lettuce leaves

Shawarma, which originated in Turkey, is a popular street food in the Middle East. It's traditionally made with spit-roasted meats, but vegan takes on this dish are also popular. All of the spices that make traditional shawarma so good go into the marinade for the tofu before it's crisped up in the pan.

MAKE THE TZATZIKI: In a small bowl, stir together the sour cream, radishes, cucumber, dill, lemon juice, salt, and garlic. Cover and refrigerate until ready to serve.

MAKE THE TOFU: In a resealable plastic bag, combine the tofu, olive oil, lemon juice, vinegar, garlic, paprika, cumin, salt, cinnamon, and red pepper flakes. Seal the bag and let marinate for 30 minutes. Drain the tofu and discard the marinade.

In a large, preferably nonstick, skillet over medium heat, heat the coconut oil. Add the tofu and cook, stirring occasionally, until cooked through, 5 to 8 minutes.

Serve: Spread some of the hummus on each of the lettuce leaves, then fill with some of the tofu and drizzle with tzatziki.

TIP: Tzatziki will keep in an airtight container in the refrigerator for up to 5 days.

THAI TEMPEH AND VEGGIE BOWL

SERVES 3 • PREP: 15 MINUTES + 30 MINUTES MARINATING • COOK: 10 MINUTES •
TOTAL: 55 MINUTES

FOR THE TEMPEH

2 (8-ounce) packages tempeh, drained

½ cup coconut aminos

¼ cup unseasoned rice vinegar

¼ cup fresh orange juice

2 teaspoons toasted sesame oil

1 tablespoon olive oil

FOR THE VEGETABLES

1 tablespoon coconut oil or extra-virgin olive oil

1½ cups broccoli florets

2 medium carrots, peeled and cut into matchsticks

1 cup snow peas, sliced in half diagonally

2 garlic cloves, minced

1 teaspoon salt

½ teaspoon black pepper

½ teaspoon red pepper flakes (optional)

FOR SERVING

¼ cup chopped peanuts

Chopped fresh cilantro and Thai basil (see Tip)

Lime wedges

Plant-Based Whole30-compatible sriracha or hot sauce (optional)

A mixture of coconut aminos, rice vinegar, orange juice, and sesame oil serves as both a marinade for the tempeh and a sauce for the meal, infusing everything with a balanced sweet, savory, toasty flavor. A squeeze of lime, a sprinkle of peanuts, and a drizzle of sriracha finish it off with a burst of acid, crunch, and heat.

MAKE THE TEMPEH: Place a vegetable steamer in a large skillet; add water to just below the steamer basket. Bring the water to a boil, then add the tempeh to the steamer basket. Reduce the heat to low, cover, and simmer for 10 minutes. Transfer the tempeh to a cutting board and dice.

In a small bowl, combine the coconut aminos, vinegar, orange juice, and sesame oil. Reserve ½ cup for serving, and pour the remaining into a resealable plastic bag. Add the tempeh, seal the bag, and marinate for at least 30 minutes, or up to 24 hours. Drain the tempeh and discard the marinade.

Heat the olive oil in a large, preferably nonstick, skillet over medium heat. Add the tempeh and cook, stirring occasionally, until browned and cooked through (an instant-read thermometer reads 165°F), 5 to 8 minutes.

MAKE THE VEGETABLES: In a large skillet, heat the coconut oil over medium heat. Add the broccoli and carrots and cook, stirring frequently, until almost tender, 3 to 5 minutes. Stir in the snow peas, garlic, salt, pepper, and red pepper flakes (if using), and cook until the vegetables are tender, about 2 minutes.

Serve: Divide the tempeh and vegetables among 3 serving bowls and drizzle each with the reserved marinade. Top with the peanuts and herbs, and serve with lime wedges and sriracha (if using)

TIP: Thai basil is native to Southeast Asia and its cuisines. Its flavor is crisp and pungent, adding a fresh, herbal flavor that is markedly bolder and spicier than its sweet Italian cousin. If you can't find Thai basil in your local grocery store, you can substitute sweet basil. You can also add a dash of fresh mint for an extra punch of flavor.

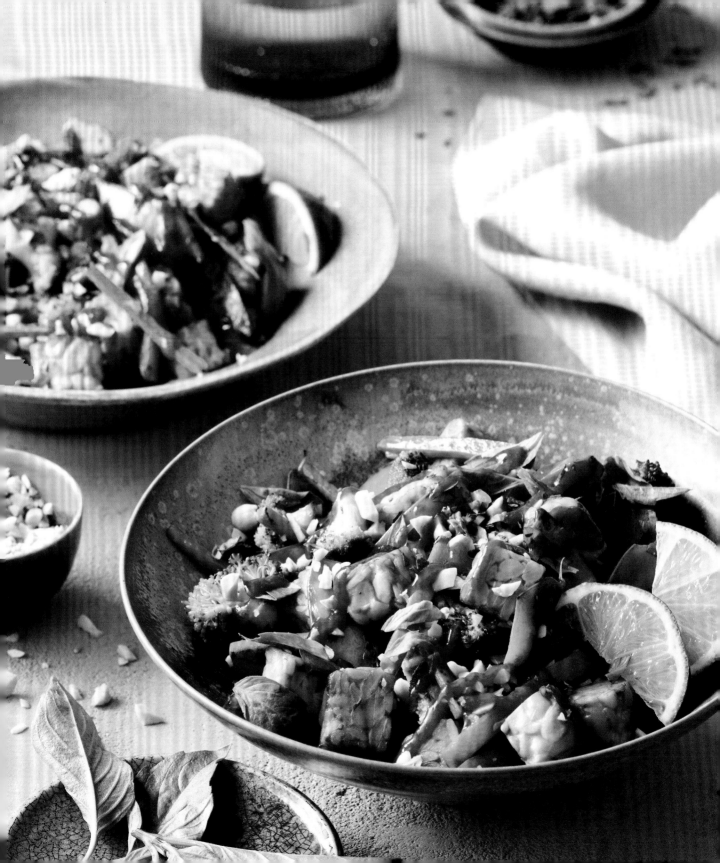

PLANT-BASED WHOLE30 SIDES

ROASTED DELICATA SQUASH
WITH SPICY CASHEW DRESSING

SERVES 3 • PREP: 10 MINUTES • BAKE: 15 MINUTES • TOTAL: 25 MINUTES

1½ to 2 pounds delicata squash, trimmed, halved, seeded, and sliced into ½-inch-thick pieces (see Tip)

2 tablespoons extra-virgin olive oil

1 teaspoon salt

½ teaspoon black pepper

½ cup roasted and salted cashews

½ cup warm water, or more as needed

¼ cup avocado oil or light olive oil

2 tablespoons unseasoned rice vinegar

¾ teaspoon coconut aminos

¾ teaspoon Aleppo pepper flakes or red pepper flakes

1 small garlic clove

2 tablespoons chopped fresh parsley

TIP: Delicata squash has a thin, edible skin, so it doesn't require peeling. (Which is great, because peeling squash can be a pain.) If you can't find delicata, substitute 4 cups of peeled and chopped butternut squash.

Delicata squash is in the same botanical family as summer squash and zucchini. Culinarily, however, it's considered more of a winter squash because of its sweet-tasting flesh. Here, it's simply sliced and roasted, then topped with a rich, lightly spicy cashew dressing.

Preheat the oven to 400°F. Line a large rimmed baking sheet with parchment.

Place the squash on the sheet pan and drizzle with the olive oil. Toss to coat and sprinkle with the salt and black pepper. Arrange in a single layer. Roast until tender and golden brown, 15 to 20 minutes.

Meanwhile, in a blender, combine the cashews, ½ cup water, avocado oil, vinegar, coconut aminos, Aleppo pepper flakes, and garlic. Blend until smooth and creamy. Add additional water, 1 teaspoon at a time, to reach desired consistency.

Arrange the squash on a serving platter and drizzle with the dressing. Sprinkle with the parsley and serve.

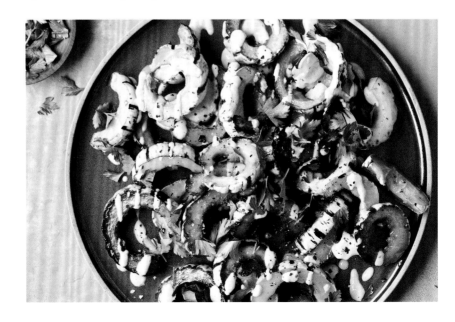

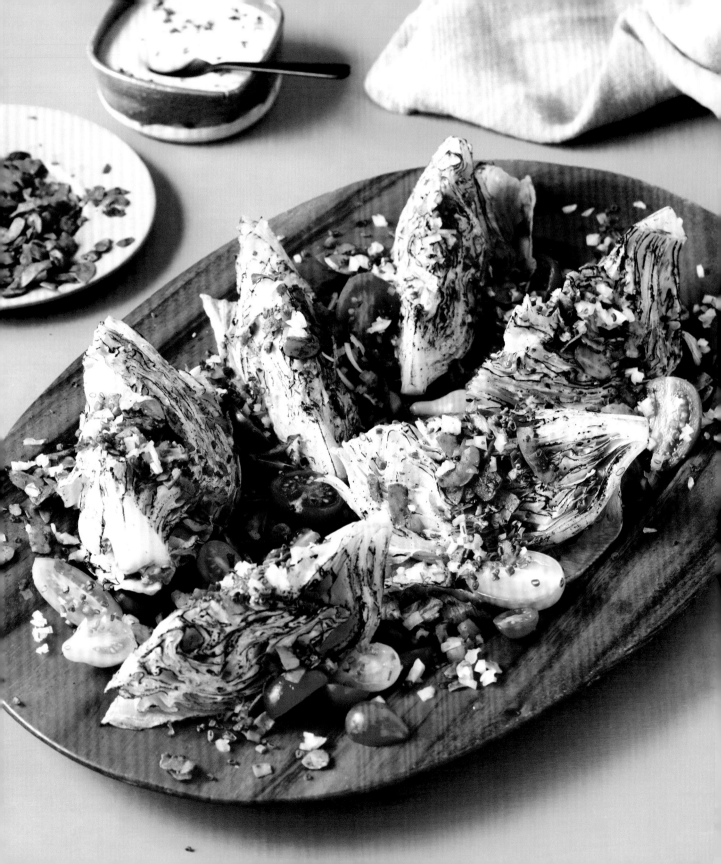

BROILED WEDGE SALAD WITH COCONUT-ALMOND BACON

SERVES 6 • PREP: 10 MINUTES • BAKE: 10 MINUTES • BROIL: 5 MINUTES • TOTAL: 25 MINUTES

FOR THE BACON

1 cup large-flake unsweetened coconut (see Tip)

½ cup sliced almonds

1 tablespoon avocado oil

2 tablespoons coconut aminos

¾ teaspoon smoked paprika

¼ teaspoon Plant-Based Whole30–compatible liquid smoke (see Tip)

¼ teaspoon black pepper

FOR THE SALAD

1 large head of iceberg or romaine lettuce, trimmed and cut into 6 wedges (see Tip)

Vegan Caesar Dressing (page 335)

1 (8-ounce) container cherry tomatoes, halved

1 small shallot, finely chopped

2 tablespoons chopped fresh chives

½ teaspoon black pepper

If you've never had grilled or broiled romaine or iceberg lettuce, you're missing out. The heat softens the exterior of the lettuce but retains its crunchy center. This riff on a traditional wedge salad is almost a full meal, with umami-rich caesar dressing, cherry tomatoes, and smoky Coconut-Almond Bacon.

MAKE THE COCONUT-ALMOND BACON: Preheat the oven to 325°F. Line a large rimmed baking sheet with parchment.

Add the coconut, almonds, avocado oil, coconut aminos, paprika, liquid smoke, and pepper to the baking sheet and toss to combine. Bake for 5 minutes. Stir and continue to bake until the coconut is golden brown, 5 to 8 minutes more (watch carefully so the coconut doesn't burn). Transfer to a plate and let cool for 10 minutes. The bacon will continue to crisp as it cools. Change the oven setting to broil. Keep the lined baking sheet handy.

MAKE THE SALAD: Adjust the top oven rack to the upper third of the oven, about 4 inches from the broiler. Place the lettuce wedges, cut side up, on the baking sheet. Brush the cut sides with some of the dressing. Broil until the lettuce is browned on the edges, rotating the baking sheet halfway through, about 3 minutes total.

Transfer the wedges to a serving platter. Top with the bacon, cherry tomatoes, shallot, chives, and pepper. Serve with the remaining dressing.

> **TIP:** For the bacon, use large coconut flakes or coconut chips, not shredded coconut. You can store leftover bacon at room temperature in an airtight container for up to 1 week.
>
> If you're using romaine, cut the lettuce in half across the middle to form two shorter portions. Then cut each half into three wedges (like orange slices).
>
> Note that liquid smoke often contains added sugar and other ingredients that don't work on the Whole30. An online search for "sugar-free liquid smoke" can turn up compatible brands. You can also skip it, or add a little chipotle powder to the smoked paprika in the recipe.

CAULIFLOWER WITH SPICY TOFU SAUCE

SERVES 6 • PREP: 10 MINUTES • BAKE/COOK: 25 MINUTES • TOTAL: 35 MINUTES

2 large (16-ounce) heads of cauliflower, trimmed and cut into florets

4 tablespoons extra-virgin olive oil

2 teaspoons salt

1 teaspoon black pepper

2 shallots, sliced

2 jalapeños, halved, seeded, and chopped (seeds reserved, optional)

½ (12-ounce) package silken tofu, drained

2 tablespoons miso

1 teaspoon grated lemon zest

2 tablespoons fresh lemon juice

Chopped fresh cilantro

Though golden-brown, caramelized cauliflower is always delicious, the real star of this dish is the creamy sauce. Made with silken tofu spiked with lemon, shallot, miso, and jalapeño, it pairs perfectly with any roasted vegetable and it is easy to customize to your desired level of heat.

Preheat the oven to 400°F. Line a large rimmed baking sheet with parchment.

Arrange the cauliflower florets on the baking sheet. Drizzle with 3 tablespoons of the olive oil, then sprinkle with 1½ teaspoons salt and the pepper. Toss to combine and spread out again on the baking sheet. Roast until the cauliflower is tender and golden brown, stirring occasionally, 25 to 30 minutes.

Meanwhile, heat the remaining tablespoon oil in a medium saucepan over medium heat. Add the shallots and jalapeños and cook until the shallots are golden brown and the jalapeños darken, about 5 minutes.

Transfer the shallots and jalapeños to a blender. Add the tofu, miso, lemon zest, lemon juice, and remaining ½ teaspoon salt. Blend until smooth. Taste the sauce and add the jalapeño seeds for more heat (if using). Pour the sauce back into the saucepan and heat over low heat until warmed through.

Spoon the sauce onto a serving platter and top with the cauliflower. Sprinkle with the cilantro and serve.

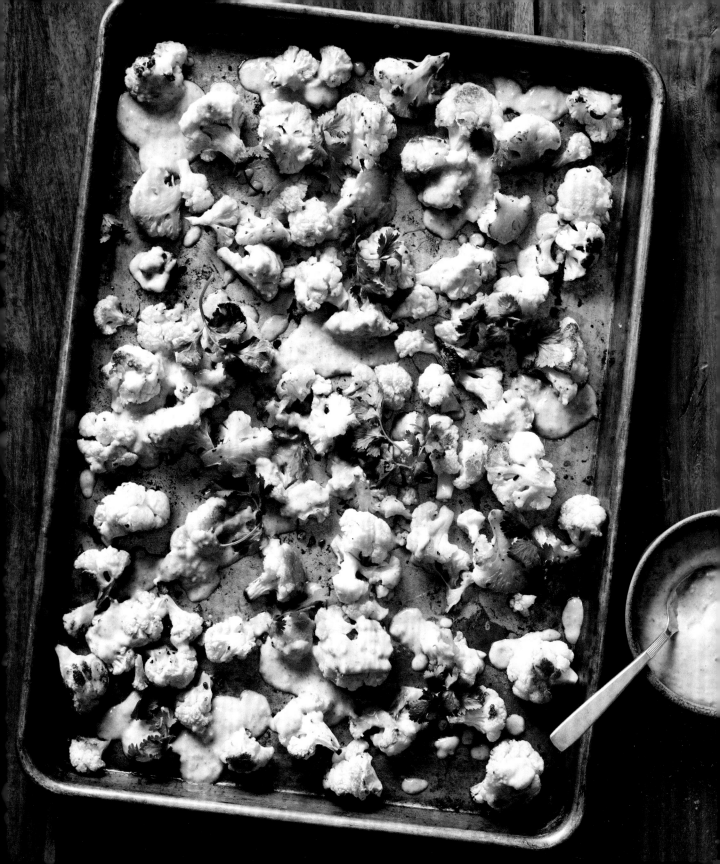

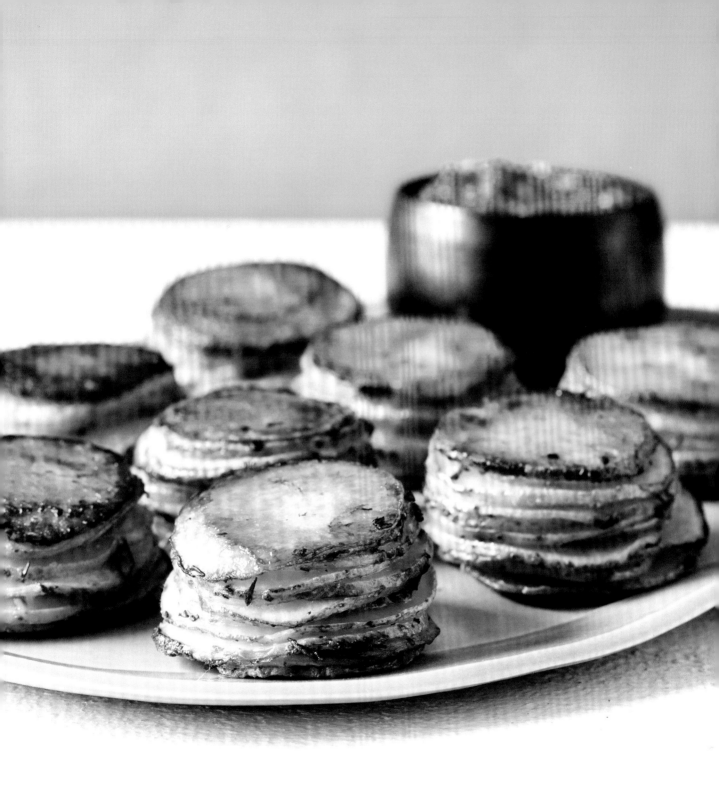

CRISPY POTATO STACK

SERVES 4 • PREP: 15 MINUTES • BAKE: 35 MINUTES • TOTAL: 50 MINUTES

4 tablespoons extra-virgin olive oil

2 pounds small Yukon Gold potatoes, scrubbed and sliced about ⅛ inch thick (see Tip)

2 tablespoons finely chopped fresh herbs, such as rosemary, parsley, thyme, and/or oregano

1 teaspoon salt

½ teaspoon black pepper

Romesco Sauce (page 329)

The ingredients and procedure here are simple, but this finished side dish looks company-worthy. It features lacy layers of potato that are crisp on the edges and tender and creamy in the center.

Preheat the oven to 375°F. Using a standard (12-cup) muffin tin, brush 8 of the cups with 1 tablespoon of the olive oil. (See Tip.)

In a large bowl, combine the potatoes, the remaining 3 tablespoons olive oil, the herbs, salt, and pepper and toss to coat the slices well. Stack the potato slices in the oiled muffin cups, laying in the larger slices first, then the smaller slices on the top. (Fill the remaining cups with water.) Bake until the potatoes are tender and golden brown, 35 to 45 minutes. Serve with the romesco sauce.

TIP: Peeling the potatoes first will provide a smoother texture, but these are sliced so thin and the edges crisp up so nicely, you really can skip that step. Use a mandoline for speedy and accurate slicing.

Alternatively, if you don't have a muffin tin with the correct size cups, place the potato slices in a single layer on a parchment-lined baking sheet, slightly overlapping each slice. Bake until potatoes are golden brown and crisp around the edges, 30 to 35 minutes.

CRUNCHY CABBAGE SALAD
WITH SPICY PEANUT DRESSING

SERVES 3 • PREP: 10 MINUTES • TOTAL: 10 MINUTES

2 cups thinly sliced napa
cabbage

2 cups thinly sliced curly kale

1 red bell pepper, seeded and
diced

1 small cucumber, diced
(½ cup)

1 ripe mango, pitted, peeled,
and chopped (see Tip)

2 green onions, thinly sliced
(green part only)

½ cup chopped fresh mint and
cilantro

Spicy Peanut Dressing
(page 332)

⅓ cup chopped peanuts

This salad covers all four sensory bases: sweet, spicy, crunchy, and creamy. If you'd like more heat, sprinkle your finished dish with red pepper flakes. If desired, make it a full meal by adding air-fried or pan-fried super-firm tofu.

In a medium serving bowl, toss together the cabbage, kale, bell pepper, cucumber, mango, green onion, and herbs. Drizzle with some of the dressing and toss to coat. Sprinkle with the chopped peanuts.

TIP: If mango isn't in season, you can use frozen! Thaw the package in the refrigerator overnight or in a bowl of cold water for 2 hours, then dice the frozen squares even smaller for this salad.

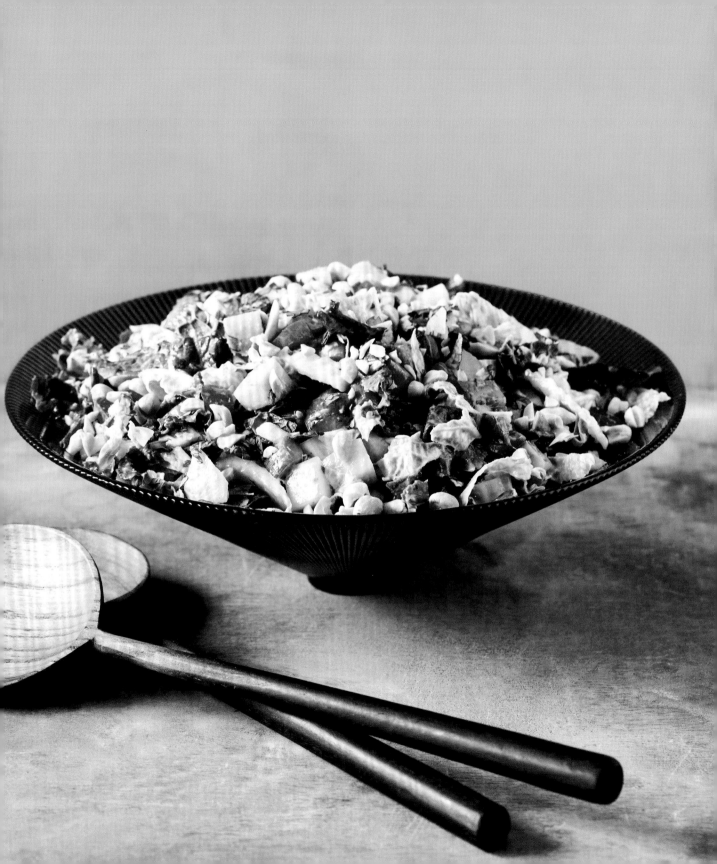

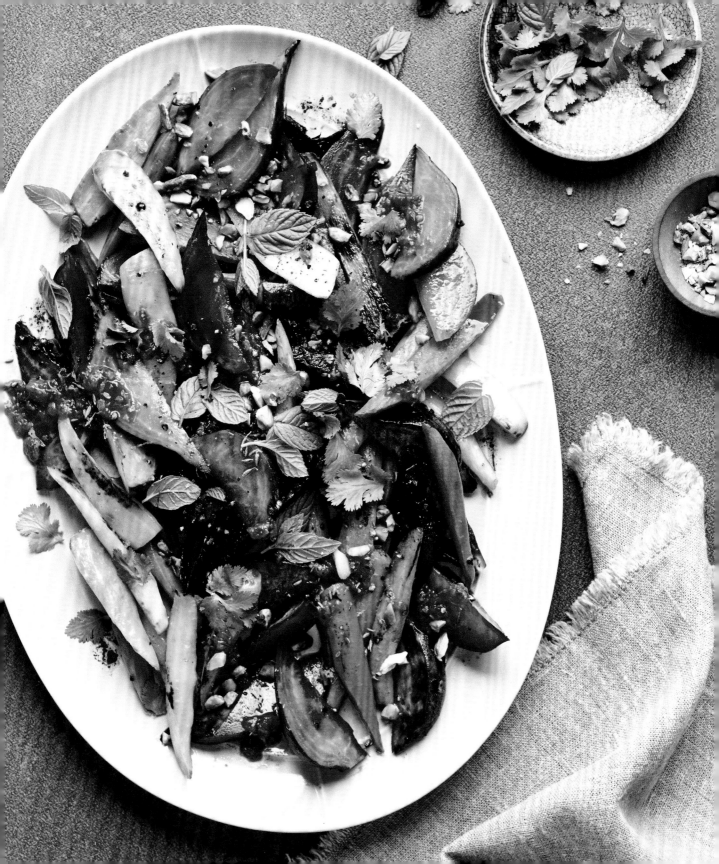

MOROCCAN CARROTS AND BEETS

SERVES 6 • PREP: 10 MINUTES • BAKE: 30 MINUTES • TOTAL: 40 MINUTES

1 pound carrots, peeled, large carrots quartered

5 beets, trimmed and cut into ½-inch-thick wedges

¼ cup extra-virgin olive oil

1 teaspoon salt

½ teaspoon black pepper

1 lemon, thinly sliced, seeds removed

2 tablespoons Plant-Based Whole30–compatible harissa (see Tip)

2 tablespoons grated orange zest

1 teaspoon cumin seeds

3 tablespoons chopped pistachios

2 tablespoons chopped fresh cilantro or mint

When arranged on a serving platter, this dish is absolutely gorgeous. Use rainbow carrots and red and golden beets to maximize the eye-popping colors. The flavors bring a perfect contrast of sweet roasted root veggies with a hint of heat from the harissa.

Preheat the oven to 450°F. Line a large rimmed baking sheet with parchment.

Arrange the carrots and beets on the baking sheet. Drizzle with 2 tablespoons of the olive oil, the salt, and pepper and toss to coat. Arrange the vegetables in a single layer, and place the lemon slices on top of the vegetables. Roast until the carrots and beets are tender, turning halfway, about 30 minutes. Discard the lemon slices.

Meanwhile, in a small bowl, whisk together the remaining 2 tablespoons oil, the harissa, orange zest, and cumin seeds.

Transfer the roasted vegetables to a serving platter. Drizzle with the seasoned harissa and sprinkle with the pistachios and cilantro.

TIP: You can find sugar-free harissa online and at many health food markets, but you can also make the sauce yourself. Combine 2 tablespoons of harissa powder with 1 tablespoon extra-virgin olive oil and 1 tablespoon water and stir. Add equal parts additional olive oil and/or water if the paste is too thick, until you achieve the desired consistency.

SEAWEED SALAD WITH MISO VINAIGRETTE

SERVES 3 • PREP: 10 MINUTES + 10 MINUTES REHYDRATING • TOTAL: 20 MINUTES

1 (1.76-ounce) package wakame seaweed (see Tip)

2 tablespoons toasted sesame oil

2 tablespoons avocado oil or light olive oil

2 tablespoons miso

2 tablespoons unseasoned rice vinegar

1 (½-inch) piece fresh ginger, peeled and grated (see Tip, page 268)

1 small garlic clove, minced

Pinch of red pepper flakes (optional)

1 medium carrot, peeled and coarsely shredded

¾ cup thinly sliced daikon radish or 3 red radishes, thinly sliced

1 small cucumber, peeled and thinly sliced

Sesame seeds, toasted

Unlike the seaweed salad you typically get in sushi restaurants, the dressing for this salad doesn't contain any sugar or mirin (a sweet rice wine). It's gingery and garlicky, with a touch of umami from the miso.

Place the wakame in a medium bowl and cover with cold water. Let stand until rehydrated, about 10 minutes. In a colander, strain the seaweed and rinse thoroughly. Squeeze out the excess water. If it still tastes salty, repeat with clean water. Roughly chop into 1-inch pieces.

In a medium bowl, whisk together the sesame and avocado oils, miso, vinegar, ginger, garlic, and red pepper flakes (if using).

In a serving bowl, combine the seaweed, the carrot, radishes, and cucumber. Drizzle with the vinaigrette and sprinkle with the sesame seeds.

TIP: Wakame is an edible seaweed best served in soups or seaweed salads. Read your labels! Surprisingly, some packages of wakame will contain added sugar. Wakame is most often sold dried, but it's easily reconstituted in water, as done here.

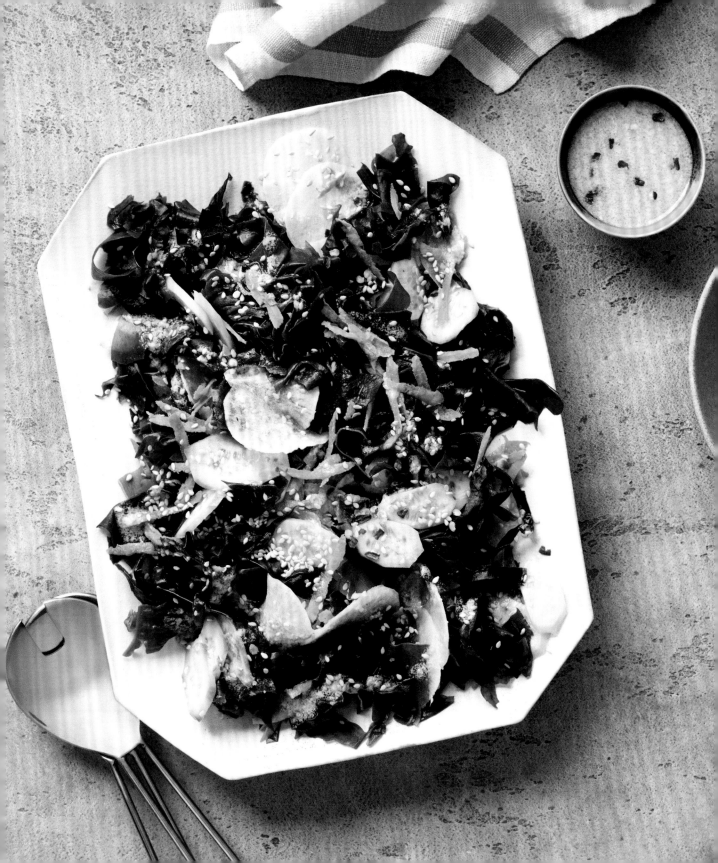

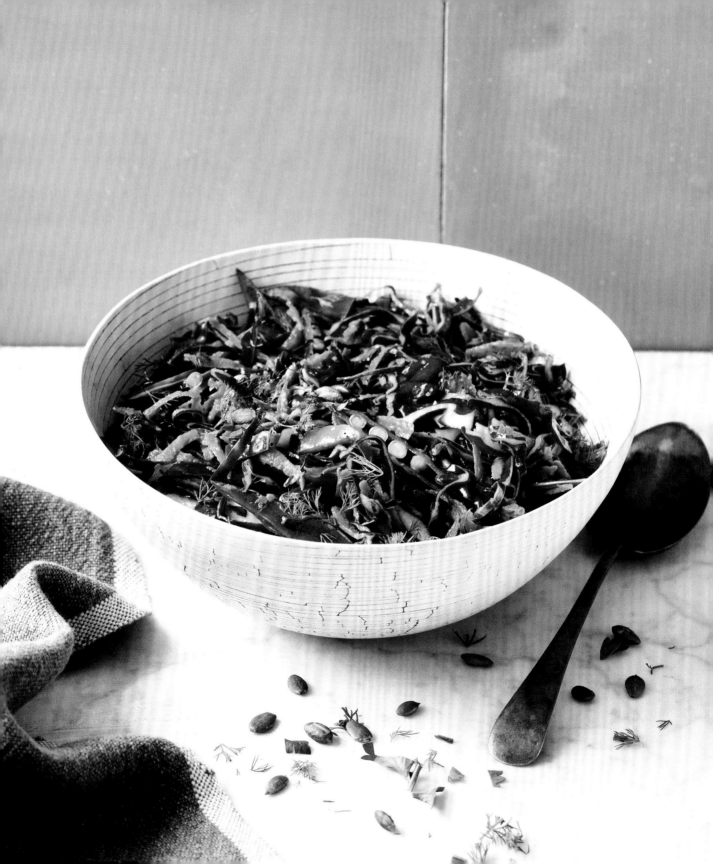

TRIPLE VEGGIE SLAW

SERVES 3 • PREP: 10 MINUTES + 2 HOURS CHILLING • TOTAL: 2 HOURS 10 MINUTES

¼ cup extra-virgin olive oil

3 tablespoons fresh lemon juice

1 teaspoon Plant-Based Whole30–compatible Dijon mustard

1 garlic clove, minced

½ teaspoon salt

⅛ teaspoon black pepper

½ (8-ounce) package shredded red cabbage or 1 small red cabbage, trimmed and shredded (about 2 cups)

2 cups coarsely shredded carrots

8 ounces sugar snap peas or snow peas, thinly sliced lengthwise

½ cup pepitas (pumpkin seeds) or sunflower seeds, toasted and lightly salted

⅓ cup chopped fresh herbs, such as parsley, dill, thyme, or chives

Fresh, crisp, and colorful, this vinaigrette-dressed slaw is the perfect side dish to accompany grilled foods. Be patient and chill the slaw for the full 2 hours before serving; this allows time for the cabbage to soften and the vegetables to pick up the flavors of the dressing.

In a small bowl, whisk together the olive oil, lemon juice, mustard, garlic, salt, and pepper.

In a large serving bowl, combine the cabbage, carrots, peas, pepitas, and herbs. Drizzle the vinaigrette over the slaw and toss to combine. Cover and refrigerate for 30 minutes to 2 hours before serving. If making ahead, store the vegetables and dressing separately and combine 2 hours before serving. (See Tip.)

TIP: To make your slaw stay crunchy longer and to mellow its somewhat bitter flavor, add the shredded cabbage to a bowl and sprinkle with a tablespoon of salt. Let sit for 10 minutes to an hour, then drain off the excess moisture. Pat the cabbage dry with paper or cloth towels, then continue making your slaw.

PLANT-BASED WHOLE30 SAUCES AND DRESSINGS

CHARRED TOMATO DRESSING

MAKES 1½ CUPS • PREP: 5 MINUTES • COOK: 5 MINUTES • TOTAL: 10 MINUTES

2 tablespoons extra-virgin olive oil

1 pint cherry tomatoes (see Tip)

1 shallot, minced

½ teaspoon Aleppo pepper flakes (see Tip, page 251)

¼ teaspoon salt

¼ teaspoon black pepper

1 tablespoon balsamic or sherry vinegar

1 tablespoon chopped fresh basil

Mildly spicy and deliciously smoky, this sauce has a nice balance of sweetness and acidity. Try it on grilled or roasted tofu, chickpea meat (see page 349), or cauliflower steaks.

In a large skillet, heat 1 tablespoon of the olive oil over medium heat. Add the tomatoes and cook, covered and undisturbed, until slightly browned on the bottom, 2 to 3 minutes. Stir in the shallot, Aleppo pepper flakes, salt, and pepper. Cook, covered, until the tomatoes collapse and release their juices, 3 to 5 minutes.

Transfer the tomato mixture to a medium bowl. Stir in the remaining tablespoon oil, the vinegar, and basil. Use immediately or refrigerate in an airtight container for up to 3 days.

TIP: You really want *cherry* tomatoes here, not grape tomatoes. Cherry tomatoes have a sweet and delicate flavor and a lighter texture, with a higher water content. Their juiciness makes them perfect for cooking down into a dressing.

FRY-STYLE SAUCE

MAKES ¾ CUP • PREP: 5 MINUTES • TOTAL: 5 MINUTES

⅔ cup Plant-Based Whole30 Mayo (page 350) or Plant-Based Whole30– compatible mayonnaise

½ cup Plant-Based Whole30– compatible ketchup

1 teaspoon fresh orange or lemon juice

¼ teaspoon cayenne

¼ teaspoon garlic powder

¼ teaspoon onion powder

¼ teaspoon chipotle powder

Fry sauce is a popular condiment with its origins in Utah. As its name implies, this simple sauce is perfection served with oven-baked or air-fried potatoes or the Crispy Potato Stack on page 317.

In a medium bowl, whisk together all the ingredients until smooth. Store, covered, in an airtight container for up to 2 weeks.

TIP: To add more heat, use more cayenne. For more of a smoky flavor, use more chipotle powder.

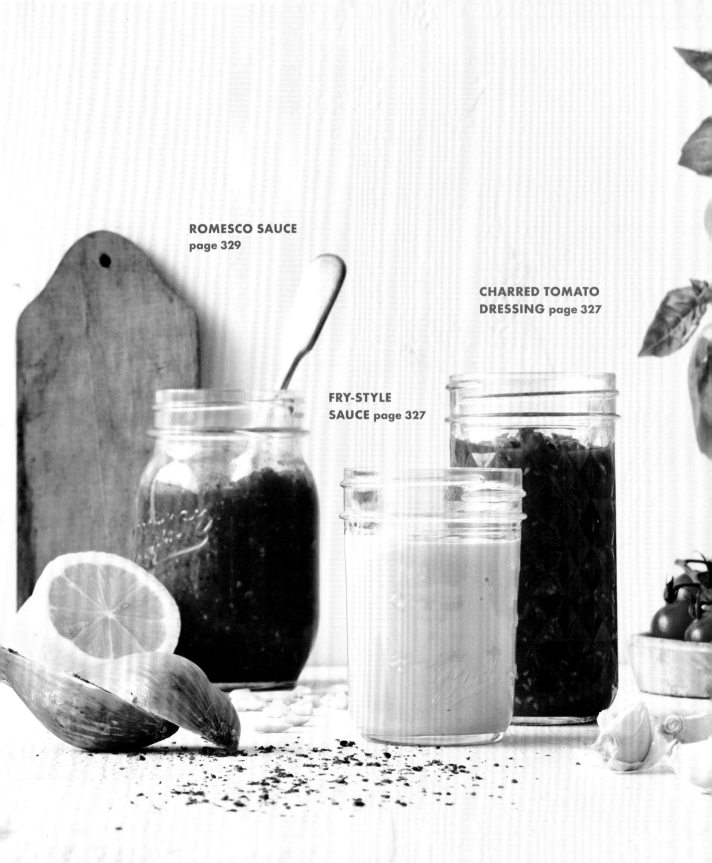

ROMESCO SAUCE
page 329

CHARRED TOMATO
DRESSING page 327

FRY-STYLE
SAUCE page 327

CREAMY ANCHO CHILE DRESSING

MAKES ¾ CUP • PREP: 5 MINUTES • TOTAL: 5 MINUTES

½ cup Plant-Based Whole30 Mayo (page 350) or Plant-Based Whole30–compatible mayonnaise

¼ cup Plant-Based Whole30–compatible almond milk (see Tip)

2 tablespoons apple cider vinegar

1 garlic clove, minced

1 teaspoon ancho chile powder

1 teaspoon grated lime zest

½ teaspoon dried oregano

½ teaspoon salt

¼ teaspoon black pepper

¼ teaspoon smoked paprika

This can be used for dipping or drizzling, based on the amount of almond milk you use. Serve it with raw veggies as a dip, or drizzle it as a dressing over a salad of mixed greens, grapefruit, avocado, and thinly sliced red onion.

In a medium bowl, whisk together all the ingredients until smooth.

Store in an air-tight container in the refrigerator for up to 1 week.

TIP: To make a thicker sauce instead of a dressing, use only 2 tablespoons of almond milk.

ROMESCO SAUCE

MAKES 4 CUPS • PREP: 10 MINUTES • TOTAL: 10 MINUTES

1 (14-ounce) can fire-roasted tomatoes

1 (12- to 16-ounce) jar roasted red bell peppers, drained and coarsely chopped

½ cup slivered or blanched almonds, toasted, or chopped roasted unsalted almonds

1 large garlic clove, coarsely chopped

1½ teaspoons red wine vinegar

1 teaspoon smoked paprika

¼ teaspoon salt

¼ teaspoon black pepper

¼ cup extra-virgin olive oil

Traditionally, this rustic Spanish sauce (with its origins in Catalonia) is a puree of tomatoes and roasted red peppers, thickened with almonds and bread. Our version omits the bread, but the result doesn't miss a beat. Serve it alongside grilled or roasted tofu, tempeh, or vegetables. It's particularly good with roasted cauliflower and potatoes (see Crispy Potato Stack, page 317).

In a food processor or high-speed blender, combine the tomatoes, peppers, almonds, garlic, vinegar, paprika, salt, and pepper. Process until well combined, leaving some texture. Slowly add the olive oil and pulse to combine.

Store, covered, in the refrigerator for up to 5 days or freeze up to 3 months.

SALSA MACHA

MAKES 2 CUPS   •   PREP: 10 MINUTES + 10 MINUTES RESTING   •   COOK: 2 MINUTES   •   TOTAL: 22 MINUTES

4 dried ancho chiles

1 dried guajillo chile

1 dried chile de arbol

1 cup extra-virgin olive oil

⅓ cup roasted unsalted peanuts

4 garlic cloves, chopped

1 tablespoon sesame seeds

1 teaspoon apple cider vinegar

1 teaspoon salt

While this sauce contains three kinds of dried chiles—ancho, guajillo, and chile de arbol—the end result isn't super spicy, just deeply flavorful. The sum of the chiles' individual qualities creates a perfect balance of heat, smokiness, and fruitiness. Serve this with plant-based Salsa Macha Tacos (page 280), drizzle over roasted sweet potato wedges, or serve as a dip for thinly sliced pan-fried plantains.

Wearing rubber gloves, remove the stems and seeds from the chiles (see Tip). Chop the chiles into small pieces; set aside.

In a medium saucepan, heat the olive oil, peanuts, garlic, and sesame seeds over medium heat. Cook until the garlic and sesame seeds are golden brown, about 2 minutes. Remove from the heat and add the chiles; let stand 10 minutes.

Stir in the vinegar and salt. Carefully transfer the chile mixture to a food processor and pulse just until combined (do not overprocess—you want to see bits in the sauce).

Store, covered, in the refrigerator for up to 1 month.

TIP: These dried chiles can be found in the produce departments of many supermarkets, or try a Latin food market.

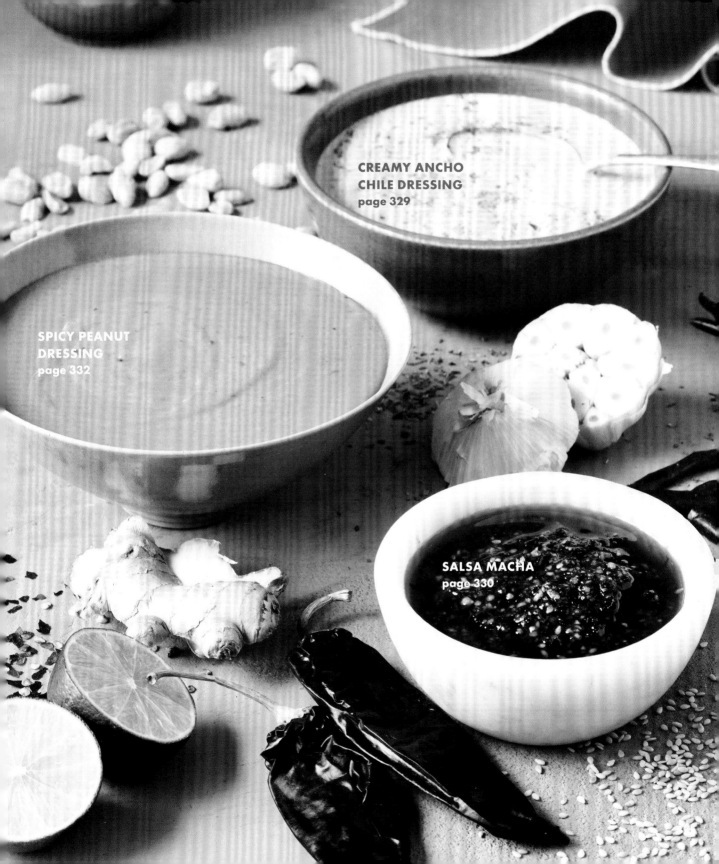

CREAMY ANCHO
CHILE DRESSING
page 329

SPICY PEANUT
DRESSING
page 332

SALSA MACHA
page 330

SPICY PEANUT DRESSING

MAKES 1 CUP • PREP: 5 MINUTES • TOTAL: 5 MINUTES

½ cup Plant-Based Whole30–compatible creamy peanut butter

⅓ cup water

1 tablespoon coconut aminos

2 tablespoons fresh lime juice

1 tablespoon unseasoned rice vinegar

1 (1-inch) piece fresh ginger, peeled and grated (see Tip, page 268)

1 garlic clove, minced

1 teaspoon toasted sesame oil

¾ teaspoon red pepper flakes

½ teaspoon salt

When the flavors of this Thai-inspired peanut sauce get together, magic happens. Try it drizzled over roasted carrots or steamed zoodles, poured onto crispy roasted or pan-fried tofu or tempeh, or thinned with water and used as a dressing for a garden salad. You can also use less water during the preparation and serve this as a dip for raw veggies.

Combine all the ingredients in a bowl. Using an immersion blender, blend until smooth.

Store, covered, in the refrigerator for up to 5 days. Bring to room temperature before serving.

TURMERIC-GINGER DRESSING

MAKES ¾ CUP • PREP: 5 MINUTES • TOTAL: 5 MINUTES

½ cup tahini

1 tablespoon water

1 tablespoon fresh lemon juice

1 (1-inch) piece fresh ginger, peeled and grated (see Tip, page 268)

1 teaspoon turmeric powder or curry powder

1 teaspoon grated lemon zest

1 garlic clove, minced

¼ teaspoon salt

The earthy, bitter, peppery taste of turmeric and the warming, spicy flavor of ginger are natural partners. The gorgeously hued golden tone here adds a pop of color to any salad, bowl, or meal. This dressing pairs beautifully with a winter salad, drizzled over Good-Day Tofu Eggs, Greens, and Hash Browns (page 252), or the Macrobiotic Bowl (page 275).

In a food processor, combine all the ingredients. Cover and process until smooth.

Store in an airtight container in the refrigerator for 5 to 7 days.

ZA'ATAR DRESSING

MAKES ¾ CUP • PREP: 5 MINUTES • TOTAL: 5 MINUTES

3 tablespoons fresh lemon juice, white wine vinegar, or apple cider vinegar

1 tablespoon fresh orange juice

2 teaspoons minced shallot

1 teaspoon za'atar

2 teaspoons Plant-Based Whole30–compatible Dijon mustard

¼ teaspoon salt

⅛ teaspoon black pepper

½ cup extra-virgin olive oil

Herby and flavorful, za'atar has its ancient roots in the Middle East and eastern Mediterranean. Like many spice blends from around the world, the nature of za'atar varies from region to region and cook to cook but traditionally includes hyssop (a wild herb in the thyme family), sumac (a popular Middle Eastern spice), and sesame seeds. Our version uses a za'atar seasoning whisked with olive oil, citrus, shallot, and Dijon mustard. Serve this dressing over roasted vegetables or tofu.

In a medium bowl, whisk together the lemon juice, orange juice, shallot, za'atar, mustard, salt, and pepper. While whisking, slowly add the olive oil until incorporated.

Store, covered, in the refrigerator for up to 1 week.

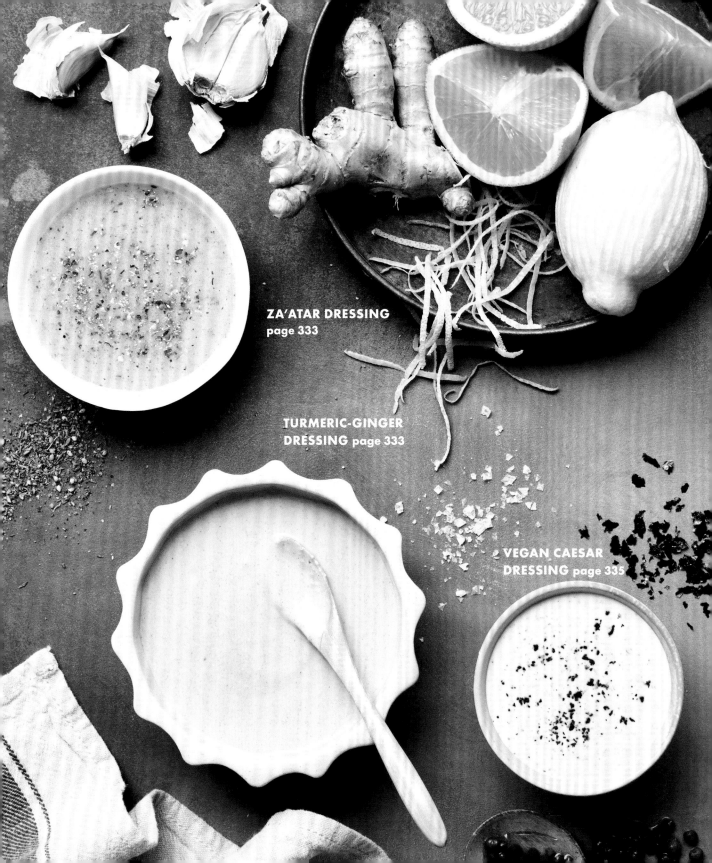

ZA'ATAR DRESSING
page 333

TURMERIC-GINGER DRESSING page 333

VEGAN CAESAR DRESSING page 335

VEGAN CAESAR DRESSING

MAKES 1 CUP • PREP: 5 MINUTES • TOTAL: 5 MINUTES

1 cup Plant-Based Whole30 Mayo (page 350) or Plant-Based Whole30–compatible mayonnaise

3 tablespoons water

1 tablespoon capers, drained and minced (1 teaspoon brine reserved)

2 teaspoons nutritional yeast

1 teaspoon nori dust (see Tip)

1 teaspoon coconut aminos

2 garlic cloves, minced

¼ teaspoon black pepper

Nori gives this dressing the briny, umami flavor of anchovy in a traditional Caesar. Its use goes well beyond salads, though! Use it as a marinade for tofu or a dressing for potato salad or slaw. You can also use it to coat vegetables before roasting, or serve it as a dip for raw veggies.

Place all the ingredients in a bowl (including the teaspoon of reserved caper brine). Using an immersion blender, blend until well combined.

Store, covered, in the refrigerator for up to 1 week.

TIP: If you want a thicker dressing, start with less water and add slowly until you've achieved the desired consistency.

To make the nori dust, place one (1-inch) strip from a nori sheet in a food processor and pulse until minced. You could also use nori powder.

ZHUG

MAKES 1½ CUPS • PREP: 5 MINUTES • TOTAL: 5 MINUTES

5 garlic cloves, roughly chopped

2 cups packed roughly chopped fresh cilantro and/or parsley (about 2 bunches total)

5 jalapeños, seeded and chopped (seeds reserved, optional)

1 tablespoon fresh lemon juice

¾ teaspoon ground cumin

½ teaspoon ground coriander

½ teaspoon salt

½ teaspoon black pepper

⅔ cup extra-virgin olive oil

Argentina has chimichurri, Mexico has salsa verde, Morocco has chermoula, and Yemen has zhug. This bright, herbaceous sauce brings a kick of heat from the jalapeño and is a flavorful addition to any dish. Pair this with grilled or roasted tofu or tempeh, drizzle over cauliflower steaks, or stir into vegan mayonnaise to make a dip for raw vegetables.

In a food processor, pulse the garlic until finely chopped. Add the cilantro, jalapeños, lemon juice, cumin, coriander, salt, and pepper. Process until well combined and finely chopped. With the food processor running, slowly drizzle in the olive oil until the sauce is mostly smooth. If a spicier sauce is desired, add the jalapeño seeds for more heat (if using), a few at a time, and pulse to combine.

Store, covered, in the refrigerator for up to 1 week. Let the sauce warm to room temperature before use.

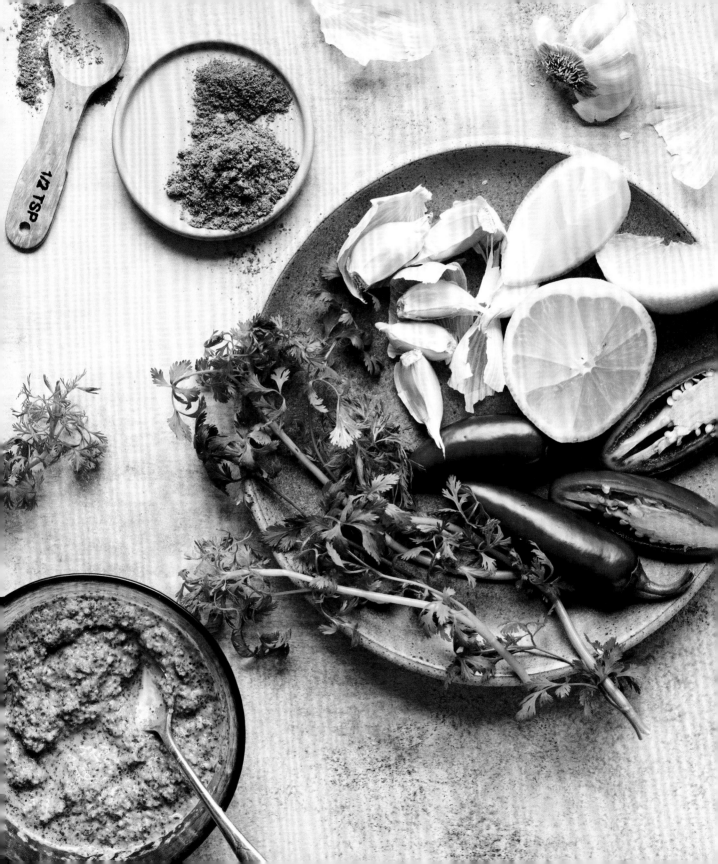

PLANT-BASED WHOLE30 SNACKS

SWEET POTATO–ROASTED GARLIC HUMMUS

SERVES 3 TO 4 • PREP: 10 MINUTES • BAKE: 45 MINUTES • TOTAL: 55 MINUTES

1 large (8- to 10-ounce) sweet potato, scrubbed

2 large garlic cloves

3 tablespoons plus 1 teaspoon extra-virgin olive oil, or more as needed

¼ cup tahini

2 tablespoons fresh lemon juice

½ teaspoon za'atar

½ teaspoon salt

Assorted sliced vegetables (cucumber, bell peppers, broccoli, carrots, sugar snap peas)

Assorted olives

This hummus has all the flavorings of traditional hummus—lemon, garlic, and tahini. But the base is sweet potato, not chickpeas, which makes for a colorful and tasty change of pace.

Preheat the oven to 350°F. Line a large rimmed baking sheet with parchment.

Prick the sweet potato with a fork and place on the baking sheet. Place the garlic in the center of a small piece of foil and drizzle with 1 teaspoon of the olive oil; seal to enclose and place on the baking sheet as well. Bake until the sweet potato and garlic are tender, 45 minutes to 1 hour.

When the sweet potato is cool enough to handle, cut it in half, scoop out the flesh, and place in a food processor. Add the roasted garlic, the remaining 3 tablespoons oil, the tahini, lemon juice, za'atar, and salt and process until smooth. Add additional olive oil, 1 tablespoon at a time if needed, to reach desired consistency.

Serve the hummus with the vegetables and olives.

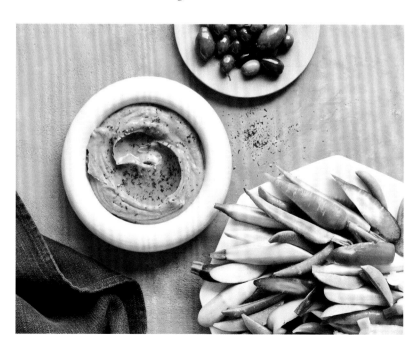

POWER-UP SMOOTHIE

SERVES 3 • PREP: 5 MINUTES • TOTAL: 5 MINUTES

1 (13.5-ounce) can full-fat coconut milk, chilled

1½ cups cold Plant-Based Whole30–compatible almond milk

1 cup frozen diced sweet potato

2 tablespoons roasted cashews

3 to 4 scoops Plant-Based Whole30–compatible protein powder

1 teaspoon vanilla extract

½ teaspoon ground cinnamon

1 Medjool date, pitted

Unsweetened coconut flakes, toasted (optional)

This is an easy way to get extra protein into your day, or an easy on-the-go meal. For the best flavor and consistency, the coconut milk, almond milk, and sweet potatoes should be cold. Keep a few cans of coconut milk in the fridge so you're always prepared.

In a blender, combine the coconut milk (both cream and water), almond milk, sweet potato, cashews, protein powder, vanilla, cinnamon, and date. (If your blender is too small to handle all the ingredients together, divide and process in batches.) Process until smooth and creamy.

Pour into 3 serving glasses and top with the coconut flakes (if using).

TIP: Store any extra smoothie in an airtight container or mason jar in the fridge for up to 1 day. Give it a shake before serving, or pop it back into the blender with a bit more fruit and/or ice to reconstitute a thick, creamy texture. You can also freeze it! Just be sure to leave enough room in your glass or plastic jar for the smoothie to expand.

MUHAMMARA

SERVES 6 • PREP: 5 MINUTES • TOTAL: 5 MINUTES

1 (12- to 16-ounce) jar roasted red bell peppers, drained

½ cup walnuts, toasted

3 tablespoons tomato paste

2 tablespoons extra-virgin olive oil, plus more for serving

2 tablespoons balsamic vinegar

1 teaspoon Aleppo pepper flakes (see Tip, page 251) or ½ teaspoon cayenne

1 teaspoon ground sumac

1 garlic clove, chopped

½ teaspoon salt

Chopped fresh parsley

Assorted roasted vegetables, such as potatoes, mushrooms, carrots, cauliflower, and asparagus

TIP: This warm red dip and accompanying roasted vegetables made for such a colorful and beautiful dish, we featured it on the cover!

This Middle Eastern roasted red pepper and walnut dip is a cousin to Spanish romesco sauce (see page 329) but is a little spicier and sweeter. Here, it's served with roasted vegetables, but it would be equally good as a dip for raw veggies. Or prepare a double batch and serve half with the Roasted Veggies and Black Beans with Muhammara (page 304), leaving plenty of dip for your next snack.

In a food processor, combine the peppers, walnuts, tomato paste, 2 tablespoons olive oil, vinegar, Aleppo pepper flakes, sumac, garlic, and salt. Process until smooth.

Transfer the dip to a serving bowl. Drizzle with additional olive oil, if desired. Sprinkle with the parsley and serve with the vegetables for dipping.

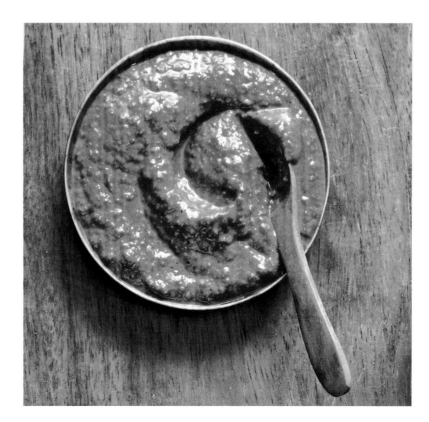

ORANGE-BERRY CHIA PUDDING

SERVES 6 TO 8 • PREP: 5 MINUTES + 15 MINUTES RESTING AND 2 HOURS CHILLING •
TOTAL: 2 HOURS 20 MINUTES

3 cups Plant-Based Whole30–
compatible soy or almond
milk

1 (6-ounce) container
Plant-Based Whole30–
compatible plain yogurt

1 tablespoon grated orange
zest

¾ teaspoon vanilla extract

⅔ cup chia seeds

Mixed fresh berries

Sliced almonds, toasted

Most chia puddings call for honey or maple syrup, neither of which
is compatible with the Whole30. This recipe, though, relies on fresh
orange zest and vanilla to add delicate flavor and a hint of sweetness.
This is the perfect snack to make ahead and keep in the fridge. Storing in
individual-sized containers makes it easy to grab and go.

In a large bowl, combine the soy milk, yogurt, orange zest, and vanilla. Stir
in the chia seeds and let stand for 15 minutes.

Stir to break up any seed clumps. Divide among serving-sized containers
with lids. Cover and refrigerate for at least 2 hours, or up to overnight.

Top the individual puddings with the berries and almonds, and serve.
Store in an airtight container in the refrigerator for up to 5 days.

TIP: If your pudding is too runny, add more chia seeds, stir, and let it sit for
another 15 minutes. If your pudding is too thick, add more milk. To boost the
protein content, add 3 to 4 scoops of a Plant-Based Whole30–compatible
protein powder and mix well to incorporate before stirring in the chia seeds.

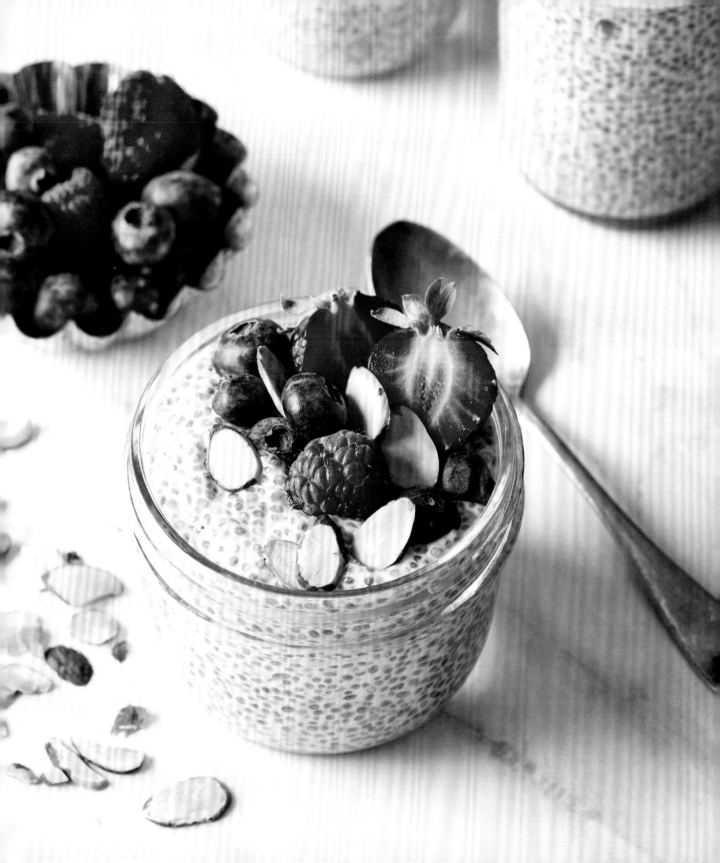

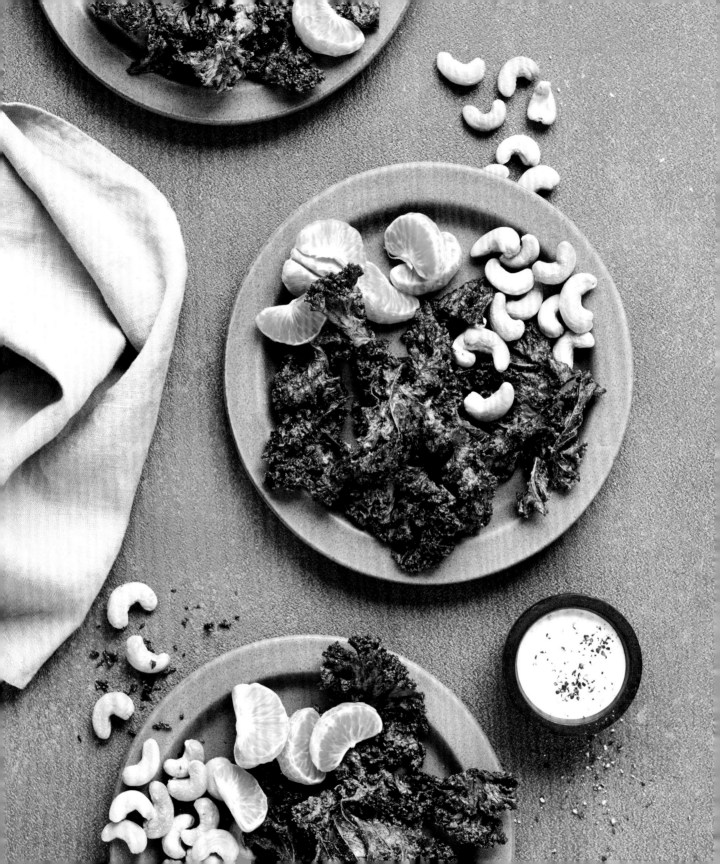

TRUFFLED KALE CHIPS

SERVES 6 • PREP: 10 MINUTES • BAKE: 25 MINUTES • TOTAL: 35 MINUTES

3 tablespoons almond flour

2 teaspoons nutritional yeast

1 teaspoon paprika

2 bunches lacinato or curly kale, stemmed and torn into 2-inch pieces

2 tablespoons extra-virgin olive oil

½ teaspoon truffle salt

Vegan Caesar Dressing (page 335)

Mandarin orange segments

Roasted cashews

Savory, crispy kale chips get the gourmet treatment with a sprinkle of truffle salt and a drizzle of dressing.

Preheat the oven to 300°F. Line 2 large rimmed baking sheets with parchment.

In a small bowl, stir together the almond flour, nutritional yeast, and paprika.

Place the kale in a large bowl. Drizzle with the olive oil and massage to soften, about 2 minutes. Sprinkle with the almond flour mixture, then toss to coat. Arrange the kale in a single layer on the baking sheets. Bake for 15 minutes. Turn and rearrange the kale on the sheets, then sprinkle with the truffle salt and continue to bake until the kale is dry and crisp, 10 to 15 minutes.

Let cool completely on the baking sheets, then transfer the kale to a serving bowl. Just before serving, drizzle with the dressing. Serve with the mandarin oranges and roasted cashews on the side.

TIP: To vary the flavor in these chips, try using smoked salt, sriracha salt, or any one of several types of chile salts.

Store in an airtight container or paper bag at room temperature for 2 to 3 days.

VEGGIE NORI ROLLS

SERVES 2 TO 3 (3 ROLLS) • PREP: 20 MINUTES • TOTAL: 20 MINUTES

FOR THE VEGGIE ROLLS

3 unseasoned nori sheets

3 tablespoons miso

¾ teaspoon nutritional yeast

¾ teaspoon grated lemon zest

1 red bell pepper, cored, seeded, and sliced

1 avocado, sliced

¾ cup coarsely shredded carrots

6 tablespoons sweet pea shoots

FOR THE SESAME DRESSING

2 garlic cloves, smashed

1 small shallot, roughly chopped

2 tablespoons coconut aminos

¼ cup unseasoned rice vinegar

1 tablespoon white miso

½ cup avocado oil or extra-virgin olive oil

2 tablespoons toasted sesame oil

½ teaspoon sesame seeds, toasted

These fresh rolls are filled with a rainbow of vegetables and are served with a tasty sesame dressing. They make a yummy midafternoon snack, but they're fancy enough to serve as an appetizer when entertaining.

MAKE THE VEGGIE ROLLS: For each roll, place the nori sheet, dull side up, on a clean work surface with the long edge close to you. Spread 1 tablespoon miso in a thin layer over the nori, then sprinkle with ¼ teaspoon nutritional yeast and ¼ teaspoon lemon zest.

On the bottom one-third of the nori, arrange 2 rows of red bell pepper slices at the edge closest to you, followed by one row of avocado slices, one row of carrots, and the pea shoots. Gently but firmly, roll the edge closest to you toward the center and into a sushi-like roll. Repeat to make 2 more veggie rolls.

MAKE THE DRESSING AND SERVE: In a food processor, combine the garlic, shallot, coconut aminos, vinegar, and miso and pulse to combine. With the food processor running, slowly add the avocado oil. Add the sesame oil and pulse to combine. Transfer to a serving bowl and sprinkle with the sesame seeds.

Slice each roll into 6 pieces and serve with the dressing.

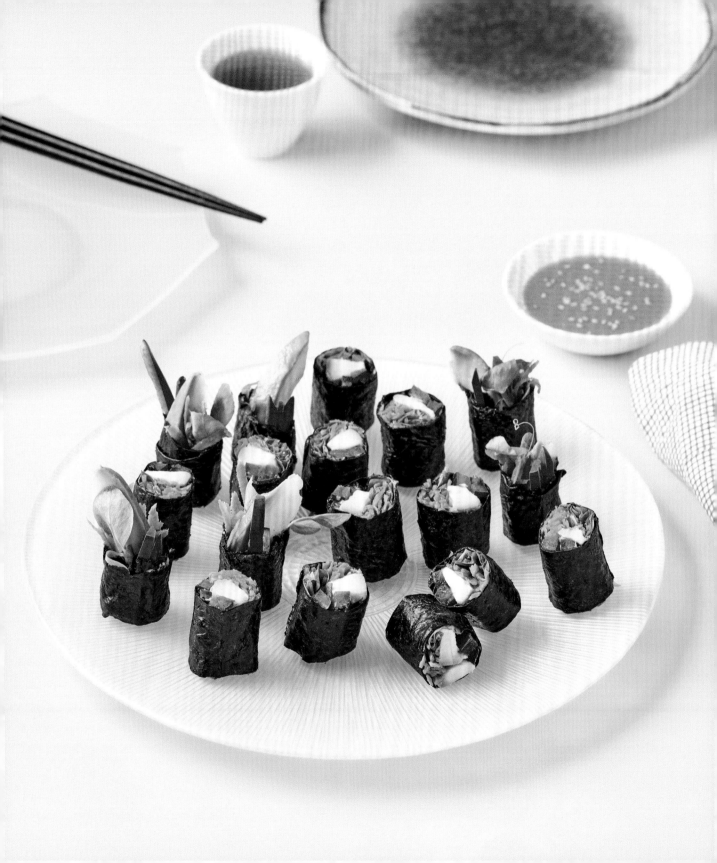

PLANT-BASED WHOLE30 FOUNDATIONAL RECIPES

ROASTED CHICKPEA MEAT

MAKES ABOUT 3 CUPS • PREP: 5 MINUTES • BAKE: 35 MINUTES • TOTAL: 40 MINUTES

2 tablespoons coconut flour or almond flour

2 tablespoons nutritional yeast

1½ teaspoons ground cumin

1 teaspoon smoked paprika

1 teaspoon salt

½ teaspoon black pepper

½ teaspoon ground coriander

2 (14-ounce) cans chickpeas, rinsed, drained, and blotted dry, or 3 cups cooked sprouted chickpeas (see Tip)

2 tablespoons extra-virgin olive oil

We love tofu and tempeh, but it's nice to have a recipe for a plant-based protein you can make at home. This chickpea meat is called for in several recipes in this book, but it can also serve as the protein source for many other dishes. Feel free to change the spices to complement your dish—you'll need 2 tablespoons total spices.

Preheat the oven to 400°F. Line a large rimmed baking sheet with parchment.

In a small bowl, stir together the coconut flour, nutritional yeast, cumin, paprika, salt, pepper, and coriander. In a medium bowl, stir together the chickpeas and olive oil. Sprinkle the seasoning over the chickpeas and toss to coat.

Spread the chickpeas in an even layer on the baking sheet. Bake until the chickpeas are golden brown and crisp, 35 to 45 minutes.

Let chickpeas cool completely. To retain crispness, store at room temperature, partially covered, or in a bowl, covered with a clean kitchen towel, for up to 3 days. Or store in an airtight container in the refrigerator for up to 2 weeks, or freeze for up to 2 months. (Chickpeas will not retain their crispness in the refrigerator or freezer, but will retain their flavor.)

TIP: To sprout chickpeas, place 1 cup dried chickpeas in a 1-quart canning jar. Add water to cover. Cover with a piece of cheesecloth, then secure the cheesecloth with the jar ring or with a tight-fitting rubber band. Let stand for 12 hours out of sunlight. Rinse and drain the chickpeas through the cheesecloth twice during this time, adding about 2 cups cool water each instance. After 12 hours, drain and rinse the chickpeas again with cool water, then let stand without water, rinsing and draining 2 or 3 times daily until you see short sprouts, usually in 3 to 4 days. Store, covered, in the refrigerator to slow further sprouting.

When cooking spouted chickpeas, begin to check for tenderness halfway during the cooking time called for in a recipe. Note that 1 cup of dried chickpeas makes about 4 cups of cooked chickpeas.

PLANT-BASED WHOLE30 MAYO

MAKES 1½ CUPS • PREP: 10 MINUTES • TOTAL: 10 MINUTES

½ cup Plant-Based Whole30–compatible soy milk (see Tip)

2 tablespoons apple cider vinegar

½ teaspoon garlic powder

½ teaspoon salt

1 teaspoon dry mustard

1 cup light olive oil, avocado oil, or high-oleic safflower or sunflower oil

You can use this mayo as a base for dressings, dips, and sauces, or to add a creamy texture to wraps. It comes together in just minutes, and is budget friendly.

In a blender or food processor, combine the soy milk, vinegar, garlic powder, salt, and dry mustard. Process for about 1 minute, until the mixture starts to thicken. Slowly pour in the oil, continuing to blend, until the mixture starts to emulsify. Blend until thickened.

Store in an airtight container for up to 2 weeks; it will thicken even more once in the fridge. If it starts to get an oily layer on top, just use a spoon to mix.

TIP: The key to this emulsion is making sure all ingredients are at room temperature. Leave your soy milk out on the counter for an hour, or microwave it for 15 to 20 seconds. Adding the oil *slowly* encourages the right texture.

VEGETABLE BROTH

MAKES 9 CUPS • PREP: 10 MINUTES • COOK: 45 MINUTES + 10 MINUTES COOLING • TOTAL: 1 HOUR 5 MINUTES

2 tablespoons extra-virgin olive oil

2 large onions, coarsely chopped

1 (8-ounce) package fresh button mushrooms, halved or coarsely chopped

2 large carrots, trimmed and coarsely chopped

2 celery stalks, coarsely chopped

6 large garlic cloves, smashed

2 ripe tomatoes, quartered and seeded

½ apple, cored and coarsely chopped

1 tablespoon salt

1 tablespoon black pepper

10 cups cool water

3 fresh parsley sprigs

3 fresh basil sprigs

3 fresh thyme sprigs

This perfectly balanced broth is packed with fresh flavors. You can also mix and match the vegetables in this recipe, which makes it a perfect way to use up those leftovers.

In a 4- to 6-quart pot, heat the olive oil over medium heat, then add the onions, mushrooms, carrots, celery, and garlic and cook until softened, about 10 minutes. Add the tomatoes, apple, salt, pepper, and then the water. Bring to a boil, then reduce the heat to low, cover, and simmer for 45 minutes.

Turn off the heat below the pot. Add the fresh herbs and let cool for 10 minutes.

Strain the soup into another large pot and discard the solids. Let cool completely before transferring to containers for freezing. Store, covered, in the refrigerator up to 5 days or in the freezer for up to 6 months.

TIP: Experiment with using different herbs, spices, and vegetables in your broth. Try adding green onions, leeks, shallots, mushrooms, chard, parsnips, garlic, red pepper flakes, bay leaves, rosemary, sage, or ginger. Avoid using broccoli, turnips, cabbage, Brussels sprouts, green peppers, kale, collard greens, or mustard greens, as they can make your broth bitter. Skip the potatoes, too, as they can leave broth cloudy.

APPENDIX : WHOLE30 RESOURCES

A simple internet search points to the *thousands* of Whole30-related recipes, articles, resources, and support groups out there—but please, reader beware. Not every article written about the Whole30 is accurate, and I've seen many a "Whole30 recipe roundup" that includes meals or ingredients that aren't actually compatible with the program.

To maximize your Whole30 success and avoid unexpected obstacles, make sure you're getting your Whole30 information from a trusted source. The Whole30 books, website, newsletter, and social media feeds are the best places to conduct research, gather resources, and find the answers to your Whole30 questions.

WHOLE30.COM

The official home of the Whole30 program. This is where you'll find our Original and Plant-Based Whole30 programs, as well as hundreds of recipes, our Whole30 Daily texts, downloadable PDFs, our Whole30 Approved® partners, our Whole30 meal delivery services, and more Whole30-related articles than you could possibly hope to read in 30 days.

WHOLE30 BOOKS

It Starts with Food: Discover the Whole30 and Change Your Life in Unexpected Ways: This book outlines a clear, balanced, sustainable plan to change the way you eat forever—and transform your life in unexpected ways. Here, Melissa details the theories behind the Whole30, summarizing the science in a simple, accessible manner, and shows you how certain foods may be having negative effects on how you feel and live.

The Whole30 Day by Day: Your Daily Guide to Whole30 Success: This book is the essential companion to your Whole30 journey, keeping you motivated, inspired, accountable, and engaged. In this guided journal-meets-handbook, Melissa shares a day-by-day timeline, personal motivation, community inspiration, habit hacks, and meal tips—plus guidance for self-reflection and tracking your Non-Scale Victories.

Food Freedom Forever: Letting Go of Bad Habits, Guilt, and Anxiety Around Food: This book offers real solutions for anyone stuck in the exhausting cycle of yo-yo dieting and the resulting stress, guilt, cravings, and health issues. In her detailed three-part plan, Melissa helps you create a lasting, self-directed Food Freedom plan that keeps you feeling your best while applying your Whole30 learnings in a satisfying, sustainable, joyful way.

WHOLE30 COOKBOOKS

Cooking Whole30: In this updated edition (previously *The Whole30 Cookbook*), Melissa delivers more than 150 recipes to help you prepare delicious, healthy meals for your Whole30 and beyond. *Cooking Whole30* also features tips that simplify meal planning and prep to save time and money, and Recipe Remixes designed to turn one dish into multiple meals.

The Whole30 Fast and Easy: This book is packed with 150 delicious Whole30 recipes, perfect for weeknight cooking, lunches in a hurry, and hearty breakfasts that get you out the door on time. It also features skillet meals, stir-fries, sheet-pan suppers, and slow-cook and no-cook meals, most of which can be made in 30 minutes or less using widely available ingredients found in any supermarket.

The Whole30 Slow Cooker: This book features delicious slow cooker and Instant Pot recipes including no-fuss dinners that cook while you work; roasts that transform into tacos, salads, and soups for easy meals; and satisfying one-pot dishes that make prep and cleanup a breeze.

The Whole30 Friends & Family: Learn how to honor your health commitments while enjoying time with the people you care about. This book is packed with recipes for all of life's special moments, providing tips and tricks to make every social situation a success.

WHOLE30-ENDORSED COOKBOOKS

Our Whole30 Endorsed cookbooks feature authors who have a long history with and close ties to the Whole30 brand and community. Each book includes over 100 delicious and flavorful Whole30 and food freedom recipes.

Whole Food for Your Family, **by Autumn Michaelis** (wholefoodfor7.com): As a busy mother of five growing boys, Autumn shares no-fuss, budget-friendly, gluten- and dairy-free family meals that are delicious and nutritious.

The Primal Gourmet Cookbook, by Ronny Joseph Lvovski (cookprimalgourmet.com): Ronny struggled with a lifetime of health issues before adopting a grain-free, dairy-free diet. He now creates gourmet-quality meals that prove healthy can be delicious.

Buck Naked Kitchen, by Kirsten Buck (bucknakedkitchen.com): Kirsten transformed her life through food and is now a certified holistic nutritionist, sharing delicious and beautiful recipes inspired by her First Nations roots.

The Defined Dish, by Alexandra Snodgrass (thedefineddish.com): *New York Times* best-selling author Alex Snodgrass shares grain-free, dairy-free recipes that sound and look way too delicious to be healthy.

No Crumbs Left, by Teri Turner (nocrumbsleft. net): Teri Turner leads readers through a discovery of new flavors and teaches people to trust their cooking instincts with her grain-free, dairy-free, and Whole30-compatible recipes.

The Whole Smiths, by Michelle Smith (thewholesmiths.com): Michelle Smith shares 150 delicious recipes designed to help anyone achieve a long-term approach to good health.

Social media

Tag Whole30 and use #whole30 or #pbwhole30 to share your Whole30 journey!

- Instagram: @whole30, @pbwhole30
- TikTok: @whole30
- YouTube.com/whole30
- Facebook.com/whole30
- Pinterest.com/whole30
- X (Twitter): @whole30

SHARE YOUR WHOLE30 SUCCESS STORY

I love nothing more than reading your Whole30 stories, celebrating your successes, and encouraging your food freedom. Share your story with us at whole30.com/share-whole30-story, or email us at headquarters@whole30.com.

Or browse through our Whole30 testimonials before you start your journey, to be inspired by people just like you who found success through the program. Read them at **whole30.com /testimonials**.

ACKNOWLEDGMENTS

The Whole30 has changed millions of lives (and will change millions more) thanks to the talents, hard work, support, and unwavering faith of the people on these pages.

I first must thank my editor at Rodale, Diana Baroni. This was our first book together, but you made me feel confident in myself and this project from our very first call. I am so proud of what we have created. Thank you for your guidance and the positive comments you left in the side-notes—they got me though this truly grueling deadline.

To my Rodale team—Jenny Davis, Tiffany Ma, Jonathan Sung, Odette Fleming, Cindy Murray, Kelly Doyle, Sarah Breivogel, Loren Noveck. Carole Berglie, Regina Castillo, Melanie Gold, Richard Elman, Nancy Inglis, Charlee Trantino, and Theresa Zoro—I am so lucky to have such a talented, inspired, motivated team! The vibes were *on* from the very first call, and I can't wait to bring this book into readers' homes and kitchens with you.

To my Penguin Canada family—Andrea Magyar, Megan Konzelman, Michelle Arbus, and Charlotte Nip—your ongoing support and faith in my work (Whole30 and otherwise) have been a dream come true over the last nine(!) years. Andrea, thank you for your vision, your direction, and your mentorship throughout the years.

To my agent, Christy Fletcher, *look how far we have come*. I will never forget the way you stood by me, nor the comfort I have taken knowing you are always in my corner. I wouldn't want anyone but you by my side through deadline after deadline.

For my team at UTA, Zoe Balestri, Melissa Chinchillo, and Yona Levin, thank you for all of your support and encouragement throughout the years. It is always a joy to bring a new book into the world with all of you.

To Ghazalle Badiozamani, your photography is almost as beautiful as your spirit. Thank you for turning our ingredients into gorgeous, vibrant, comforting meals. Being with you in the studio is my happy place.

To Barrett Washburne, Brett Regot, Vanessa Vazquez, EJ Muniz, Chris Smith, Brett Statman, Paul Wang, Yoora Kim, and Evan McWeeny, y'all are the *dream team*! I've never had so much fun on set, nor learned so much about food styling, props, and creativity in the process. I cannot wait to work with all of you again.

To Clara Nosek, RD; Stephanie Greunke, RD; Rhyan Geiger, RD; Jennifer Anderson, RD; Eliza Kingsford, LPC; Vickie Bhatia, PhD; and Phil Koberlein, FFL: thank you for your contributions to the Whole30 community and my work. Your voices here are important and valued.

To my Whole30 HQ team, you are the beating heart of Whole30. I am grateful every day to work with people who are so talented, passionate, and committed to helping people find success with the program. I would work with all of you forever if I could—and I hope I do.

To my husband, your unwavering faith in me, relentless support of my goals, and special brand of encouragement have convinced me that I won the partner lottery. I didn't blow it, babe.

To my sister, you'll always be the first one I call when I need to make a small but paralyzing decision, need permission to rest, or am tempted to chop my hair. I love you; you are my person.

To my son, I remember taking you to the bookstore every weekend when you were little, where you'd point at my books on the shelf and say, "Mama's book!" I love you more than anything.

Finally, to my Whole30 community. I've said this a million times, and it remains true—every good idea I've ever had has come from you. You *are* Whole30, and I see each and every one of you. For your support, enthusiasm, generosity, and many contributions to the program and the brand . . . thank you, thank you, thank you.

INDEX

Note: Page numbers in *italics* indicate photos.

A

alcohol (wine, beer, cider, liquor, etc.)
  eliminating, 30, 36, 38, 97, 233
  exceptions, 30, 37, 39, 97, 233
  food choices affected by, 102
  reintroducing, 37, 39, 97, 233
  research on triggering cravings, 40
  systemic inflammation and, 102
  why Whole30 eliminates this, 102, 238
animal protein (meat, seafood, and eggs)
  included in Original Whole30, 10, 36
  no mix-and-match, 29
  not included in Plant-Based Whole30, 29, 38
  reintroducing in Plant-Based Whole30 (optional track), 39, 233

B

blood sugar (blood glucose)
  alcohol and, 102, 238
  crashes and "head on desk" feeling, 87
  grain consumption and, 103, 239
  NSVs checklist and, 44
  Plant-Based Whole30 and, 11
  reintroduction of foods and, 83
  snacks/smoothies and, 75
  sugar consumption and, 102, 238
  Whole30 and, 21, 63, 73
Book of Boundaries, The (Urban), 77
botanical extracts, 30, 37, 39, 97, 233

C

caffeine/coffee, 17, 32, 45, 52, 73, 81
calorie restriction or calorie counting, 19, 20, 70, 72–73
  creating a dysfunctional relationship with food and, 20, 69
  discouraged by Whole30, 19, 52, 60, 63, 72–73, 233
  tracking calories or macros, 72–73
"Can I have?" information, 57–59
  food labels and, 57
  reading the Whole30 Program rules and, 57
  recipe ingredients and, 57
  smoking or using nicotine patches, 59
  taking supplements, 57–59
  using marijuana or THC, 59
  website for a detailed list, 57
carrageenan, 33
challenges of Whole30, 49–50, 77–78
coconut aminos, 30, 37, 39, 97, 233
cooking oils
  allowed on Original and Plant-Based Whole30, 34–35, 37, 39, 97, 233
  most versatile, 94–95
  which to choose for recipes, 94
cooking Whole30, 91–95
  cooking and recipe tips, 93–95
  cooking oils, 94–95
  cooking times, 94
  mise en place, 94
  reading the recipe and labels, 93–94
  tools and gadgets, 91–93
  See also Recipe Index
Cooking Whole30 (Urban), 352
cravings, 16, 20, 21–22, 32–33
  caused by problematic foods, 30

Days 1–7 on the elimination diet, 52
  finding your "why" and, 46
  food as a coping mechanism and, 16
  hunger vs., 81
  new habits and, 82
  reducing cravings, 40
  reintroduction phase and, 86, 87
  stress and, 81, 82
  sugar cravings, 40, 81, 102
  thirst vs., 82
  tips for distracting yourself and, 82
  when to seek help for, 82

D

dairy
  choosing Original Whole30 and, 29
  dining out and, 77
  eliminating, 23–24, 36, 97
  exceptions, 36, 37, 97
  food sensitivities, lactose intolerance, digestive issues, and adverse food reactions to, 17, 21, 24, 77, 88, 102, 103
  Pancake Rule and, 32, 40
  reintroducing, 29, 37, 39, 61, 85, 86, 97, 233
  in supplements, 59
  why Whole30 eliminates this, 103
diabetes and pre-diabetes, 63, 66, 102, 238
"diet culture," 19, 20, 60–61
  definition, 60
  eating disorders and, 60
  fasting, keto, and cleanses, 73
  as harmful, 20
  quick-fix diets, 20
  unhealthy behaviors and, 60, 61
  Whole30 as an alternative, 60
  yo-yo dieting, 20

V

vegetables
FODMAP vegetables, 31, 66, 67
for Original Whole30, 28
for Plant-Based Whole30, 28

W

WANDA (Women Advancing
Nutrition Dietetics and
Agriculture), 12
wearables (WHOOP band, Apple
watch, Oura ring)
improvement of HRV during
Whole30 elimination, 87
staying motivated and, 42
Whole30 community, 12, 54–55
Whole30 Day by Day, The (Urban),
51, 54, 352
Whole30 Fast and Easy, The
(Urban), 352
Whole30 Friends & Family
(Urban), 353
Whole30 meal delivery, 50, 72
website for, 77
Whole30/Original Whole30
as alternative to "diet culture,"
60
author's history and, 15–17
benefits, 21, 22
as a body "reset," 19, 26
clinical evidence to support
Whole30, 63
commitment to, 23, 28, 63
commonly problematic foods,
23–24
cooking, 91–95
diet doesn't fix everything, 67
elimination diet basics, 21–26,
28
FAQ, 102–4
Food Freedom Plan, 26
foods allowed during Phase 1,
36, 37
foods eliminated during Phase
1, 36, 97
goals of, 19
"on-the-go" food ideas, 104

hardest days and tips for
sticking with the program, 53
how to choose Original or
Plant-Based, 29
how to share with your family
and friends, 48
how to talk about the program
to kids, 68
identifying food sensitivities
and adverse food reactions, 21,
25, 60
keeping a promise to yourself,
23
meal planning as critical for, 48
Meal Template, 98, *98*
Mindset checklist, 28
new healthy eating and food
habits, 20, 22
no mix-and-match options, 29
not recommended for those
with a history of disordered
eating, 69
physiological benefits, 20, 21,
22, 23, 24, 25, 26, 52, 53, 60, 63
planning and preparation,
46–50
Plant-Based Whole30 vs.
Original Whole30, 28–29
psychological and emotional
benefits, 53, 65
repeating the Whole30, 26
Rules, 36–37, 97
Rules, Quick Reference guide,
97
rules changed since 2015, 29–36
satiety and fat adaptation, 70
Shopping List, 99–101
snack ideas, 104
for special populations, 66–69
strict adherence, importance
of, 62
"This is not hard," 65
Timeline, 51–55
troubleshooting, 79–82
website (whole30.com), 57
weight loss and, 19, 20, 42,
60–61

what it is and isn't, 19, 20
your Whole30 "elevator pitch,"
47–48
See also Plant-Based Whole30;
Rules for Original Whole30
Phase 1: elimination; Rules
for Original Whole30 Phase 2:
reintroduction
Whole30 Slow Cooker, The
(Urban), 353
Whole30 Resources, 352–53
website, 352

RECIPE INDEX

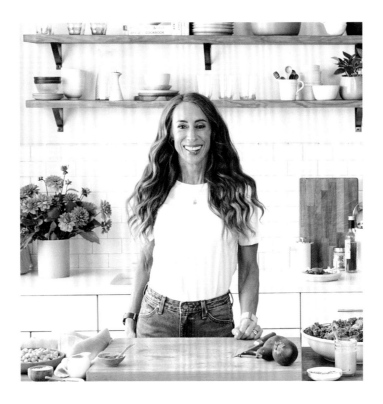

ABOUT THE AUTHOR

MELISSA URBAN is the co-founder and CEO of Whole30, a seven-time *New York Times* bestselling author, and an authority on helping people create lifelong healthy habits. She lives in Salt Lake City, Utah with her husband, son, and a poodle called Henry.

CONNECT WITH MU

I love hearing your Whole30 success stories, answering your questions, and offering support. I talk about the Whole30 (and a whole lot more) on my personal channels:

- Website: melissau.com
- Instagram: @melissau
- TikTok: @melissa_u
- Facebook.com/melissau.author
- X (Twitter): @melissa_urban